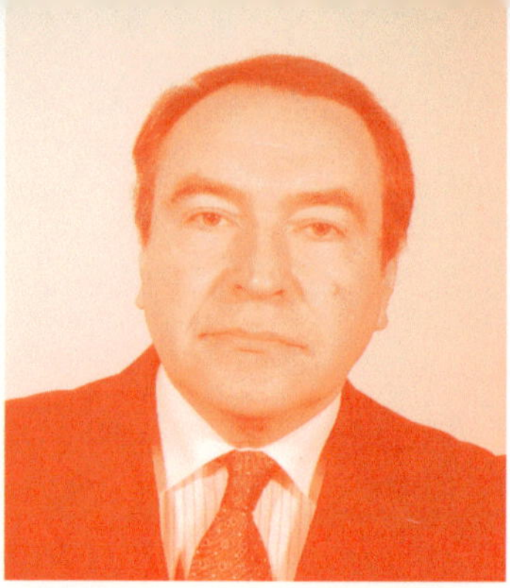
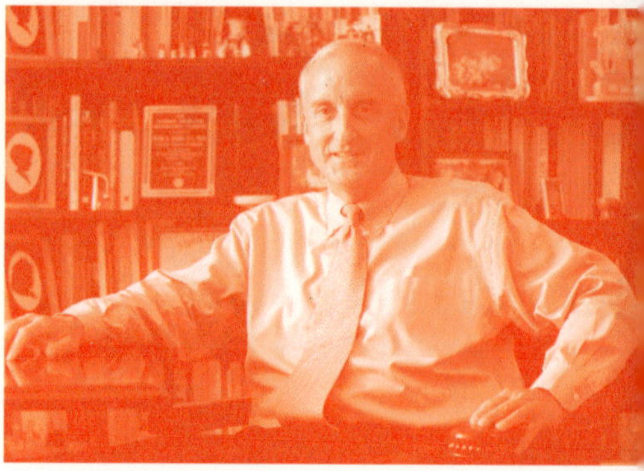
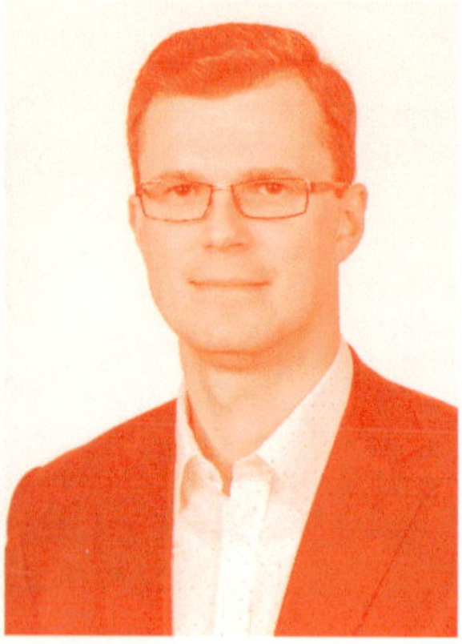
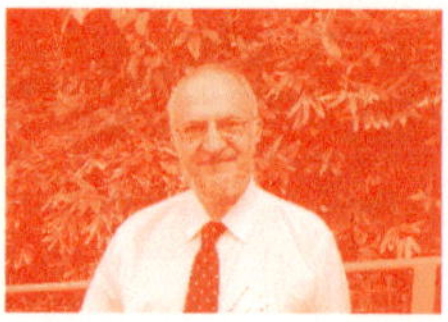
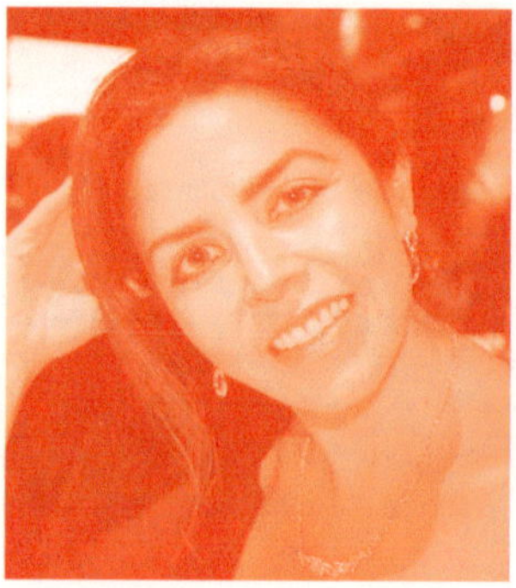

*Supporting open minds since 2005*

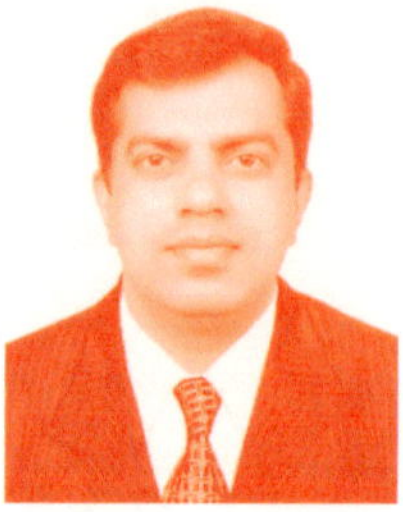
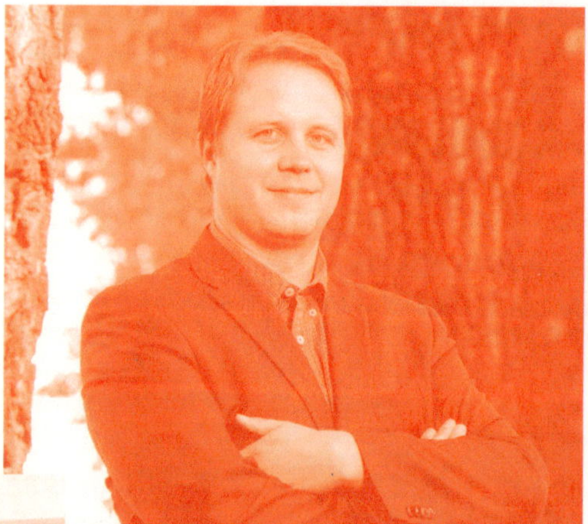
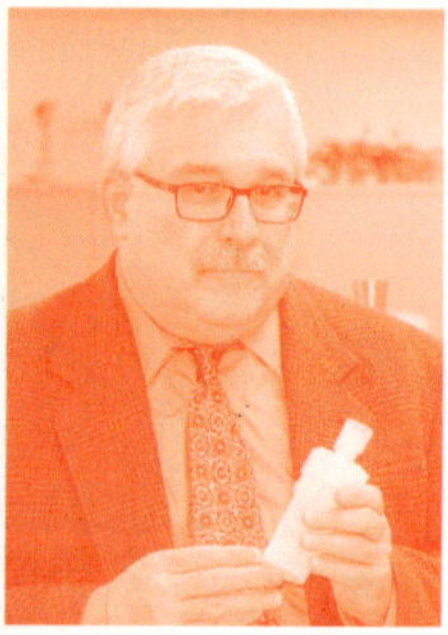
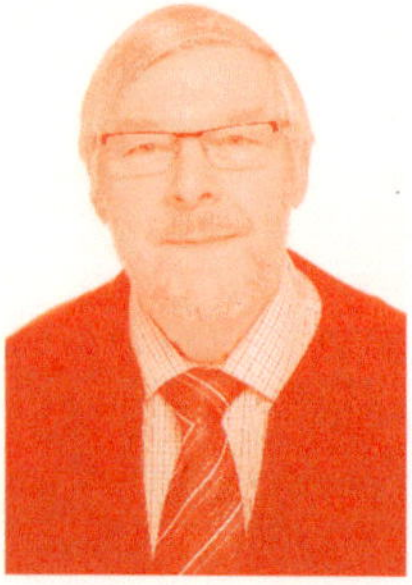
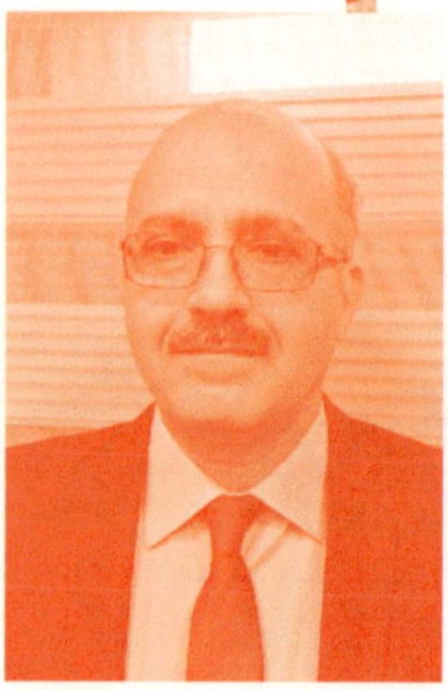
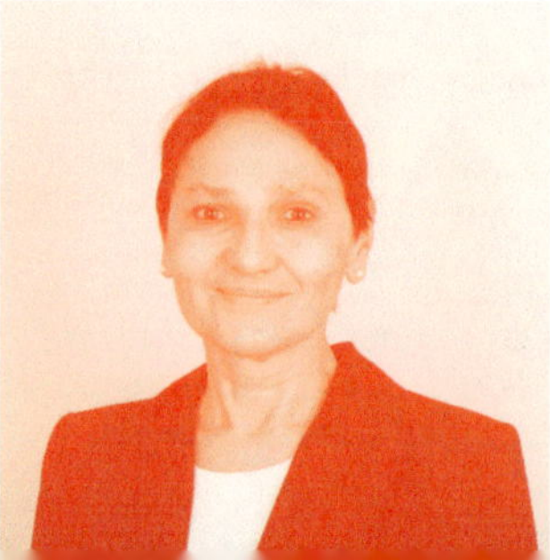
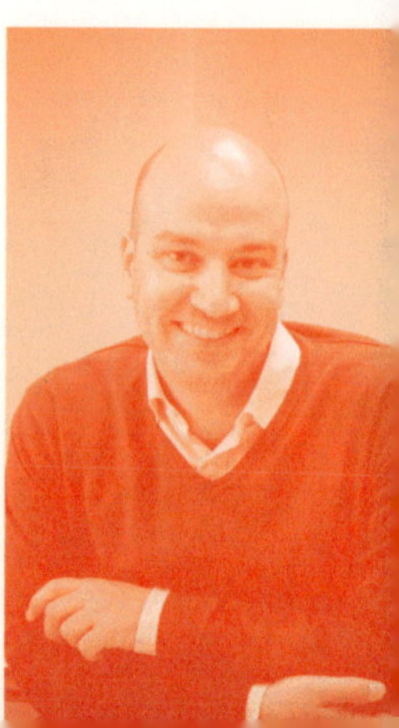

Central Nervous System Tumors
http://dx.doi.org/10.5772/intechopen.94607
Edited by Scott George Turner

Contributors
Liam Chen, Raghunadharao Digumarti, Venkata Pradeepbabu Koyyala, Nikos Tapinos, David Karambizi, Michiko N. Fukuda, Motohiro Nonaka, Misa Suzuki-Anekoji, Roberto Garcia-Navarrete, Alfonso Marhx-Bracho, Natael Olvera González, Ericka León-Alvárez, Cointa Arroyo Jiménez, Javier Terrazo-Lluch, Beatriz Alvarez-Mora, Luz Maria Cordero, Daniel Magos Rodríguez, Ana Niembro-Zúñiga, Vianey Maceda Morales, Rosario Aguilar Silva, Juan Alberto Díaz Ponce Medrano, Sandra Luz Lizarraga-Lopez, Thien Nhat Nu Tran, Jorge Ocon Rodríguez, Judy Castañeda Goyes, Constantino Contreras Vázquez, José Luis Pérez Gómez, Kanwalpreet Kaur, Nu Thien Nhat Tran, Rajesh Alugolu, Sumitra Sivakoti, Beatrice Anne, Abhishek J. Arora, Bibha Choudhary, Tanvi R. Parashar, Febina Ravindran, Andres Cardona, Alvaro Munoz, Lucia Zatarain Barron, Christian Rolfo, Juan Esteban Garcia-Robledo, Camila Ordóñez Reyes, Oscar Arrieta, Diana Carolina Sotelo-Rodríguez, Ahmad Ozair, Erum Khan, Vivek Bhat, Anil Nanda, Arjumand Faruqi, Scott Turner, Alejandro Ruíz-Patiño



First published in London, United Kingdom, 2022 by IntechOpen
IntechOpen is the global imprint of INTECHOPEN LIMITED, registered in England and Wales, registration number: 11086078, 5 Princes Gate Court, London, SW7 2QJ, United Kingdom
Printed in Croatia

British Library Cataloguing-in-Publication Data
A catalogue record for this book is available from the British Library

Additional hard and PDF copies can be obtained from orders@intechopen.com

Central Nervous System Tumors
Edited by Scott George Turner
p. cm.
Print ISBN 978-1-83969-306-9
Online ISBN 978-1-83969-307-6
eBook (PDF) ISBN 978-1-83969-308-3

For EU product safety concerns:
IN TECH d.o.o., Prolaz Marije Krucifikse Kozulić 3, 51000 Rijeka, Croatia, info@intechopen.com or visit our website at intechopen.com.

# Meet the editor

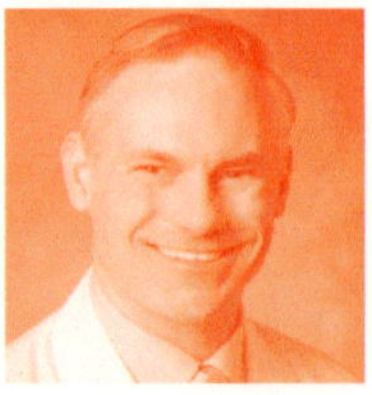

Dr. Turner received his medical degree from the Medical College of Wisconsin and completed a neurology residency at Stony Brook University, the State University of New York. He subsequently completed a neuro-oncology fellowship at Duke University, North Carolina. He has been practicing neuro-oncology for over ten years and has served as the director of the neuro-oncology programs at Geisinger Medical Center in Pennsylvania and at Saint Luke's Hospital in Kansas City. He has worked to develop a multidisciplinary treatment paradigm, which integrates clinical trials with chemo and radiation therapy, intrathecal chemotherapy, and stereotactic radiosurgery. He created a comprehensive care plan that includes physical and occupational therapy, nutritional planning, psychiatric and neuropsychologic evaluation, and palliative care. He is currently a neuro-oncologist at the University of California, Irvine.

# Contents

# Preface

The book *Central Nervous System Tumors* represents the contribution of many experts in the field, each with his own specialty and interests. The management of patients with tumors of the central nervous system (CNS) is complex and involves the expertise of many disciplines including neuro-oncology, neuroradiology, neurosurgery, radiation oncology, neuropathology, and more. Many of our patients are quite debilitated and require the aid of physical and occupational therapy, spiritual counseling, pain management, and palliative care. Our field has changed greatly over the past several years as we gain a better understanding of the mechanisms of tumorigenesis and the genes involved. Many of them can be targeted with new pharmaceuticals, and immunotherapy is a very active area of research. We rely heavily on new breakthroughs from basic science research labs around the world.

I am grateful for the wonderful and exciting contributions from the many authors that have helped with the publication of this book, and I remain hopeful for the future of the field with the many new advances that are sure to come in the years ahead. I also would like to thank our *IntechOpen* colleagues for their help and support in bringing the most up-to-date findings to its readers.

**Dr. Scott George Turner**
Associate Professor of Neurology,
Department of Neuro-Oncology,
University of California,
Irvine, Orange, CA

Section 1

# Introduction

Chapter 1

# Introductory Chapter: The Current State of the Treatment of CNS Malignancies

*Scott George Turner*

## 1. Introduction

The management of patients with malignancies of the central nervous system (CNS) has presented a challenge for many years. For benign tumors such as pituitary adenomas or low-grade meningiomas, surgery is often adequate to ensure a good outcome, whereas for high-grade gliomas, maximal surgery followed by radiation and chemotherapy is the standard of care. Newer modalities such as immunotherapy and tumor-treating fields have shown benefit, and have been added to the armamentarium that neuro-oncologists employ to care for patients with challenging high-grade tumors.

## 2. WHO classification

In 2016, the World Health Organization (WHO) revised its classification scheme for tumors of the central nervous system. The 2000 [1] and 2007 [2] classification schemes relied on histologic findings, including immunohistochemistry, to determine tumor type based on similarities to the cell of origin, as well as tumor grade. The 2016 [3] changes combined the histologic findings with genetic information in order to better characterize these tumors and to establish data on prognosis. An updated classification scheme is coming this year [4] and builds on the 2016 version, incorporating updated molecular and genetic biomarkers.

## 3. Pediatric CNS tumors

CNS tumors are the most common solid tumors in children. The ones most commonly found in the posterior fossa are medulloblastoma, juvenile pilocytic astrocytoma, ependymoma, diffuse pontine glioma, and atypical teratoid-rhabdoid tumor [5]. Medulloblastomas [6] are characterized by molecular features and histopathology, and there are four subtypes: WNT-activated, SHH-activated, and Group 3 and Group 4 non-WNT/non-SHH. Each subtype has its own molecular and histologic characteristics, and all are considered WHO Grade 4. Ependymomas [7] occur in both adults and children and can occur in the brain and spinal cord. The majority occur in the posterior fossa and can be WHO Grade 2 or 3. A supratentorial RELA-fusion-positive variant was first described in 2016. Astrocytomas, oligodendrogliomas, craniopharyngiomas, gangliogliomas, primitive neuroectodermal tumors, and meningiomas are most often found supratentorially. Often these are low-grade, slow-growing tumors that can be treated with surgery alone.

## 4. Adult CNS tumors

Meningiomas [8] arise from the meninges and are most often benign, Grade I tumors, though there are rare higher-grade meningiomas that can invade into the brain tissue. As mentioned above, ependymomas can occur in both children and adults. A myxopapillary variant is commonly found at the filum/cauda equina and is more common in adults. The new 2021 WHO classification has changed this sub-type from a Grade 1 tumor to Grade 2 due to its more aggressive clinical course. The two glands within the brain also can develop tumors: Pituitary adenomas [9] arise from the pituitary gland within the sella turcica and can cause endocrinopathies and visual field loss. Tumors of the pineal gland [10] can lead to symptoms from hydrocephalus, among others. However, the most common primary CNS tumor is also the most aggressive, glioblastoma multiforme, which are classified as IDH mutant or wildtype with very different survival outcomes. Maximal surgical resection correlates with better survival [11], and surgical advances have led to improved outcomes. Following surgery, post-operative radiation and chemotherapy are the standard of care. Only temozolomide chemotherapy [12] and Optune tumor-treating fields [13] have been shown to improve overall survival in these patients, though new therapies are being investigated.

Neuro-oncology remains a very exciting field with new therapies being developed based on our better understanding of the genetics and molecular characteristics of these tumors. Targeted therapies [14] and immunotherapy [15], including vaccines, are being developed. This is truly a very exciting time for the field, and I am sure that, as our understanding of the most aggressive types of primary brain tumors grows, we will make even greater strides toward successfully treating these deadly malignancies.

## Author details

Scott George Turner
Department of Neuro-Oncology, University of California, Irvine, Orange, CA, USA

*Address all correspondence to: sgturne1@hs.uci.edu

## References

[1] Kleihues P et al. The WHO classification of tumours of the central nervous system. Journal of Neuropathology & Experimental Neurology. 2002;**3**:15-225

[2] Louis DN et al. The 2007 WHO classification of tumours of the central nervous system. Acta Neuropathologica. 2007;**114**(2):97-109

[3] Louis DN et al. The 2016 WHO classification of tumours of the central nervous system: A summary. Acta Neuropathologica. 2016;**131**(6):803-820

[4] Louis DN et al. The 2021 WHO classification of tumors of the central nervous system: A summary. Neuro-Oncology. 2021;**23**(8):1231-1251

[5] Udaka Y, Packer R. Pediatric brain tumors. Neurologic Clinics. 2018;**36**(3): 533-556

[6] Quinlan A, Rizzolo D. Understanding medulloblastoma. JAAPA. 2017;**30**(10): 30-36

[7] Gerstner ER, Pajtler KW. Ependymoma. Seminars in Neurology. 2018;**38**(1):104-111

[8] Apra C et al. Current treatment options for meningioma. Expert Review of Neurotherapeutics. 2018;**18**(3): 241-249

[9] Penar P et al. Pituitary tumor diagnosis and treatment. Current Neurology and Neuroscience Reports. 2002;**2**(3):236-245

[10] Mottolese C et al. History of the pineal region tumor. Neurochirurgie. 2015;**61**(2-3):61-64

[11] Lacroix M et al. Extent of surgery correlates with survival and surgical advances have led to improved survival. We include a discussion of awake craniotomies and new neuro-navigation and brain mapping techniques for surgical planning. Journal of Neurosurgery. 2001;**92**(2):190-198

[12] Stupp R et al. Radiotherapy plus concomitant and adjuvant temozolomide for glioblastoma. NEJM. 2005;**352**:987-996

[13] Stupp R et al. Effect of tumor-treating fields plus maintenance Temozolomide vs maintenance temozolomide alone on survival in patients with glioblastoma. JAMA. 2017;**318**(23):2306-2316

[14] Mercer R et al. Targeted therapies for malignant glioma. BioDrugs. 2009;**23**(1):25-35

[15] Kamran N et al. Current state and future prospects of immunotherapy for glioma. Immunotherapy. 2018;**10**(4): 317-339

Section 2

# Pediatric Brain Tumors

Chapter 2

# Pediatric Brain Tumors: From Modern Classification System to Current Principles of Management

*Ahmad Ozair, Erum Khan, Vivek Bhat, Arjumand Faruqi and Anil Nanda*

## Abstract

Central nervous system (CNS) malignancies contribute significantly to the global burden of cancer. Brain tumors constitute the most common solid organ tumors in children and the second most common malignancies of childhood overall. Accounting for nearly 20% of all pediatric malignancies, these are the foremost cause of cancer-related deaths in children 0–14 years of age. This book chapter provides a state-of-the-art overview of pediatric brain tumors. It discusses their morbidity and mortality and introduces the WHO 2021 classification of CNS tumors, which is critical to therapeutic decision-making. It then describes the modern understanding of tumor grading and its clinical implications, followed by the general principles of diagnosis and management. The chapter then discusses, in detail, those brain tumors which have the highest disease burden in children, including medulloblastoma, astrocytoma, ependymoma, schwannoma, meningioma, amongst others. The landscape of treatment of pediatric brain tumors has been rapidly evolving, with several effective therapies on the horizon.

**Keywords:** CNS tumor, oncology, neuro-oncology, pediatric oncology, malignancy, neurology, neurosurgery, neuroradiology, brain tumor

## 1. Introduction

Central nervous system (CNS) malignancies contribute significantly to the global burden of cancer. The average annual age-adjusted incidence rate (AAAIR) of all CNS tumors, as estimated in the US population was 23.79 according to the most recent report of the Central Brain Tumor Registry of the United States (CBTRUS) [1]. Amongst individuals aged 15–39 years, CNS tumors constitute the third most common tumor overall, while amongst individuals aged 40 and above, they are the third most common cause of cancer death.

Brain tumors find an overwhelmingly high representation in the pediatric age group. They constitute the most common solid organ tumors in children and the second most common malignancies of childhood overall, accounting for nearly 20% of all pediatric malignancies [1]. The CBTRUS 2020 report estimated that the AAAIR of CNS tumors amongst children aged 0 to 14 was 5.83 per 100,000 individuals. The annual age-adjusted mortality rate (AAAMR) of CNS tumors in this age group was determined to be 0.71 per 100,000, leading to brain tumors being the biggest cause of cancer death

amongst 0 to 14 years of age. Despite the advances of the last few decades in imaging, molecular diagnostics, surgical techniques, and adjuvant therapy, unfortunately, less than required improvement has occurred in rates of survival in the pediatric age group.

Girardi et al., in a systematic review published in 2019, determined that little data from low and low-middle-income countries (LMICs) is available regarding long-term survival from pediatric brain tumors [2]. This sobering data stands amidst the backdrop of studies demonstrating that the nations with lower economic development deliver a significantly poorer quality of care [3].

Adult survivors of pediatric brain tumors face significant challenges. Several factors come together to drastically impact their neurocognitive and psychosocial outcomes. These include but are not limited to, the clinical features of the tumor itself, its treatment especially radiotherapy to a developing brain, access to support systems and quality of rehabilitative services, individual factors, amongst others [4].

The pediatric landscape is significantly different from the adult landscape with regard to brain tumors. Pediatric brain tumors have differing common sites of origin, histology, genetics, which lend themselves to dissimilar diagnostic and therapeutic considerations. As a rule of thumb, two-thirds of tumors in adults arise from sites above the tentorium cerebelli, while two-thirds of tumors in children arise from structures below the tentorium cerebelli. Several genetic syndromes also include pediatric brain tumors as one of their clinical manifestations. These include but are not limited to tuberous sclerosis, Li-Fraumeni syndrome, Turcot syndrome, Type 1 and 2 Neurofibromatosis, Gorlin syndrome, Cowden syndrome, amongst others.

Brain tumors that have the highest disease burden in children include medulloblastomas, astrocytomas, ependymomas, schwannomas, meningiomas, amongst others. Their details, along with their specific epidemiology, will be discussed in greater depth in further sections.

## 2. Classifying brain tumors: an evolving paradigm

The classification of tumors in the central nervous system (CNS) is the critical factor driving treatment decisions, given the wide variation amongst different tumors in response to each anti-cancer modality. For instance, some like midline pontine gliomas do not respond well to chemotherapy and are only partially amenable to radiotherapy.

Several classification schemas for CNS tumors exist. These range from those solely based on histology alone to those relying primarily on genetic and epigenetic features. While microscopic diagnosis finds utility in its low cost and accessibility, its insufficiently high inter-rater reliability along with the advancements in molecular biology have led to it not being the sole basis for classification [5].

Other simpler classification systems divide tumors based on the major site of origin. Supratentorial tumors are those which are located above the tentorium cerebelli and therefore may involve cerebral hemispheres. In children, these commonly include high-grade gliomas, low-grade gliomas, embryonal tumors, atypical teratoid/rhabdoid tumors, meningiomas, choroid plexus tumors, and pineal tumors. In contrast, infratentorial tumors are located below the tentorium and, therefore, originate from the brainstem, the cerebellum, and the 4th ventricle. In children, these commonly include medulloblastomas, cerebellar astrocytomas, ependymomas, brainstem gliomas, atypical teratoid/rhabdoid tumors, and rarely choroid plexus tumors. The sellar region is a region at the base of the skull around the sella turcica where the major tumors of note in children include pituitary adenomas, craniopharyngiomas, gliomas, and germ cell tumors.

## 3. The WHO 2021 classification of CNS tumors

The World Health Organization (WHO) has developed and published updated versions of the most widely used classification system for CNS tumors for decades. The WHO 2007 classification schema was the last iteration to primarily be based on histology [6]. Very recently, the WHO 2021 classification (WHO CNS5) has been published, which functions as an integrated histo-molecular classification system [7].

### 3.1 Key updates in the WHO 2021 classification

The WHO CNS5 classification, a broad overview of which is given in **Figure 1**, adheres to the landmark recommendations made by the cIMPACT-NOW group, especially the ones made at the Utrecht Meeting in 2019. The Consortium to Inform Molecular and Practical Approaches to CNS Tumor Taxonomy—Not Official WHO (cIMPACT-NOW) is an influential group of neuro-oncologists and neuropathologists which was established in 2016 to provide recommendations regarding the upcoming WHO classification [8]. Based on the cIMPACT-NOW recommendations, WHO CNS5 makes new categories, merges a few ones, and introduces new entities. These updates include the following:

I. Greater integration of histology has been done with immunohistochemical, ultrastructural, and molecular features of tumors.

II. Arabic numerals (1, 2, 3, and 4) for tumor grade have replaced Roman numerals (I, II, III, and IV) to have CNS tumor grading consistent with other systems and prevent typographical errors.

III. Grading of tumors is to be done *within* tumor types (rather than across different tumor types).

IV. Gliomas have been separated into pediatric-type and adult-type, with several subcategories. This change carries several key clinical implications.

V. The term 'glioblastoma' is reserved for IDH wild-type tumors and only refers to grade 4 tumors

VI. IDH-mutant astrocytoma will be graded based on histo-molecular features

VII. Layered reporting of medulloblastoma is recommended:

   a. Integrated Diagnosis (combining histology and biology)

   b. Histological Diagnosis

   c. CNS WHO Grade

   d. Molecular Information

VIII. Ependymomas have new sub-categories including Posterior Fossa A Ependymoma, Posterior Fossa B type Ependymoma, etc.

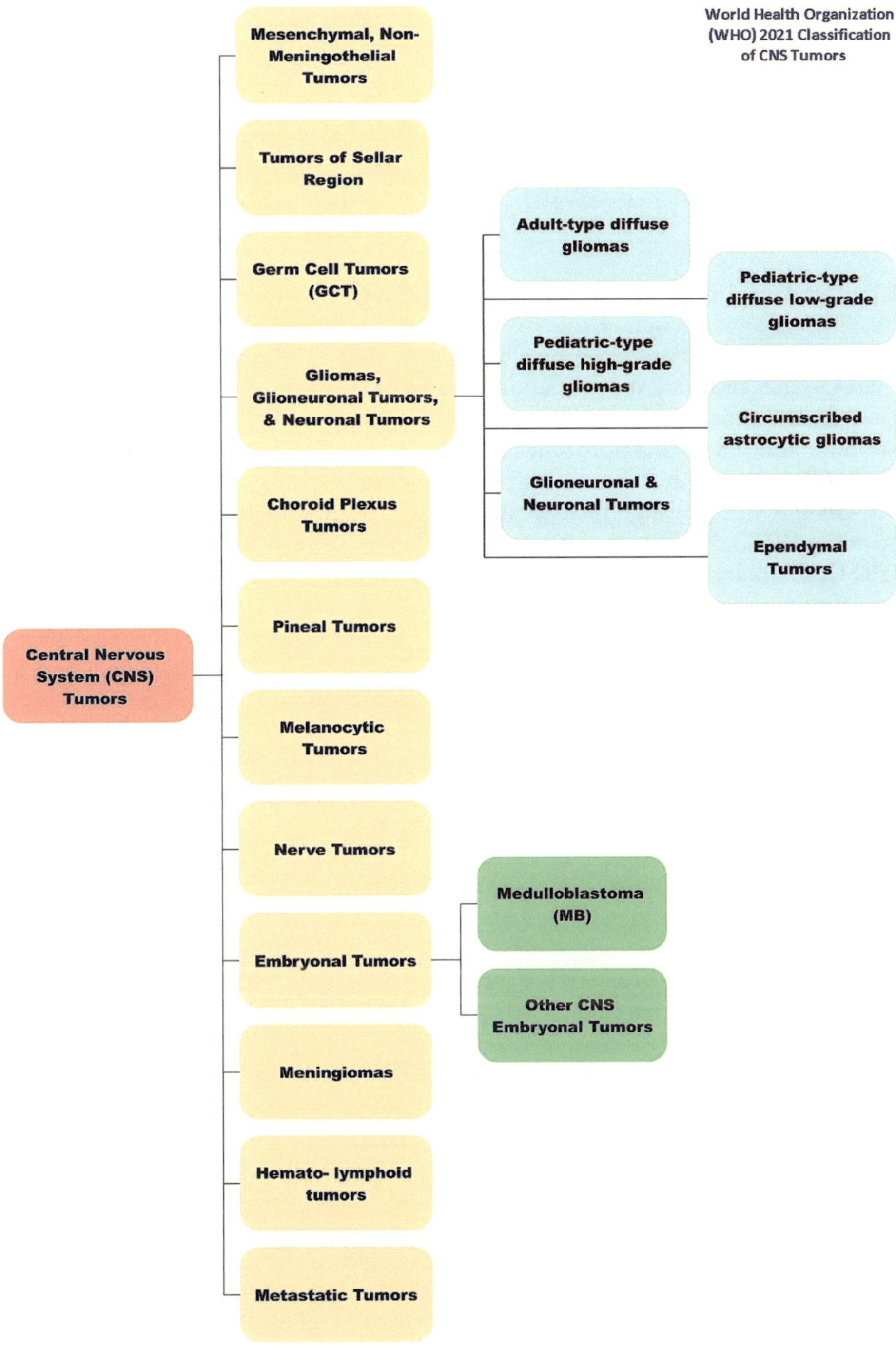


**Figure 1.**
*A broad overview of the World Health Organization (WHO) 2021 classification of central nervous system (CNS) tumors. This original figure has been drawn from [34], published online ahead of print, 2021 Jun 29, noab106, where the full classification is available.*

## 3.2 Modern understanding of tumor grading and its clinical implications

CNS tumor grading has been long-known to be linked closely with clinical-biological features, and this has been augmented with recent works in genomics and

methylomics. Tumor grading guides treatment decisions and the four WHO tumor grades have been historically essential in determining prognosis.

Previously, WHO used to assign a grade to one tumor type (e.g. anaplastic astrocytoma to grade 3), and grading was done across tumor types. With WHO CNS5, this has been radically shifted to grading within tumor types, similar to non-CNS tumors where the latter had been the norm for decades. This approach, while enhancing flexibility while grading, also highlights the pathobiological similarities within tumor types, rather than simply trying to crudely approximate clinical behavior across entities [7].

The current grading paradigm is a combination of histological and molecular featusres, rather than solely being based on microscopic features alone. Key examples of this are reflected in the Update 3 and 5 of cIMPACT-NOW [8]. The newly introduced integrated grading system continues to retain some features from prior WHO classification editions. For instance, meningiomas can only go from grade 1–3, and therefore it is not possible to have a '*CNS WHO Grade 4 Meningioma*'. Additionally, because these malignancies were traditionally graded based on their natural history as well, therefore, current therapeutic options lead to a conflict between the grade and the expected outcome. For instance, a medulloblastoma can be assigned a CNS WHO grade 4, yet a WNT-activated medulloblastoma has good survival outcomes when given effective therapies [7].

## 4. Clinical features of pediatric brain tumors

Pediatric brain tumors are usually suspected based on their specific clinical features. Details regarding the clinical presentation of some common tumors are given in their respective sections. However, in general, these tumors find their manifestation in two major ways, one due to raised intracranial pressure, and the other due to the specific location of the tumor involving adjacent neural structures [9].

In children, raised intracranial pressure may be due to the tumor mass itself, or secondary to hydrocephalus, or maybe a consequence of cerebral edema. Acutely, this may manifest as headache, nausea and vomiting, altered sensorium, irritability, papilledema, hypertension, abnormal breathing, seizures, etc. In the long-term, this may manifest as macrocephaly, loss of appetite, delayed psychomotor development, personality changes, etc. [10].

Brain tumors also may manifest through the involvement of adjacent structures. Focal neurological deficits such as arm or leg weakness in case of cerebral tumors, ataxia and torticollis in posterior fossa tumors, endocrinopathies such as precocious puberty, obesity in case of sellar/parasellar tumors, vision impairment due to cranial nerve involvement, etc. [10].

## 5. Principles of diagnosis and treatment of pediatric brain tumors

An experienced, multidisciplinary team is essential for the management of pediatric CNS tumors, consisting of pediatrician, neuro-radiologist, neuro-oncologist, neurosurgeon, radiation oncologist, physiatrist, and other ancillary services.

### 5.1 Diagnosis

Brain imaging is the mainstay of diagnosis. Computed tomography (CT) and magnetic resonance (MR) imaging are both often required. While the former allows a better assessment of bony involvement and tumoral calcifications, the latter helps

to closely delineate the tumor and the involved anatomy of the region, along with helping predict the type of tumor. MR imaging with gadolinium contrast is often the single most valuable diagnostic test for CNS tumors.

MR Angiography (MRA) is useful for visualizing blood vessels, which helps determine the surgical approach. MR Spectroscopy allows for non-invasive determination of tissue properties of intracranial structures, helping differentiate between neoplastic and non-neoplastic lesions. MR Perfusion helps visualize blood flow to the involved areas [11].

Advances in imaging in the last few decades have led to increasing utilization of additional imaging methods. Diffusion tensor imaging (DTI) for evaluating the involvement of white matter tracts, can be combined with functional MRI to help in preoperative surgical planning. Positron emission tomography (PET) helps to visualize small metastases which may be missed, along with helping differentiate between normal postoperative changes and residual tumor.

Preoperative biopsy serves as the confirmatory tool in determining the presence and the type of tumor. Additionally, in some cases, the preoperative biopsy is not performed and diagnosis is made only based on MR imaging, for instance in diffuse pontine glioma. In other cases, the imaging allows narrowing down to few differentials, the surgery is begun and intraoperative frozen section is viewed to arrive at a tentative diagnosis, after which the definitive surgery is completed.

In addition, coupled with the advent of histo-molecular classification, immunohistochemistry, molecular genetics, and molecular profiling arrays, have all become a key tools of management, especially in well-resourced regions globally. Methylome profiling, which refers to the utilization of broad arrays to find out genome-wide methylation patterns in the DNA, has taken on a greater role as well in helping determine an integrated diagnosis and, thereby, provide effective targeted treatment. The WHO CNS5 provides for the specific methylation signatures for the vast majority of CNS tumors.

Finally, electroencephalography (EEG), audiological and ophthalmological testing, pituitary hormone profile, etc. also are useful tools in the clinician's armamentarium. Lumbar puncture and CSF analysis also serve as an adjunct in some cases, for instance, in the detection of tumor markers in germ cell tumors of the CNS.

## 5.2 Treatment approaches

3 major anti-cancer approaches, in various combination treatment protocols, are the pillars of treatment in pediatric brain tumors: surgery, radiotherapy, and chemotherapy. As discussed prior, these three approaches have extremely varying efficacy in different tumor types and grades.

### *5.2.1 Surgery*

When undertaken with curative intent, surgery often serves as a major player in reducing the bulk of the tumor. It is extremely valuable in tumors with low grade e.g. a CNS Tumor Grade 1 Meningioma. However, its utility is reduced in tumors that lie close to critical structures such as diffuse pontine glioma.

Surgery may be done through the conventional open approache or a microsurgical approach or an endoscopic endonasal approach. The latter may prove invaluable for selected tumors, as in tumors of the sellar/parasellar region [11]. When resecting a tumor, the surgery may be classified based on the residual tumor into subtotal resection, gross total resection, supra-maximal resection, etc. While the subtotal approach leaves behind residual neoplastic tissue to avoid damage to critical structures, a supramaximal resection aims at reducing the tumor burden as much as

possible grossly. Global consensus continues to evolve into the exact definition of these terms and the varying utility of these different resections in different tumors.

Newer methods are pushing the boundaries of safe and effective surgery. Combined with MR Angiography, DTI, and fMRI, along with intraoperative neuromonitoring, surgery can be performed in challenging locations, such as those close to eloquent areas. Furthermore, awake surgery with intra-operative stimulation may be utilized for tumors in eloquent areas in older children [11]. Additionally, 5-Amino Levulinic Acid (5-ALA) based techniques are allowing better intraoperative visualization of residual tumor, thereby assisting in enhanced resection, especially in high-grade gliomas.

A small surgical procedure to insert a ventriculoperitoneal shunt remains a key measure for alleviating hydrocephalus, which is a common complication of brain tumors in the pediatric age group, especially those of the posterior fossa.

#### 5.2.2 Chemotherapy

It finds less value in the brain than in other organs due to the blood–brain barrier which prevents adequate permeation of drugs administered. However, it is still a useful adjuvant approach for several common pediatric tumors, such as medulloblastoma. Notably, intrathecal chemotherapy based on methotrexate and cytarabine is significantly useful in intracranial lymphomas/leukemias [12]. The Ommaya Reservoir is a useful tool for repeated chemotherapy administration as well as repeated CSF withdrawal for either diagnostic and/or therapeutic purposes [13].

#### 5.2.3 Radiotherapy

It has been a cornerstone of preventing recurrence after surgery and in treating tumors that are not amenable to resection. It may be given as teletherapy, in the form of conventional beam radiotherapy, or can be given as brachytherapy, via surgical delivery of emitters into the brain. Radiotherapy is especially valuable in tumors with rapidly dividing cells and/or those having high tumor grade. However, radiotherapy carries significant risks in the growing brain, where it can adversely impact neuronal development and hamper long-term cognitive outcomes. Proton therapy, albeit significantly more expensive, is slowly replacing conventional photon beam therapy [11].

#### 5.2.4 Newer approaches

In addition, other therapeutic approaches have been coming up but are yet to become the standard of care for most tumors. Immunotherapy has been less than successful in pediatric brain tumors [14]. Meanwhile, targeted biological therapies have found greater utility in specific tumors, such as the role of BRAF-inhibitors in tumors with BRAF V600E mutation [15].

#### 5.2.5 Supportive care

Amidst all of this, the role of supportive care, including physiotherapy and rehabilitation cannot be understated. Brain tumors rob children of the joy of their life and their devastating symptoms cause immense stress to both children and their guardians. Corticosteroids for managing cerebral edema, opioids for pain management, antiemetics, anticonvulsants for prophylaxis and treatment of seizures, baclofen for management of spasticity, adequate nutritional support, psychosocial care, etc. all help enhance the quality of life of brain tumor patients [11].

### 5.3 Summary

Having covered the general principles of management, this chapter now proceeds to examine specific brain tumors that have a high burden amongst children.

## 6. Medulloblastoma

Medulloblastoma (MB) is an embryonal tumor of the cerebellum having discrete origins from the neuronal stem or progenitor cell populations during early life. The peak age of diagnosis is 6–8 years. MBs are rarely seen in infancy or during adulthood [16].

### 6.1 Epidemiology and genetics

Medulloblastoma is the most common childhood malignancy of the brain accounting for 20–30% of all pediatric tumors and 64% of all intracranial embryonic tumors [17, 18]. The overall annual incidence rate is approximately 5 cases per million, which does not vary substantially across ethnicities or geographical regions [19, 20]. The male to female ratio is 1.8:1 [21, 22]. A wide range of syndromes like Gorlin syndrome, FAP syndrome, ataxia-telangiectasia, Bloom syndrome, Fanconi's anemia, Li-Fraumeni syndrome and Xeroderma pigmentosum have been implicated in MB pathogenesis [23].

Four subgroups of MB have been defined based on the age of onset, genetic alterations, and prognosis. These are the WNT subgroup MB (10% of MB), the SHH subgroup MB (10–15% of MB), the Group 3 MB (25% OF MB), and the Group 4 MB (50% of MB) [23]. Activating mutations of CTNNB1 stabilize Beta-catenin leading to the constitutional activation of WNT signaling in 85–90% of the WNT subgroup MB, which has a good prognosis in children [24, 25]. Germline/somatic mutations in genes of the SHH signaling pathway (PTCH1, SUFU, SMO, GLI1/2, and MYC) lead to its constitutional activation in SHH subgroup. MYC activation is characteristic for Group 3 MB. Several mutations are implicated in Group 4 MB with no clear majority, including transcriptional repressors like PRDM6 and histone modifiers like KDM6A and KMT2C [26].

### 6.2 Clinical features

The various manifestations of MB are largely attributed to an increase in ICT and cerebellar dysfunction. These include nocturnal or morning headache, nausea, vomiting, and altered mental status. These symptoms evolve over a period of a few weeks to months. Specific cerebellar symptoms include ataxia, visual disturbances (eg. strabismus), impacted fine motor skills (eg. clumsy handwriting) that reflect in the patient's school performance [26]. These commmon clinical features may be accompanied by syndrome-specific presentations. If spinal drop metastasis has occurred, presenting features may include back pain, gait disturbances, bladder and bowel abnormalities. The tumor grows rapidly, worsening the symptoms. If accelerated growth occurs before 18 months, macrocephalus can delay diagnosis in a subset of children owing to the non-fusion of skull sutures [9].

### 6.3 Diagnosis

The diagnosis of MB is based on clinical features, radiology, and histopathology. CSF cytology for microscopic metastasis and molecular analysis for prognostication

are done. MRI shows a midline mass involving the vermis or the fourth ventricle, rarely seen laterally encroaching the cerebellar hemispheres [27, 28]. T1-weighted imaging finds a hypodense to isodense lesion and T2/FLAIR yields a hyperdense tumor. On diffusion-weighted imaging, the lesion shows reduced diffusion due to high cellularity and nucleus-to-cytoplasm ratio [29]. Imaging the spine is more fruitful in detecting drop metastasis than CSF analysis. MB subgroups show characteristic localizations. For instance, the WNT subgroup is usually located in cerebral peduncle/cerebellopontine angle, the SHH subgroup in cerebellar hemispheres, the Group 3 and Group 4 MBs usually located along the midline with extension into the 4th ventricle [30–32].

Medulloblastoma is a round blue cell tumor, having characteristic microscopic appearance. Histopathology and molecular diagnosis distinguish it from other posterior fossa tumors like ependymoma, pilocytic astrocytoma, and other embryonal tumors. These reveal a combination of patterns including classic, desmoplastic/ nodular, MB with excessive nodularity, large cell, and anaplastic [33]. A combination of histologic and genetic variants is integrated for diagnosis.

### 6.4 Treatment and prognosis

The treatment approach includes a combination of maximal safe surgical resection, radiotherapy, and systemic chemotherapy [34]. Though gross total resection remains the mainstay of surgery, patients with minimal residual tumor can be expected to have similar outcomes. The morbidity of a complete resection should be adequately assessed by the surgeon against leaving a part of the tumor [35, 36]. Since MB usually pushes the vermis in a posterior direction, there are high chances of damaging it with tumor removal. Telovelar and transvermian approaches are used to preserve vermis and deep cerebellar nuclei as much as possible. Neuronavigation and neuroimaging are useful in identifying the anatomy correctly to avoid entry into the brainstem and preserve the large draining veins to prevent significant bleeding [37]. Complications following resection include cerebellar mutism syndrome or posterior fossa syndrome possibly due to splitting of the inferior vermis [38].

Adjuvant radiation therapy is initiated 3–4 weeks after surgery. It should involve the entire craniospinal axis and is termed craniospinal irradiation [39]. Focal radiation to surgical bed is not inferior to entire posterior fossa radiation, hence it should be preferred due to less exposure. Outcomes that are based on genomic drivers and prognostic indicators warrant an individualized approach [36]. Proton beam and volumetric arc/ intensity-modulated radiation therapy are being evaluated [39].

Histological subtypes have varying sensitivity for chemotherapy in patients $<3$ years old and $\geq 3$ years old groups. Conventional chemotherapy was found sufficient for patients after gross total resection but not with metastasis or incomplete resection [40]. However, adjuvant chemotherapy and radiotherapy have better outcomes in patients who have undergone partial resection [41].

The overall survival rate is approximately 75% [40]. Age, disseminated or metastatic disease, residual disease after resection, MYC amplification, and large cell anaplastic pathology are all associated with poor prognosis. Infants and children less than 3 years of age have a poor prognosis with a 40–50% survival rate [42].

## 7. Craniopharyngiomas and pituitary tumors

Craniopharyngiomas (CPs) are benign tumors that develop along the hypothalamo-hypophyseal tract, constituting 6–9% of pediatric brain tumors [43]. They arise from remnants of the Rathke's pouch - the craniopharyngeal duct epithelium and may be sellar or suprasellar [44].

## 7.1 Epidemiology and genetics

The incidence of CPs worldwide has been estimated to be 1.33–1.56 per million children per year worldwide [45]. In the United States, the incidence is approximately 2.0–2.3 per million children per year [1], while Japan has a much higher incidence of 3.8 per million children per year [20].

There are two histologic subtypes of CPs - papillary CP (PCP) and adamantinomatous (ACP). Both subtypes have highly specific mutations - ACPs are characterized by somatic mutations in CTNNB1 (encoding β-catenin) that increase β-catenin stability, leading to the activation of the WNT pathway, while PCPs are characterized by BRAF V600E mutations. PCPs are mostly restricted to adults, so our discussion here will be restricted to ACPs [44].

## 7.2 Clinical features

Childhood CPs most commonly occur in the age groups of 6–10 years, followed by 11–15 years [46]. The diagnosis of CP is usually delayed, even by a few years, after symptom onset [47]. Symptoms reflect the location of the tumor, and usually progress with time, due to slow growth.

Features by which these tumors of the sellar region clinically present include:

- Headache is seen in approximately half of all CP patients [47, 48].

- Endocrine deficiencies due to disturbances of the hypothalamo-hypophyseal tract - diminished growth hormone (GH), gonadotropin, thyroid-stimulating hormone (TSH), or adrenocorticotropic hormone secretion (ACTH), in that order of frequency [44]. In children, this most commonly manifests as growth failure. Central diabetes insipidus is also common. At least one endocrine deficit as the first symptom is reported in nearly 87% of all cases [44]

- Visual deficits - symptoms are present, or deficits are unearthed on formal ophthalmologic examination, in 70–80%. The classical bitemporal hemianopia is seen in about half the cases [43].

- Others - depression, regardless of any hormonal deficiency, may occur [48]. Diencephalic syndrome leading to cachexia is a rare manifestation [44].

## 7.3 Diagnosis

A simple rule of thumb is that nearly 90% of pediatric CPs demonstrate calcification, approximately 90% of tumors are predominantly cystic, and about 90% take up the contrast in the cyst walls [47] CT remains the gold standard for the identification of calcifications [44]. The mixed solid and cystic components appear hypodense compared to surrounding cerebral parenchyma. Fluid within the cysts will be of slightly greater density than cerebrospinal fluid due to the higher protein content. CT can also illustrate secondary skull base changes useful for surgical planning [43].

MR Imaging and MR Angiography provide greater clarity regarding the relationship of the tumor with vascular structures. MR spectroscopy (MRS) can identify characteristic elevated peaks of lactate or lipids, to differentiate them from gliomas and pituitary adenomas [43]. Finally, an endocrinological evaluation also reveals deficient hypothalamic function, which is particularly relevant preoperatively [43].

### 7.4 Treatment and prognosis

Each case must be decided on its own merit [43] as there is no consensus. Surgery is indicated in almost all cases. Two broad approaches are used - aggressive surgery at diagnosis, or more conservative surgery with radiotherapy [48].

The choice of surgical approach i.e. endoscopic or open or combined depends on the surgeon's level of comfort, and the location of the tumor. Teams that prefer limited surgical resection only use surgery to alleviate visual or other neurologic deficits, and prevent further progression, with RT used for long-term control. Proton beam therapy for CP has shown great promise [47]. For cysts specifically, repeated aspiration and/ or injection of a sclerosant, or local radiation may be attempted [44, 47, 48]. These may help in postponing RT, particularly in younger children [44].

Postoperative sequelae include panhypopituitarism and hypothalamic obesity, which can be challenging to treat [48]. Others include neurocognitive deficits, sleep disorders, and exacerbated visual deficits [48]. Patients remain at greater risk of ischemic stroke, and secondary malignancy owing to radiation exposure.

Overall, the survival rates are high, around 90%, but due to postoperative sequelae, quality of life is impaired [49]. With recent advances clarifying the pathogenesis of adamantinomatous CPs, there is hope for the development of targeted therapies [50].

## 8. Astrocytoma

Astrocytoma is a tumor arising from the astrocytes, which are a type of glial cells found in the central nervous system (CNS).

### 8.1 Epidemiology and genetics

According to the WHO CNS5 classification, astrocytomas (IDH mutant) are categorized under the broad heading of adult-type diffuse gliomas. Meanwhile diffuse astrocytomas (MYB or MYLB-1 altered) are classified into pediatric type diffuse low-grade gliomas; circumscribed astrocytic glioma encompasses pilocytic astrocytoma, high-grade astrocytoma with piloid features, pleomorphic xanthoastrocytoma, subependymal giant cell astrocytoma, choroid glioma and astroblastoma (MN1-altered) [34]. Astrocytomas do not have any racial or ethnic inclination and are usually sporadic.

### 8.2 Clinical features

Clinical features include headache, seizures, and focal neurological deficit, as discussed in previous tumors [51]. In few cases, these tumors may be associated with Li-Fraumeni syndrome and Lynch syndrome.

### 8.3 Diagnosis

Contrast-enhanced MRI is the mainstay of diagnosis. High-grade gliomas are usually associated with hypointensity on T1-weighted imaging and heterogenous contrast-enhancement. They have increased choline and reduced N-acetyl aspartate on magnetic resonance spectroscopy due to their higher vascularity as well as increased metabolism [52]. Histologically, astrocytomas include cells with irregular, hyperchromatic nuclei and glial fibrillary acidic protein (GFAP) in the cytoplasm, and increased mitotic

activity. Molecular testing plays a key role in the diagnosis, treatment, and prognosis of the patient [52, 53]. IDH mutation testing and, 1p/19q codeletion testing is done.

### 8.4 Treatment

Treatment in most cases is a combination of surgery followed by radiotherapy. Surgery for astrocytoma has benefitted greatly from recent advances, including 5-ALA based resection, awake surgery, intraoperative stimulation, and neuronavigation, allowing for tumor resection close to eloquent structures and critical vessels.

## 9. Ependymomas

Ependymomas are a subset of glial tumors arising from radial glial cells in the subventricular zone, located in or adjacent to the ependymal lining. Most commonly, they are associated with the fourth ventricle [54].

### 9.1 Epidemiology and genetics

Ependymomas account for 10% of all brain tumors making them the third most common intracranial pediatric malignancy, with a sex ratio of 1.77:1 [54]. The annual incidence rate amongst children is 0.46 per million in the United States [1].

WHO classifies ependymomas according to a combination of histopathological and molecular features into supratentorial ependymomas with ZFTA, RELA, YAP1 or MAML2 mutation, posterior fossa ependymomas with H3K27-mutation, EZHIP mutations, and spinal ependymomas with NF2, MYCN mutations. Molecular classification of myxopapillary ependymoma and subependymoma do not add to clinical utility, hence they are studied as separate entities [7].

### 9.2 Clinical features

The age and the site of origin determine presentation. Failure to thrive, lethargy, and irritability like non-specific clinical features are observed in very young children. Posterior fossa tumors present with increased intracranial pressure, nerve palsies, neck pain, and/or ataxia. Supratentorial tumors present with limb weakness, bowel bladder dysfunction, paraesthesia, and pain [55].

Seizures with or without focal neurological deficits are also commonly seen in supratentorial tumors. This may be due to the surrounding edema and mass effect. Spinal cord tumors involve ascending or descending tracts and manifest as specific anatomical lesions. Very rarely, CSF seeding may accompany both infratentorial and supratentorial ependymomas [56].

### 9.3 Diagnosis

The imaging modality of choice is an MRI scan of the brain and spine to evaluate for leptomeningeal dissemination [57]. T1 hypointensity and T2 hyperintensity with heterogeneous enhancement on T1 sequences post-gadolinium enhancement is seen in both spinal and intracranial tumors. Cysts and calcification can be observed, usually with supratentorial tumors. Spinal ependymomas can be differentiated from astrocytomas by a sharp margin and central location. Leptomeningeal spread can be suspected by smooth enhancement along the surface of the spinal cord, nerve root thickening, or irregular thecal sac, and confirmed by cytological assessment post lumbar puncture. Testing for the mutations discussed prior can be done if resources are available.

### 9.4 Treatment and prognosis

Pediatric ependymomas are treated with surgery and radiotherapy [58]. The surgeon's decision about the extent of resection is the most important prognostic factor. Posterior fossa tumors may limit the extent of resection due to involvement of lower cranial nerves and brainstem, thus incomplete resection warrants a second look surgery since overall survival for incomplete resection is much lower than gross total resection [59].

Postoperative radiotherapy is recommended for children as young as 18 months but dose modifications to reduce toxicity should be done [60]. Hypofractionated stereotactic boost in addition to conventional radiotherapy, especially for incomplete surgery, is being studied and shows promise [59]. To avoid radiation exposure to children, chemotherapy use has been investigated but its role remains equivocal [61]. Though long-term follow-up studies of radiotherapy toxicity are pending, the higher progression-free survival with radiotherapy has led to the abandonment of radiotherapy deferral strategies for children below 12 months [62].

Patients with intracranial ependymomas usually have a significant risk of recurrence and decreased 5-year overall survival, nearing approximately 50–70% [62].

## 10. Germ cell tumors

According to the W.H.O. CNS tumor 2021 classification, germ cell tumors are classified into mature teratoma, immature teratoma, teratoma with somatic-type malignancy, germinoma, embryonal carcinoma, yolk sac tumor, choriocarcinoma, and mixed germ cell tumor [34].

### 10.1 Epidemiology and genetics

The incidence of all types of CNS germ cell tumors (GCT) is greater in males of 10–14 years of age. These tumors also possess a racial inclination towards Asians and Pacific Islanders [63]. Although GCTs can arise anywhere in the CNS, the pineal gland is most commonly involved, followed by the suprasellar/ neurohypophyseal area and the basal ganglia. A bifocal tumor is one where both the pineal gland and the neurohypophyseal region are involved [64].

### 10.2 Clinical features

Obstructive hydrocephalus can result from the compression of the cerebral aqueduct by the tumor, often manifested as headache [65]. The damage to the optic nerve due to the mass effect of the tumor can cause visual field defects and decreased visual acuity [66]. Neurophypophyseal tumors can often lead to hypopituitarism, diabetes insipidus [66]. GCT of the basal ganglia can present with hemiparesis. Intracranial hemorrhage is also a complication of GCTs [66]. Due to the involvement of the optic nerve, often the ophthalmologists are the first ones to interact with the patients of CNS GCT, and play a crucial role in the diagnosis.

### 10.3 Diagnosis

The tumor markers associated with CNS GCTs are the following: beta subunit of human chorionic gonadotropin (β -HCG), alpha-fetoprotein (AFP), and placental alkaline phosphatase, which are raised in different types of GCTs differently. In choriocarcinoma, the β-HCG value is >500 mIU/mL, while in germinoma with

syncytiotrophoblastic giant cells, β-HCG is <100 mIU/mL. β-HCG is also increased in mixed germ cell tumors. AFP is raised in yolk sac tumors and mixed germ cell tumors.

The findings on imaging include a typical pineal mass on MRI or CT, usually with calcifications, and signs of obstructive hydrocephalus on CT. Germinomas are generally of uniform intensity with blurred margins. Pineal teratomas appear as heterogeneous well-demarcated masses with occasional calcifications, irregular cysts, or fatty tissue and thus show a peculiar pattern on both CT and MRI [64]. For GCTs occurring in the basal ganglia, enhancement is minimal, and the only detectable abnormality is an occasionally increased signal intensity on FLAIR [64].

### 10.4 Treatment and prognosis

According to the Japanese Pediatric Brain Tumor Study Group, patients with CNS non-seminamatous GCT may be divided into three categories (based on their prognosis): good (mature teratoma and pure germinoma), intermediate (e.g. immature teratoma), and poor (e.g. choriocarcinoma, yolk sac tumor). The 5-year overall survival rate varies as per the histologic type from 10 to over 98%. As for non-seminomatous germ cell tumors, the group reported a 5-year survival rate of 67% with platinum-based chemotherapy followed by surgical resection and craniospinal irradiation together with focal boost [67, 68].

## 11. Brain stem gliomas

Brainstem gliomas constitute 10–20% of all pediatric CNS malignancies and can be broadly divided into focal brainstem gliomas (FBGs) and diffuse intrinsic pontine gliomas (DIPGs) [1, 69].

### 11.1 Epidemiology and genetics

#### *11.1.1 FBG*

FBGs usually arise in the midbrain or the medulla and are well-circumscribed, low-grade tumors – usually being pilocytic or diffuse astrocytomas. These may be associated with Neurofibromatosis 1 (NF1). Characteristic mutations include chromosome 7q34 duplications, resulting in a KIAA1549-BRAF fusion, in pilocytic astrocytomas, and a BRAF V600E mutation in fibrillary astrocytomas, the majority of pleomorphic xanthoastrocytomas, and nearly half of the gangliocytomas [69–71].

#### *11.1.2 DIPG*

DIPGs constitute 80% of all pediatric brainstem tumors and are diffuse, high-grade, and infiltrative. 80% of these have H3K27 mutations on two histone H3 genes, identified primarily through autopsy studies [69]. EGFR mutations are also common [72]. Histologically, these are usually high grade, although a significant proportion may appear low grade, which is ultimately irrelevant for prognosis.

### 11.2 Clinical features

#### *11.2.1 FBG*

These usually present insidiously over many years [69–71]. Isolated cranial nerve deficits, neck stiffness, and pain, contralateral hemiparesis are common [69–71].

Medullary tumors may cause dysphagia or apnea, while cervicomedullary tumors may present with ataxia and/ or lower motor neuron signs. Hydrocephalus is uncommon, except in posteriorly extending tumors and tumors of tectal origin [69–71].

#### *11.2.2 DIPG*

Patients typically present around the age of 7 years, with a short history, sometimes for less than a month [69, 73, 74]. The classical triad of (1) cranial nerve palsies, most commonly VI and VII - facial asymmetry and diplopia (2) long tract signs - upgoing Babinski, and hyperreflexia, and (3) cerebellar signs - ataxia, dementia is seen in over 50% [73]. Symptoms and signs of raised ICT are seen in less than 10% at diagnosis and are more typical in the end stages of the disease [73].

### **11.3 Diagnosis**

#### *11.3.1 FBG*

On MRI, these usually have well-defined borders, no edema, iso- or hypointensity on T1, and hyperintensity on T2 weighted images, with homogeneous contrast enhancement [69–71]. MR Spectrography can support the diagnosis, with the estimation of choline-to-N-acetylaspartate (Choline:NAA) ratios differentiating high grade from low-grade tumors. Diffusion Tensor Imaging (DTI) can also provide estimates of long tract disruption [69].

#### *11.3.2 DIPG*

DIPGs are typically hypointense on T1 and hyperintense on T2 weighted MRI [69, 73]. Contrast enhancement is variable. A diffuse expansion of the pons is typical. This may involve adjacent areas, such as the cerebellum and midbrain; the medulla is usually spared [69–71]. There is usually an exophytic component, and the tumor may surround the basilar artery. However, a serial assessment may be difficult due to their heterogeneous signal characteristics and interobserver variability. Here too, MR spectrography with Choline:NAA ratio estimation can support the tentative diagnosis and may provide prognostic information [71].

### **11.4 Treatment and prognosis**

#### *11.4.1 FBG*

In surgically accessible regions, resection is performed. While complete resection is curative, it should not be performed at the cost of neurologic deficit, as even incomplete resection has excellent long-term outcomes [75].

Chemotherapy is preferred for inoperable tumors, symptom progression, or persistence after surgery. Tumor growth can at least be stabilized, delaying or even eliminating the need for RT in young children [69–71]. Two popular, effective combinations are that of vincristine and carboplatin, and another of 6-thioguanine, procarbazine, lomustine, and vincristine (TPCV) [69]. TPCV has improved progression-free survival, but carries long-term risks associated with alkylator use [69]. Radiotherapy is an option for surgically inaccessible tumors but should be reserved for older children given the potential for significant morbidity [69–71]. Long-term overall survival approaches 100% [70], but chronic disability is common, resulting from both tumor expansion and RT [70].

### 11.4.2 DIPG

Surgery is usually not recommended [71]. The mainstay of treatment is fractionated radiotherapy alone [73]. There is still uncertainty regarding the mode of RT to be delivered, with future trials comparing fractionated and conventional RT encouraged [76]. Monotherapy or combination chemotherapy have proven ineffective.

With greater clarity regarding the genetic make-up and microenvironment of these tumors, immunotherapy and molecular targets, such as anti-GD2 chimeric antigen receptor (CAR) T-cell therapy and histone deacetylase (HDAC) inhibitors are showing promise [71, 73].

The prognosis remains dismal, with less than 3% surviving at 5 years [71]. Long-term survivors usually have neurological deficits and cognitive impairment [76].

## 12. Meningiomas

Meningiomas arise from arachnoidal cap cells in CNS.

### 12.1 Epidemiology and genetics

They are rare in children, representing only 2–3% of pediatric CNS tumors [77]. Their incidence is markedly greater in syndromes like Neurofibromatosis 2, Schwannomatosis, Gorlin syndrome, and familial meningioma syndrome [77, 78]. Exposure to irradiation in childhood predisposes to the development of meningiomas [77, 78].

### 12.2 Clinical features

Mostly, they present in the second decade of life [78]. The most common presenting symptoms are headache, seen in almost half, followed by seizures, seen in almost 30%. Focal findings such as visual deficits, cranial nerve signs may also be present.

### 12.3 Diagnosis

CT and MRI demonstrate a well-defined, extra-axial, dural-based mass, that displaces the normal brain. It is isointense or hypointense to gray matter on T1 and isointense or hyperintense on T2-weighted images [77]. Contrast enhancement is strong and uniform on both CT and MRI [78]. On histology, most are WHO Grade I. The best-characterized mutation is that of the NF2 gene, with other molecular mechanisms in the pediatric age group poorly characterized. Tumors in this age group are genetically distinct from their adult counterparts [78].

### 12.4 Treatment and prognosis

Symptomatic meningiomas require resection. The extent of initial resection is a prognostic factor, so total resection must be done where possible. Adjuvant RT is recommended for WHO Grade III tumors, while inoperable WHO Grade I and Grade II tumors require a case-by-case consideration [78]. The 5-year survival is approximately 90%. Those who undergo gross-total resection, those without NF2, and those with lower-grade tumors have higher survival rates.

## 13. Schwannoma

Schwannomas or neurilemmomas are tumors originating from schwann cells around the axons of the cranial nerves. They are encapsulated and do not transform into malignancies [79].

### 13.1 Epidemiology and genetics

Though schwannomas are more commonly seen in adults between the ages of 50-60 years, 89% of nerve sheath tumors are schwannomas even in children [79], the incidence of which is 0.44 cases per 100,000/ year [80, 81]. Most (90%) of the schwannomas are sporadic and others occur as part of syndromes like NF2 and Carney complex. Inactivation of gene NF2 coding for the merlin protein (schwannomin) has been implicated in both sporadic and syndromic schwannomas. Spinal schwannomas may have SMARCB1 mutations [82].

### 13.2 Clinical features

These tumors grow slowly and may present much later with location-specific symptoms. Vestibular schwannomas may present with headache, imbalance, tinnitus, cranial nerve deficits and motor weakness. Spinal schwannomas may present with pain, paresthesia, and/or motor weakness [83].

### 13.3 Diagnosis

MRI is preferred over CT for diagnosis since plain radiographs are not specific. They usually show an oval or round mass with an isointense or hypointense signal on T1 and hyperintense, heterogeneous signal on T2 images [82]. Classically, microscopic findings include Antoni A and Antoni B areas, with Verrocay Bodies.

### 13.4 Treatment and prognosis

The benign course of these tumors may allow for observation and serial MRI scans for periodic assessment. Biopsy to confirm histology before resection is recommended. Surgical approaches include the retro-sigmoid, middle fossa, or translabyrinthine approach [84]. Stereotactic radiosurgery may be of benefit if complete resection cannot be done. Usually, these tumors have an excellent prognosis, however, postoperative complications which are more common in the pediatric population may worsen it [85].

## 14. Other tumors

### 14.1 Choroid plexus tumor

Choroid plexus tumors arise from neuroepithelial tissue that makes CSF in the ventricles, and therefore their distribution corresponds to the amount of the choroid plexus present in different ventricles [86]. Nearly 50% occur in the lateral ventricles, 40% in the 4th ventricle and merely 5% in the third ventricle. Meanwhile, multifocal occurrence is seen in around 5% of tumors. Overall, they are merely 1% of all pediatric brain tumors, but make up 15% of tumors in children aged <1 year. Headache and/or hydrocephalus are two common clinical presentations [87].

They are of two major varieties:

#### *14.1.1 Choroid plexus papilloma (CPP)*

These are likely hamartomas and therefore appear similar to normal choroid plexus tissue histologically. Classified as WHO grade I in general, they contain uniform cellularity with little/no atypia and KI-67 index <2%. Atypical CPPs have higher mitotic count (≥2 mitoses/high power field) and are classified as grade II [86]. They are calcified and enhance with contrast. On MR imaging they have flow voids due to their vascularity, with enlarged choroidal arteries on MR angiography. Asymptomatic tumors can be monitored conservatively and only resected if producing symptoms or enlarging. Surgery is the modality of choice for symptomatic and/or large CPPs. Adjuvant radiotherapy is usually not required and prognosis is excellent, with 10-year survival exceeding 80% [88, 89].

#### *14.1.2 Choroid plexus carcinoma (CPC)*

These are rarer than CPPs and can be a part of manifestation of Li-Fraumeni Syndrome. They are aggressive tumors, with their invasion making gross total resection insufficient. Radiotherapy is useful but prognosis is poor with median survival of <3 years [87].

### 14.2 Atypical teratoid/rhabdoid tumor

These are highly aggressive tumors which occur in children <3 years of age, with nearly two third occurring in the cerebellum, and nearly a fourth being supratentorial.

These have specific diagnostic criteria, of which the characteristic 'Rhabdoid Cells' are not a part. The criteria are (A) loss of INI1 nuclear staining (corresponding to biallelic inactivation of SMARCB1) and (B) loss of BRG1 staining (corresponding to inactivation of SMARCB4) [90, 91]. On MRI, they are hypo-intense on both T1 and T2, with several cysts and hemorrhages, leading to a heterogeneous appearance. Leptomeningeal enhancement may be visualized. Surgery has little role here. Combination chemotherapy followed by radiotherapy is utilized but is challenging to implement given the very young age of patients at the time of diagnosis. Therapy has to be closely matched to the child's age, AT/RT's location, and disease extent [92]. Prognosis is unsatisfactory, with nearly 30% 5-year survival [93].

### 14.3 Neuronal and mixed neuronal-glial tumors

Neuroepithelial tissues in the CNS give rise to mixtures of glial and/ or neuronal differentiated tumors. These are rare tumors in children.

#### *14.3.1 Ganglioneuromas*

These account for 0.3–1.4% of all CNS tumors, usually occurring in adolescents [94]. Focal motor seizures are the most common presentation involving the temporal lobe [95]. They are diagnosed by MRI and gross total resection is usually preferred for better survival rates [94].

#### *14.3.2 Desmoplastic infantile ganglioglioma or desmoplastic infantile astrocytoma*

They are supratentorial cystic tumors usually affecting children less than 2 years [96]. Frontal and parietal lobes are the most common locations which present as head enlargement, seizures, vomiting, and headache are observed. Diagnosed with

MRI, they are slow-growing tumors. They have a good prognosis after complete removal, rarely requiring radiotherapy and chemotherapy [97].

*14.3.3 Dysembryoplastic neuroepithelial tumor*

These tumors cause early-onset epilepsy in children with an incidence of 0.03 person-year per 100,000 and have slight male predominance [98]. The mesial temporal lobe is the most common location identified on imaging. Favorable outcomes are reached in 70–90% of cases after complete resection [99].

*14.3.4 Papillary glioneuronal tumor*

Characterized by papillary architecture and bipartite (astrocytic and neurocytic) cellularity, these tumors mostly occur near the lateral ventricles [100]. Imaging shows them as circumscribed lesions with frequent cystic alterations. Patients are either asymptomatic or complain of mild symptoms. Their benign course rarely warrants complete resection [101].

*14.3.5 Rosette-forming glioneuronal tumor*

Usually seen in children above 6 years of age, with a female predominance, their location in the 4th ventricle is one of the defining features [102]. Headache, nausea/vomiting, ataxia, and visual disturbances are common manifestations. MRI reveals solid or cystic or mixed solid and cystic masses rarely with calcifications. Full resection prevents recurrence [102].

*14.3.6 Myxoid glioneuronal tumor*

These are extremely rare tumors. They present as seizures and other focal deficits. A histopathological feature of myxoid stroma, somatic next-generation sequencing showing PDGFRA gene mutation, and MRI findings help in diagnosis. They have a benign course [103].

*14.3.7 Diffuse leptomeningeal glioneuronal tumor*

These tumors have variable neuronal components including neurocytes and ganglion cells [104]. The median age of presentation is five years with slight female predominance [105]. MRI shows meningeal enhancement in spinal cord and basilar [106]. Symptoms mimic meningitis and hydrocephalus. Chemotherapy and radiotherapy are first-line options [107].

*14.3.8 Gangliocytoma*

These account for 1–5% of all pediatric CNS tumors [108]. Majority of them occur in the temporal lobe, causing epilepsy, varied neurological signs/symptoms including cranial nerve deficits, focal weakness, and hydrocephalus [109]. Gross total resection yields a good prognosis.

*14.3.9 Multinodular and vacuolating neuronal tumor*

Very few cases have been reported diagnosing this new entity. Non-specific clinical features like chronic headache, paresthesias, and cognitive impairment are reported. MRI is used for diagnosis and studies of treatment modalities are yet unavailable [110].

#### *14.3.10 Dysplastic cerebellar gangliocytoma or Lhermitte-Duclos disease*

This is a rare entity in children that mimics low-grade glial tumors or infectious diseases. A slow-growing pattern and late clinical manifestations allow for conservative treatment and outpatient follow-up for asymptomatic children [111].

#### *14.3.11 Neurocytomas*

Depending on their location, these are divided into central, extraventricular, and cerebellar. They often mimic oligodendrogliomas and the confirmation of diagnosis rests on immunohistochemistry, histology and genetic studies. Safe maximal resection is considered the ideal option for a good prognosis. Adjuvant radiotherapy benefits incomplete resection [110].

### 14.4 Hemangiomas

Infantile CNS hemangiomas are rare benign tumors composed of endothelial cells. They are seen in about 1% of children with cutaneous hemangiomas and have a female predilection [112, 113]. They may be associated with PHACES (posterior fossa malformations, hemangioma, arterial anomalies, coarctation of the aorta/ cardiac defects, and eye abnormalities) syndrome, and are more common in the posterior fossa [112]. GLUT1 represents a reliable marker. They have a rapid, early stage of proliferation followed by one of involution that usually extends from 1 year of age to 5 to 7 years of life [112]. Many are asymptomatic or undiscovered, but others can present with seizures, focal deficits, or symptoms of raised ICP [112].

During the proliferative phase, CT and MRI show a well-circumscribed lobular homogeneous soft-tissue mass with intense and persistent enhancement, with Doppler showing features of fast flow. In the involuting phase, they enhance to a lesser degree, have fewer radiographic signs of fast-flow vascularity, and appear heterogeneous. The final involuted phase is represented by fibrofatty tissue [112]. Imaging can establish continuity between the CNS tumor and the extra CNS component. Corticosteroids represent the mainstay of treatment. Interferon-alpha and propranolol may also be used [112]. For biopsy, or mass effect alleviation, excision may be tried.

## 15. Conclusions

Pediatric brain tumors have an immense disease burden, given their status as the most common solid organ tumors of children. The WHO 2021 Classification is a landmark change in the approach to diagnosing and treating these tumors. The landscape of their treatment has been rapidly evolving, with effective therapies on the horizon. In current clinical practice, surgery, radiotherapy and chemotherapy continue to be the mainstay of management.

## Conflict of interest

The authors declare no conflict of interest.

## Author details

Ahmad Ozair[1*], Erum Khan[2], Vivek Bhat[3], Arjumand Faruqi[1] and Anil Nanda[4]

1 Faculty of Medicine, King George's Medical University, Lucknow, India

2 Faculty of Medicine, B. J. Medical College, Ahmedabad, India

3 Faculty of Medicine, St. John's Medical College, Bangalore, India

4 Department of Neurosurgery, Rutgers Robert Wood Johnson Medical School, New Brunswick, New Jersey, USA

*Address all correspondence to: ahmadozair@kgmcindia.edu

## References


[1] Ostrom QT, Patil N, Cioffi G, et al. CBTRUS statistical report: Primary brain and other central nervous system tumors diagnosed in the United States in 2013-2017. Neuro Oncol. 2020;22(12 Suppl 2):iv1-96

[2] Girardi F, Allemani C, Coleman MP. Worldwide trends in survival from common childhood brain tumors: A systematic review. J Glob Oncol. 2019;(5):1-25

[3] Mohammadi E, Ghasemi E, Azadnajafabad S, et al. A global, regional, and national survey on burden and Quality of Care Index (QCI) of brain and other central nervous system cancers; global burden of disease systematic analysis 1990-2017. PLoS One. 2021;16(2):e0247120

[4] Stavinoha P, Askins M, Powell S,. Neurocognitive and psychosocial outcomes in pediatric brain tumor survivors. Bioengineering (Basel). 2018;5(3):73.

[5] Priesterbach-Ackley LP, Wesseling P, Snijders TJ, et al. Molecular tools for the pathologic diagnosis of central nervous system tumors. Neurooncol Pract. 2019;6(1):4-16.

[6] Louis DN, Ohgaki H, Wiestler OD, et al. The 2007 WHO classification of tumours of the central nervous system. Acta Neuropathol. 2007;114(5):547-547.

[7] Lyon: International Agency for Research on Cancer. World Health Organization Classification of Tumours of the Central Nervous System. 5th ed. WHO; 2021.

[8] Gonzalez Castro LN, Wesseling P. The cIMPACT-NOW updates and their significance to current neuro-oncology practice. Neurooncol Pract. 2021; 8(1):4-10.

[9] Wilne S, Collier J, Kennedy C, et al. Presentation of childhood CNS tumours: a systematic review and meta-analysis. Lancet Oncol. 2007;8(8):685-695.

[10] Wilne SH. The presenting features of brain tumours: a review of 200 cases. Arch Dis Child. 2006;91(6):502-506.

[11] Richterová R, Kolarovszki B. Primary brain tumors in childhood. In: Agrawal A, Moscote-Salazar LR, editors. Brain Tumors - An Update. London, England: InTech; 2018.

[12] Pui C-H, Howard SC. Current management and challenges of malignant disease in the CNS in paediatric leukaemia. Lancet Oncol. 2008;9(3):257-268.

[13] Zubair A, De Jesus O. Ommaya Reservoir. In: StatPearls. Treasure Island (FL): StatPearls Publishing; 2021

[14] Foster JB, Madsen PJ, Hegde M, et al. Immunotherapy for pediatric brain tumors: past and present. Neuro Oncol. 2019;21(10):1226-1238.

[15] Kieran MW, Hargrave DR, Cohen KJ, et al. Phase 1 study of dabrafenib in pediatric patients (pts) with relapsed or refractory BRAF V600E high- and low-grade gliomas (HGG, LGG), Langerhans cell histiocytosis (LCH), and other solid tumors (OST). J Clin Oncol. 2015;33(15_suppl):10004-10004.

[16] Northcott PA, Robinson GW, Kratz CP, et al. Medulloblastoma. Nat Rev Dis Primers. 2019;5(1):11

[17] Curran EK, Sainani KL, Le GM. Gender affects survival for medulloblastoma only in older children and adults: a study from the surveillance epidemiology and end results registry. Pediatr Blood Cancer. 2009;52(1).

[18] Liu X, Ding C, Tan W, Zhang A. Medulloblastoma: Molecular understanding, treatment evolution, and new developments. Pharmacol Ther. 2020;210(107516):107516.

[19] Ezzat S, Kamal M, El-Khateeb N, et al. Pediatric brain tumors in a low/middle income country: does it differ from that in developed world? J Neurooncol. 2016;126(2):371-376.

[20] Makino K, Nakamura H, Yano S, Kumamoto Brain Tumor Group. Population-based epidemiological study of primary intracranial tumors in childhood. Childs Nerv Syst. 2010;26(8):1029-1034.

[21] Ramaswamy V, Remke M, Bouffet E, et al. Risk stratification of childhood medulloblastoma in the molecular era: the current consensus. Acta Neuropathol. 2016;131(6):821-831.

[22] Johnston DL, Keene D, Kostova M, et al. Incidence of medulloblastoma in Canadian children. J Neurooncol. 2014;120(3):575-579

[23] Northcott PA, Korshunov A, Witt H, et al. Medulloblastoma comprises four distinct molecular variants. J Clin Oncol. 2011; 29(11):1408-1414.

[24] Thompson MC, Fuller C, Hogg TL, et al. Genomics identifies medulloblastoma subgroups that are enriched for specific genetic alterations. J Clin Oncol. 2006;24(12):1924-1931.

[25] Gajjar A, Chintagumpala M, Ashley D, et al. Risk-adapted craniospinal radiotherapy followed by high-dose chemotherapy and stem-cell rescue in children with newly diagnosed medulloblastoma (St Jude Medulloblastoma-96): long-term results from a prospective, multicentre trial. Lancet Oncol. 2006;7(10): 813-820.

[26] Northcott PA, Buchhalter I, Morrissy AS, et al. The whole-genome landscape of medulloblastoma subtypes. Nature. 2017;547(7663):311-317.

[27] Fruehwald-Pallamar J, Puchner SB, Rossi A, et al. Magnetic resonance imaging spectrum of medulloblastoma. Neuroradiology. 2011;53(6):387-396

[28] Koeller KK, Rushing EJ. From the archives of the AFIP: medulloblastoma: a comprehensive review with radiologic-pathologic correlation: Medulloblastoma: A comprehensive review with radiologic-pathologic correlation. Radiographics. 2003;23(6):1613-1637.

[29] Rumboldt Z, Camacho DLA, Lake D, et al. Apparent diffusion coefficients for differentiation of cerebellar tumors in children. AJNR Am J Neuroradiol. 2006;27(6):1362-1369.

[30] Perreault S, Ramaswamy V, Achrol AS, et al. MRI surrogates for molecular subgroups of medulloblastoma. AJNR Am J Neuroradiol. 2014;35(7):1263-1269.

[31] Gibson P, Tong Y, Robinson G, et al. Subtypes of medulloblastoma have distinct developmental origins. Nature. 2010;468(7327):1095-1099.

[32] Teo W-Y, Shen J, Su JMF, et al. Implications of tumor location on subtypes of medulloblastoma: Tumor location in medulloblastoma subtypes. Pediatr Blood Cancer. 2013;60(9): 1408-1410.

[33] Ellison DW, Dalton J, Kocak M, et al. Medulloblastoma: clinicopathological correlates of SHH, WNT, and non-SHH/WNT molecular subgroups. Acta Neuropathol. 2011;121(3):381-396.

[34] Louis DN, Perry A, Wesseling P, et al. The 2021 WHO classification of tumors of the Central Nervous System:

A summary. Neuro Oncol. 2021;23(8):1231-1251

[35] Pomeroy Scott. Treatment and prognosis of medulloblastoma. In: UpToDate, Post TW (Ed), UpToDate, Waltham.MA. (Accessed on July 17,2021).

[36] Taylor MD, Northcott PA, Korshunov A, et al. Molecular subgroups of medulloblastoma: the current consensus. Acta Neuropathol. 2012;123(4):465-472.

[37] Kline CN, Packer RJ, Hwang EI, et al. Case-based review: pediatric medulloblastoma. Neurooncol Pract. 2017;4(3):138-150.

[38] Gudrunardottir T, Sehested A, Juhler M, et al. Cerebellar mutism: review of the literature: Review of the literature. Childs Nerv Syst. 2011;27(3):355-363

[39] St Clair WH, Adams JA, Bues M, et al. Advantage of protons compared to conventional X-ray or IMRT in the treatment of a pediatric patient with medulloblastoma. Int J Radiat Oncol Biol Phys. 2004;58(3):727-734

[40] Grill J, Sainte-Rose C, Jouvet A, et al. Treatment of medulloblastoma with postoperative chemotherapy alone: an SFOP prospective trial in young children. Lancet Oncol. 2005;6(8): 573-580.

[41] Deng Z, Wang Y, Li X, et al. Different prognostic effect of surgery, radiation and chemotherapy in pediatric medulloblastoma less and over three years old: A SEER analysis [Internet]. Research Square. 2021 [cited 2021 Aug 30]. Available from: https://www.researchsquare.com/article/rs-614952/latest

[42] Archer TC, Mahoney EL, Pomeroy SL. Medulloblastoma: Molecular classification-based personal therapeutics. Neurotherapeutics. 2017;14(2):265-273.

[43] Drapeau A, Walz PC, Eide JG, et al. Pediatric craniopharyngioma. Childs Nerv Syst. 2019;35(11):2133-2145.

[44] Müller HL, Merchant TE, Warmuth-Metz M, et al. Craniopharyngioma. Nat Rev Dis Primers. 2019;5(1):75.

[45] Nielsen EH, Feldt-Rasmussen U, Poulsgaard L, et al. Incidence of craniopharyngioma in Denmark (n = 189) and estimated world incidence of craniopharyngioma in children and adults. J Neurooncol. 2011;104(3): 755-763.

[46] Müller HL. Childhood craniopharyngioma: current controversies on management in diagnostics, treatment and follow-up. Expert Rev Neurother. 2010;10(4): 515-524.

[47] Müller HL, Merchant TE, Puget S, et al. New outlook on the diagnosis, treatment and follow-up of childhood-onset craniopharyngioma. Nat Rev Endocrinol. 2017;13(5):299-312.

[48] Harsh GR, Recht LD, Marcus KJ. Craniopharyngioma. In: UpToDate, Post TW (Ed), UpToDate, Waltham, MA. (Accessed on July 16, 2021.)

[49] Sterkenburg AS, Hoffmann A, Gebhardt U, et al. Survival, hypothalamic obesity, and neuropsychological/psychosocial status after childhood-onset craniopharyngioma: newly reported long-term outcomes. Neuro Oncol. 2015;17(7):1029-1038.

[50] Gupta S, Bi WL, Giantini Larsen A et al. Craniopharyngioma: a roadmap for scientific translation. Neurosurg Focus. 2018;44(6):E12.

[51] Chang SM, Parney IF, Huang W, et al. Patterns of care for adults with

newly diagnosed malignant glioma. JAMA. 2005;293(5):557-564.

[52] Scott JN, Brasher PMA, Sevick RJ, et al. How often are nonenhancing supratentorial gliomas malignant? A population study. Neurology. 2002;59(6):947-949.

[53] Velázquez Vega JE, Brat DJ, Ryken TC, et al. The role of neuropathology in the management of newly diagnosed glioblastoma: a systematic review and evidence-based clinical practice guideline. J Neurooncol. 2020;150(2):143-164.

[54] Purdy E, Johnston DL, Bartels U, et al. Ependymoma in children under the age of 3 years: a report from the Canadian Pediatric Brain Tumour Consortium. J Neurooncol. 2014;117(2): 359-364.

[55] Allen JC, Siffert J, Hukin J. Clinical manifestations of childhood ependymoma: a multitude of syndromes. Pediatr Neurosurg. 1998;28(1):49-55.

[56] Benesch M, Mynarek M, Witt H, et al. Newly diagnosed metastatic intracranial ependymoma in children: Frequency, molecular characteristics, treatment, and outcome in the prospective HIT series. Oncologist. 2019;24(9):e921–e929.

[57] Colosimo C, Celi G, Settecasi C, et al. Magnetic resonance and computerized tomography of posterior cranial fossa tumors in childhood. Differential diagnosis and assessment of lesion extent. Radiol Med. 1995;90(4):386-395.

[58] Pejavar S, Polley M-Y, Rosenberg-Wohl S, et al. Pediatric intracranial ependymoma: the roles of surgery, radiation and chemotherapy. J Neurooncol. 2012;106(2):367-375.

[59] Massimino M, Solero CL, Garrè ML, et al. Second-look surgery for ependymoma: the Italian experience: Clinical article. J Neurosurg Pediatr. 2011;8(3):246-250.

[60] Koshy M, Rich S, Merchant TE, et al. Post-operative radiation improves survival in children younger than 3 years with intracranial ependymoma. J Neurooncol. 2011;105(3):583-590.

[61] Khatua S, Ramaswamy V, Bouffet E. Current therapy and the evolving molecular landscape of paediatric ependymoma. Eur J Cancer. 2017;70:34-41.

[62] Merchant TE, Li C, Xiong X, et al. Conformal radiotherapy after surgery for paediatric ependymoma: a prospective study. Lancet Oncol. 2009;10(3):258-266.

[63] Gittleman H, Cioffi G, Vecchione-Koval T, et al. Descriptive epidemiology of germ cell tumors of the central nervous system diagnosed in the United States from 2006 to 2015. J Neurooncol. 2019;143(2):251-260.

[64] Fujimaki T. Central nervous system germ cell tumors: classification, clinical features, and treatment with a historical overview. J Child Neurol. 2009;24(11): 1439-1445.

[65] Echevarría ME, Fangusaro J, Goldman S. Pediatric central nervous system germ cell tumors: a review. Oncologist. 2008;13(6):690-699.

[66] Crawford JR, Santi MR, Vezina G, Myseros JS, Keating RF, LaFond DA, et al. CNS germ cell tumor (CNSGCT) of childhood: presentation and delayed diagnosis. Neurology. 2007;68(20): 1668-1673.

[67] Matsutani M, The Japanese Pediatric Brain Tumor Study Group. Combined chemotherapy and radiation therapy for CNS germ cell tumors--the Japanese experience. J Neurooncol. 2001;54(3): 311-316.

[68] Calaminus G, Bamberg M, Jürgens H, Kortmann RD, Sörensen N, Wiestler OD, et al. Impact of surgery, chemotherapy and irradiation on long term outcome of intracranial malignant non-germinomatous germ cell tumors: results of the German Cooperative Trial MAKEI 89. Klin Padiatr. 2004;216(3):141-149.

[69] Green AL, Kieran MW. Pediatric brainstem gliomas: new understanding leads to potential new treatments for two very different tumors. Curr Oncol Rep. 2015;17(3):436.

[70] Karajjanis MA, Marcus KJ. Focal brainstem glioma. In: UpToDate, Post TW (Ed), UpToDate, Waltham, MA. (Accessed on July 17, 2021.)

[71] Marcus KJ, Karajjanis MA. Diffuse intrinsic pontine glioma. In: UpToDate, Post TW (Ed), UpToDate, Waltham, MA. (Accessed on July 17, 2021.)

[72] Li G, Mitra SS, Monje M, Henrich KN, et al. Expression of epidermal growth factor variant III (EGFRvIII) in pediatric diffuse intrinsic pontine gliomas. J Neurooncol. 2012;108(3):395-402.

[73] Srikanthan D, Taccone MS, Van Ommeren R, et al. Diffuse intrinsic pontine glioma: current insights and future directions. Chin Neurosurg J. 2021;7(1):6.

[74] Donaldson SS, Laningham F, Fisher PG. Advances toward an understanding of brainstem gliomas. J Clin Oncol. 2006;24(8):1266-1272.

[75] Bandopadhayay P, Bergthold G, London WB, et al. Long-term outcome of 4,040 children diagnosed with pediatric low-grade gliomas: an analysis of the Surveillance Epidemiology and End Results (SEER) database: PLGG SEER Long-Term Outcome. Pediatr Blood Cancer. 2014;61(7):1173-1179.

[76] Hoffman LM, Veldhuijzen van Zanten SEM, et al. Clinical, radiologic, pathologic, and molecular characteristics of long-term survivors of Diffuse intrinsic pontine glioma (DIPG): A collaborative report from the international and European society for pediatric oncology DIPG registries. J Clin Oncol. 2018;36(19):1963-1972.

[77] Park JK. Epidemiology, pathology, clinical features, and diagnosis of meningioma. In: UpToDate, Post TW (Ed), UpToDate, Waltham, MA. (Accessed July 17, 2021.)

[78] Szychot E, Youssef A, Ganeshan B, Endozo R, Hyare H, Gains J, et al. Predicting outcome in childhood diffuse midline gliomas using magnetic resonance imaging based texture analysis. J Neuroradiol. 2021;48(4): 243-247.

[79] Bhattacharyya AK, Perrin R, Guha A. Peripheral nerve tumors: management strategies and molecular insights. J Neurooncol. 2004;69(1-3): 335-349.

[80] Propp JM, McCarthy BJ, Davis FG, et al. Descriptive epidemiology of vestibular schwannomas. Neuro Oncol. 2006;8(1):1-1.

[81] Smith JP. The functions of the nurse in an integrated national health service. J Adv Nurs. 1979;4(4):439-452.

[82] Sheikh MM, De Jesus O. Schwannoma. StatPearls [Internet]. 2021 [cited 2021 Aug 31]; Available from: https://www.statpearls.com/ArticleLibrary/viewarticle/28766

[83] Yu NH, Lee SE, Jahng T-A, et al. Giant invasive spinal schwannoma: Its clinical features and surgical management. Neurosurgery. 2012;71(1):58-67.

[84] Majumdar S, Kameshwar A, Sreekanth K, Alekhya B. Pediatric

intraosseous schwannoma in maxillary sinus: A case report with review of literature. J Oral Maxillofac Pathol. 2020;24(3):542-547.

[85] Hirai T, Kobayashi H, Akiyama T, et al. Predictive factors for complications after surgical treatment for schwannomas of the extremities. BMC Musculoskelet Disord. 2019;20(1):166.

[86] Quinones-Hinojosa A, Jun P, Jumper J, et al. Choroid Plexus Tumors. In: Textbook of Neuro-Oncology. Elsevier; 2005. p. 199-207.

[87] Bahar M, Hashem H, et al. Choroid plexus tumors in adult and pediatric populations: the Cleveland Clinic and University Hospitals experience. J Neurooncol. 2017;132:427-432.

[88] Hosmann A, Hinker F, Dorfer C, et al. Management of choroid plexus tumors-an institutional experience. Acta Neurochir (Wien). 2019;161(4):745-754.

[89] Bahar M, Hashem H, Tekautz T, et al. Choroid plexus tumors in adult and pediatric populations: the Cleveland Clinic and University Hospitals experience. J Neurooncol. 2017;132(3): 427-432.

[90] Woehrer A, Slavc I, Waldhoer T, et al. Incidence of atypical teratoid/ rhabdoid tumors in children: A population-based study by the Austrian Brain Tumor Registry, 1996-2006. Cancer. 2010;116(24):5725-5732.

[91] Nesvick CL, Nageswara Rao AA, Raghunathan A, et al. Case-based review: atypical teratoid/rhabdoid tumor. Neurooncol Pract. 2019;6(3):163-178.

[92] Reddy AT, Strother DR, Judkins AR, et al. Efficacy of high-dose chemotherapy and three-dimensional conformal radiation for Atypical teratoid/rhabdoid tumor: A report from the children's oncology group trial ACNS0333. J Clin Oncol. 2020;38:1175-1185.

[93] Athale UH, Duckworth J, Odame I, et al. Childhood atypical teratoid rhabdoid tumor of the central nervous system: a meta-analysis of observational studies. J Pediatr Hematol Oncol. 2009;31(9):651-663.

[94] Blümcke I, Wiestler OD. Gangliogliomas: an intriguing tumor entity associated with focal epilepsies. J Neuropathol Exp Neurol. 2002;61(7): 575-584.

[95] Chatrath A, Mastorakos P, Mehta GU, et al. Ganglioglioma arising from the septum pellucidum: Case report and review of the literature. Pediatr Neurosurg. 2019;54(1):36-45.

[96] Pommepuy I, Delage-Corre M, Moreau JJ, et al. A report of a desmoplastic ganglioglioma in a 12-year-old girl with review of the literature. J Neurooncol. 2006;76(3): 271-275.

[97] Avci E, Oztürk A, Baba F, et al. Desmoplastic infantile ganglioglioma: case report. Turk J Pediatr. 2008;50(5): 495-499.

[98] Nguyen HS, Doan N, Gelsomino M, et al. An analysis from the Surveillance, epidemiology, and End Results program, 2004-2013. World Neurosurg. 2017;103:380-385.

[99] Minkin K, Klein O, Mancini J, et al. Surgical strategies and seizure control in pediatric patients with dysembryoplastic neuroepithelial tumors: a single-institution experience. J Neurosurg Pediatr. 2008;1(3):206-210.

[100] Carangelo B, Arrigucci U, Mariottini A, et al. Papillary glioneuronal tumor: case report and review of literature. G Chir. 2015;36(2): 63-69.

[101] Adam C, Polivka M, Carpentier A, et al. Papillary glioneuronal tumor: not always a benign tumor? Clin Neuropathol. 2007;26(3):119-124.

[102] Schlamann A, Bueren AO, Hagel C. An individual patient data meta-analysis on characteristics and outcome of patients with papillary glioneuronal Glial Tumors with Neuronal Differentiation 135tumor, rosette glioneuronal tumor with neuropil-like islands and rosette forming glioneuronal tumor of the fourth ventricle. PLoS One. 2014;9:e101211.

[103] Richard G, Fearon C, Alan B. Incidental chiasmal rosette-forming glioneuronal tumour at post-mortem (1757). Neurology [Internet]. 2021 [cited 2021 Aug 31];96(15). Available from: https://n.neurology.org/content/96/15_Supplement/1757

[104] Carletti F. Neuronal and Mixed Glioneuronal Tumors. In: Clinical Neuroradiology. Cham: Springer International Publishing; 2019. p. 1075-1103.

[105] Rodriguez FJ, Perry A, Rosenblum MK, et al. Disseminated oligodendroglial-like leptomeningeal tumor of childhood: a distinctive clinicopathologic entity. Acta Neuropathol. 2012;124(627):641.

[106] Tiwari N, Tamrazi B, Robison N, et al. Unusual radiological and histological presentation of a diffuse leptomeningeal glioneuronal tumor (DLGNT) in a 13-year-old girl. Childs Nerv Syst. 2019;35(9):1609-1614.

[107] Aguilera D, Castellino RC, Janss A, et al. Clinical responses of patients with diffuse leptomeningeal glioneuronal tumors to chemotherapy. Childs Nerv Syst. 2018;34:329-334.

[108] Becker AJ, Wiestler OD, Figarella-Branger D, et al. Ganglioglioma and gangliocytoma. In: Louis DN, Ohgaki H, Wiestler OD, Cavenee WK, editors. 4th ed. Lyon: International Agency for Research on Cancer; 2007. p. 103-105.

[109] Khajavi K, Comair YG, Prayson RA, et al. Childhood ganglioglioma and medically intractable epilepsy. A clinicopathological study of 15 patients and a review of the literature. Pediatr Neurosurg. 1995;22(4):181-188.

[110] Sharma MC, Deb P, Sharma S, et al. Neurocytoma: a comprehensive review. Neurosurg Rev. 2006;29(4):270-285; discussion 285.

[111] Pregúntegui-Loayza I, Apaza-Tintaya A, Ramírez-Espinoza A, et al-Duclos disease in pediatric population: Report of 2 cases. Pediatr Neurosurg. 2021;56(3):279-285.

[112] Viswanathan V, Smith ER, Mulliken JB, et al. Infantile hemangiomas involving the neuraxis: clinical and imaging findings. Am J Neuroradiol. 2009;30(5):1005-1013.

[113] Goyal P, Mangla R, Gupta S, et al. Pediatric congenital cerebrovascular anomalies: Congenital cerebrovascular anomalies. J Neuroimaging. 2019;29(2): 165-181.

Chapter 3

# Patterns of Care of Childhood Cancers in India

*Raghunadharao Digumarti*
*and Venkata Pradeepbabu Koyyala*

## Abstract

Management of childhood cancers in India has seen a new high in last few decades due to collaborative efforts of Physicians and organizations- both governmental and non-governmental. However, care is still heterogenous in this vast country. The problems span from a lack of data to programs for tackling cancers at the community level and lack of awareness among parents and physicians on childhood cancers, along with a nihilistic attitude and stigma attached to cancers even in this digital era. In this article, we describe the milestones in the development of Pediatric Oncology as a specialty, of cancer registries, of diagnostic armamentarium, access to affordable drugs, and, palliative care for children with cancers in India, that perhaps reflects care in other developing countries.

**Keywords:** childhood cancers, patterns of cancer care, cancers in India, pediatric cancer care, cancers in developing nations

## 1. Introduction

### 1.1 Epidemiology of childhood cancers in India

Pediatric cancers have never been an area of attention of cancer control in India, as majority of cancers occur in adults. Globally, it is reported that up to 85% of pediatric cancers occur in the developing world with a 5-year survival rate of less than 10%. On an average, in India, pediatric cancers account for less than 5% of all cancer cases. Nearly 45,000 new cancer cases are diagnosed in children every year in India. The main focus in pediatric care has been on control and reduction of infectious disease related mortality, which is in striking contrast with the developed world [1].

More than 0.2 million cases of childhood cancers are diagnosed across the globe every year. In the developed world, majority of these are cured, with a 5- year survival rate of 95%. However, the first step towards the control of childhood cancers in developing countries like India is to find out the incidence of cancers, to take directed measures in terms of control and treatment facilities. The main sources of such data are cancer registries [2].

Compared to the West, with average incidence of 75 to 150 childhood cancers per million children, the average incidence of childhood cancers in India is high. The age standardized incidence of cancers in India in the age group 0–14 years is highest in the Chennai Urban registry (124/million children) and lowest in the Ahmedabad rural registry (38/million children). The reasons for higher incidence

in urban areas as compared to rural areas are not clear. However, cancer contributes to only 2% of cancer related deaths in childhood as per available data. It was never a priority, in comparison to infectious diseases control, the main cause of mortality among children in India. Another contrast with developed world is the preponderance of cancers in boys, except in North-East India. The main reason is probably gender bias in seeking healthcare. However, the reasons for disproportionately higher rate of Hodgkin's disease in male children, up to 20 times more incidence than in females, are not known [3, 4].

### 1.2 The challenge: the great divide and an unmet need

One decade ago, the estimated gap between the developed and developing world in the survival rates in pediatric cancers was about 60–70% - a great divide. The reasons are many.

Because of high prevalence and mortality due to infectious diseases in children in India than cancer mortality - 58% of all deaths in the age group of 5–14 years, and half of these are due to diarrhea and pneumonia - and improved outcomes of infectious diseases by simple medication that can be delivered at peripheral centers, the emphasis has been high in this domain.

The Pediatric Hematology and Oncology (PHO) chapter of Indian Academy of Pediatrics (IAP) was established in 1987, with a focus on capacity building through training initiatives across all aspects of childhood cancers. Its flagship program was the *Indian National Trainining Program in Practical Paediatric Oncology*.

In order to foster collaborative efforts in childhood cancers, both in terms of uniformity of care as well as shared databases, Dr Bharat Agarwal, Dr Purna Kurkure and Dr Anupam Sachdeva formed *Indian Paediatric Oncology Group* InPOG in 2008. The emphasis now was clearly on clinical trials and research.

The Indian Pediatric Hematology Oncology Group (IPHOG) was formed in 1987 at the 24th Annual Conference of the *Indian Academy of Paediatrics* at Madras, with an intention of identifying and overcoming the barriers and to bridge the gap, by addressing factors leading to the decreased survival of children with cancers.

Some of the identified barriers were: delayed diagnosis, nihilism about childhood cancers, abandonment of treatment, lack of experience, inadequate infrastructure to treat emergent toxicities, expectation of cure, and, unwillingness to opt for retreatment at relapse [5].

Practical solutions that are already being followed by some institutions in India are as follows:

i. Educating primary care providers, especially pediatricians, about the diagnosis of childhood cancers and early referral to specialized centers

ii. Twinning, a process of collaboration between a hospital in a developing country with another in the developed world

iii. Establishing a reliable blood component support system

iv. Training nursing staff and other valuable trained human resources like social workers

v. Measures to prevent abandonment after diagnosis of cancer in a child by providing logistic support in the form of transportation and free shelter to the family as well as employment with modest wages to parents

vi. A systems for reminding and follow up with the parents of a child shortly after missing the scheduled visit

vii. Fellowship and other training programs in medical colleges with well-established pediatrics departments

viii. Countering nihilism and misinformation by untrained or improperly trained health care workers, emphasizing curability in the majority

## 2. Cancer registries

Cancer registration, an essential part to decipher patterns presentation, care and outcomes research, was started in India only in 1960s, in a small way. Until 1964, data was gathered through cancer surveys to estimate the incidence and trends. This was grossly inadequate for any conclusions and meaningful planning of need based services.

The first registry in India was started in Bombay (current Mumbai) in 1964 followed by Pune in 1973 and then in Aurangabad in late seventies [6]. However, cancer registration as a complete coordinated program was started only in 1982, with the Indian Council for Medical Research (ICMR) taking steps towards establishing the National Cancer Registry Program (NCRP).

The beginning was humble with three population based and three hospital-based registries, which is now expanded to 36 population based and over a hundred hospital-based cancer registries.

We have come a long way in these 6 decades. The existing registries cover about only 15% of the country's population [7]. We still lack population-based registries in some of the bigger states like Andhra Pradesh, Uttar Pradesh, Odisha and Rajasthan, where we depend on hospital-based registries. Cancer registration is not mandatory in our country. Collection in population-based registries is also through active methods, involving lot of time and manpower.

To overcome these hurdles, ICMR, through the establishment of National Centre for Disease Informatics and Research (NCDIR), initiated a program called, Cancer Atlas, to fill in these gaps, by abstracting information directly from pathology labs in Hospitals and Medical colleges, where, up to 85% of the cancer cases are confirmed microscopically. Another welcome step is that cancer case reporting is now mandatory in the states like Kerala, Karnataka, Gujarat and Manipur.

Relying on Population Based Cancer registries may be grossly insufficient to estimate the burden of cancer in children. Lack of awareness among public, particularly parents, to recognize and report symptoms likely to be from cancer in children, lack of accessible pediatric cancer services in many parts of the country, financial constraints of the family, resulting in dropout from treatments or even death before being seen at a specialized facility for treatment, are some glaring lacunae. As such, the burden estimated may not reflect the actual scenario in Indian society. India shares this common problem with other countries. The same is detailed in UICC's outreach program for childhood cancers called "My Child Matters"™.

To help in this aspect, a few Voluntary and non-governmental organizations (NGO) are reaching out to maintain databases of pediatric cancers in India, such as the Jiv Daya Foundation from Dallas, USA, that funds a cloud based program called "Indian Pediatric Oncology Database" [8].

| Type of cancer | Most common presentation Symptoms and Features of disease | Reason for late diagnosis and Barriers in completion of treatment | Estimated 5-year Survival in India from available data |
|---|---|---|---|
| Acute Lymphocytic Leukemia and Acute Myeloid Leukemia [9–11] | • 40-50% of all pediatric malignancies<br>• Anemia, Fever<br>• Late age at Diagnosis, Poor prognostic T cell type and High-risk cytogenetics are common compared to west | • Symptoms often mistaken for more common nutritional Deficiency<br>• Misconceptions about word, Blood cancer<br>• Fear of invasive procedures like Intrathecal chemo and Bone marrow examination | ALL: 45–81%<br>AML: 35.5% (North India)<br>Induction Mortality: 18% |
| Lymphoma<br>• Hodgkin's and Non-Hodgkin's lymphoma [12–14] | • HL: Lymph nodal swellings<br>• NHL: Abdominal symptoms, Constitutional Symptoms and lymphadenopathy<br>• Mixed cellularity type is most common in Hodgkin's disease and Burkitts is most common in NHL | • Often mistaken for more common disease, Tuberculosis<br>• Many patients are empirically started on ATT<br>• Steroids are often used in peripheral centers without a diagnosis | Hodgkin's Lymphoma:90%<br>NHL:<br>Early stage: 91%<br>Advanced stage 61% |
| Central Nervous system tumors [15] | • Headache, vomiting and seizures<br>• Most common types are Astrocytoma and medulloblastoma<br>• Higher incidence of Craniopharyngioma compared to West. | • Non-specific in younger children<br>• Symptoms are missed and misdiagnosed as Meningo-Encephalitis and treated in those lines before referral to oncology centers<br>• Very limited number of centers with Pediatric Neuro imaging and reporting facilities | Data Not available |
| Retinoblastoma [16] | • 6-10% of all childhood tumors<br>• Mean age at presentation is 29–34 months<br>• Leukocoria, strabismus, proptosis, visual loss and red eye. | • Lack of awareness of symptoms among parents leads to delay in medical attention<br>• Not willing of enucleation | 5 years OS:<br>South India: 92%<br>North India: 63% |
| Neuroblastoma [17] | • 4-8% of all pediatric malignancies<br>• Predominant abdominal disease | • Delay in presentation<br>• up to 80% present in advanced stage | 3 year OS:<br>Early stage:60.7%<br>Advanced stage: 35.7% |
| Wilms Tumor [18] | • Abdominal mass | • Late presentation and advanced stage at diagnosis<br>• Lack of expertise and trained staff in peripheral centres, specially pediatric surgery | 5 year OS: 70–85% |

**Table 1.**
*Charateristics of common childhood cancers in India.*

### 2.1 Pediatric oncology as a sub-specialty

Although India is making rapid strides in the development in several areas like agriculture and space technology, there is glaring deficiency and disparity in delivering much needed primary medical care. While this is in part due to the difficult to reach terrain of this vast sub-continent, the main reasons appear to be a reluctance of the well trained doctor to serve remote areas due lack of basic civic amenities. Lack of political will, compounded by lack of awareness of the curability and pessimism about cancer in both law makers themselves, as well the medical fraternity further worsen the problem (**Table 1**).

This pessimism is predominant in pediatric cancers as there are insufficient points of care. Most cancers are under diagnosed due to lack of adequate diagnostic facilities, and, when diagnosed, are treated by pediatricians with limited knowledge about oncology, or adult oncologists with limited knowledge about pediatric cancers.

### 2.2 Specialized childhood cancer centers

The first pediatric oncology center was established in 1970, at the Cancer Institute, Chennai, by Professor V Shanta, a great visionary in the field of cancer education and training. Another landmark is the establishment of first dedicated Pediatric Oncology Unit in Mumbai at the Tata Memorial Hospital, in the 1990s, by Prof. Shripad Banavali. This center also pioneered the training program and award of a sub-specialty doctoral degree pediatric oncology. The main advantage of such dedicated centers is access to advanced diagnostic services like Immunophenotyping, PET CT, cytogenetics, blood component therapy and trained nurses manning clinics catering to venous access devices [19].

In early 2000, pediatric oncology developed as a specialized branch in India. It is the combined responsibility of academicians in various pediatric departments to build and develop a sustainable pediatric oncology program. The reasons are obvious: it is still not sustainable for a pediatric oncologist to restrict practice to just pediatric oncology, in the community. The earnings from care of only childhood cancer patients being meager, most practice non-malignant hematology as well as general pediatrics. Medical Oncologists with a training in pediatric oncology happily practice both adult and pediatric oncology.

### 2.3 Development of pediatric cancer society – and ISMPO

The Indian Association of Cancer Chemotherapists was founded in the early 60s by surgeons who practiced adjuvant chemotherapy for their operated patients. Most of its members were eminent cancer surgeons like Dr. Roy Choudhury of Kolkata and Dr. N C Mishra of Lucknow. It was renamed as the Indian Society for Medical and Pediatric Oncology at an annual conference of the Society in Ahmedabad, Gujarat, in late 80s (personal communication, Professor Pankaj M Shah – Former Director, Gujarat Cancer and Research Institute). Cancer oriented pediatricians still band together as the pediatric oncology sub chapter of the Indian Academy of Pediatrics.

Along with ISMPO, several other Oncology Networks like ICON (Indian Cooperative Oncology Network), and INPOG (Indian National Pediatric Oncology Group) help of pediatric oncologists in collaborating across the nation and with experts abroad to share ideas, knowledge, and expertise.

**Childhood cancer care in India - then and now.**

There is a drastic improvement in the outcomes of childhood cancers over the past two decades ago. The reasons are many, including dedicated training programs,

establishment of pediatric cancer centers, and, most importantly adoption and collaboration of treatment protocols from the developed world.

One such example of collaboration is adoption of the acute lymphoblastic leukemia and lymphoma protocols developed by Prof Ian Magrath of the National Cancer Institute, USA, specifically for the developing world [MCP 841 & MCP 842 protocols]. With the guidance from Prof. Magrath's International Network for Cancer Treatment and Research (INCTR), the outcomes of the patients on this protocol improved by three times from 20 to 60%. The protocol also paved the way for adequate platelet transfusion protocols mandating intramuscular l-asparaginase as well as immunophenotyping of acute lymphoblastic leukemia and lymphoma into cALLa positive and T cell leukemias [20, 21].

### 2.4 Volunteers and non-governmental agencies

There are several volunteer groups and non-governmental organizations (NGOs) that provide much needed help to the patient and family who travel to a city from the moffusil. The St. Jude's Children Homes specialize in establishing homes in or near the premises of major childhood cancer treatment centers, in cities, for housing the child with family as a unit, throughout the course of its treatment. Several organizations also provide technical, logistic and financial assistance with travel, food, shelter, paperwork as well as drugs.

### 2.5 Awareness programs for pediatricians

The Pediatric Oncology sub-chapter of the Indian Academy of Pediatrics created a training program for pediatricians, called NTP-PPO (National Training Program – Practical Pediatric Oncology). Over the years, through this program, nearly 50 workshops have been conducted and about 2000 pediatricians have been trained to identify, diagnose, and refer children with cancers to appropriate centers. Pediatricians are also trained in management of febrile neutropenia, venous access and maintenance chemotherapy. Since most of them practice in the community, their services are often of paramount importance in ensuring continuity of care.

There are other programs for intensive pediatric oncology training, such as a one-year program by IAP and 2-year Fellowship by the National Board of Examinations, which works under the aegis of Ministry of Health and Family Welfare, Government of India [22].

### 2.6 Overcoming delay in referral

Delay in referral is a big hindrance for timely management of pediatric cancers. Some delay is due to logistics: not so easy to negotiate monsoon inundated roads in remote rural areas. A sheer lack of awareness even among radiologists and orthopedic specialists is one reason for delay in diagnosis of Ewing's Sarcoma and Osteosarcoma, which are often treated as tubercular osteomyelitis [22].

### 2.7 Access to medicines - generics

There are several early obstacles in access to essential medications for cancer patients in India. Several attempts were made by the government to bridge this gap. One such successful attempt was providing access to generics. The other big step is

inclusion of some of antineoplastic drugs like imatinib in the Essential Medicines List (EML). In many states, such as Andhra Pradesh, Tamil Nadu, Rajasthan and Kerala, the government has evolved schemes like the *Arogyasri*, which ensure that the entire treatment of all childhood cancers is completely free for all those below the poverty line by all modalities. The state of Andhra Pradesh has even included free hematopoietic stem cell transplantation in its program for children below poverty line. The recently introduced Health Scheme of the Government of India, *Ayushman Bharat*, will hopefully be of help to children with cancer in states where this is operational. A major drawback of both these schemes is the large amount of paperwork and prior sanction that is needed for preauthorisation, for the mode of treatment as well as for every new cycle. Another drawback is the limitation both in the choice of regimen as well as the cost of drugs. A final drawback is lack of subsidy for the tests needed to prove the diagnosis and stage the disease. Since there is no health insurance cover for the child from the 'middle class', the financial impact on the parent's pocket is unusually heavy – leading to abandonment [23].

### 2.8 Development in palliative care

Pediatric palliative care is in a naïve state in most parts of the world, and so is in India. With very few dedicated pediatric palliative care centers and many cultural barriers, provision of palliative care is still mostly rudimentary [24].

A bright example for such development in India is collaboration between Nawaj Mehdi Jung (MNJ) Hospital in Telangana State with the Canadian branch of International Network for Cancer Treatment and Research in 2007 [25]. Such an exercise to prevent and treat pain in the children diagnosed with cancer irrespective of the end point resulted in enrolment of more pediatric patients, reduction in dropouts from treatment and those lost to follow up, with an increase in survival. In India, it is estimated that 1.6 million pediatric patients with various ailments are in need of pediatric palliative care. However, it will be a difficult task to train enough personnel to be able to serve this population. A first step towards such goal is the initiation of training program in MNJ hospital. In 2010, the Indian Association of Palliative Care (IAPC) established a separate pediatric palliative care unit in the state of Maharashtra, in collaboration with the International Children Palliative Care Cetwork (ICPCN) [26].

## 3. Conclusions

India, along with other low and middle income countries, has been the hub spot for leading the developments in management of pediatric cancers. Together, these countries account for nearly 90% of all diagnosed childhood cancers across the globe. In India, majority of population is from rural areas, where, awareness about symptoms of childhood cancer symptoms, the knowledge of diagnosis and even referral among physicians is low, contributing to avoidable delays in instituting treatment, with resultant inferior cure rates. Prohibitive costs in private sector coupled with unavailability of facilities in public sector, render outcomes to be very poor even in cancers like Hodgkin's lymphoma that are otherwise curable by simple protocols. Although there are policies at national level addressing the prevention and control of cancers as a whole, there is no special emphasis on pediatric cancers. However, there is light at the end of tunnel in the form of several schemes, like coverage of pediatric cancers under the newly -launched *Ayushman Bharat* scheme, a universal health policy initiated by central government, and several central

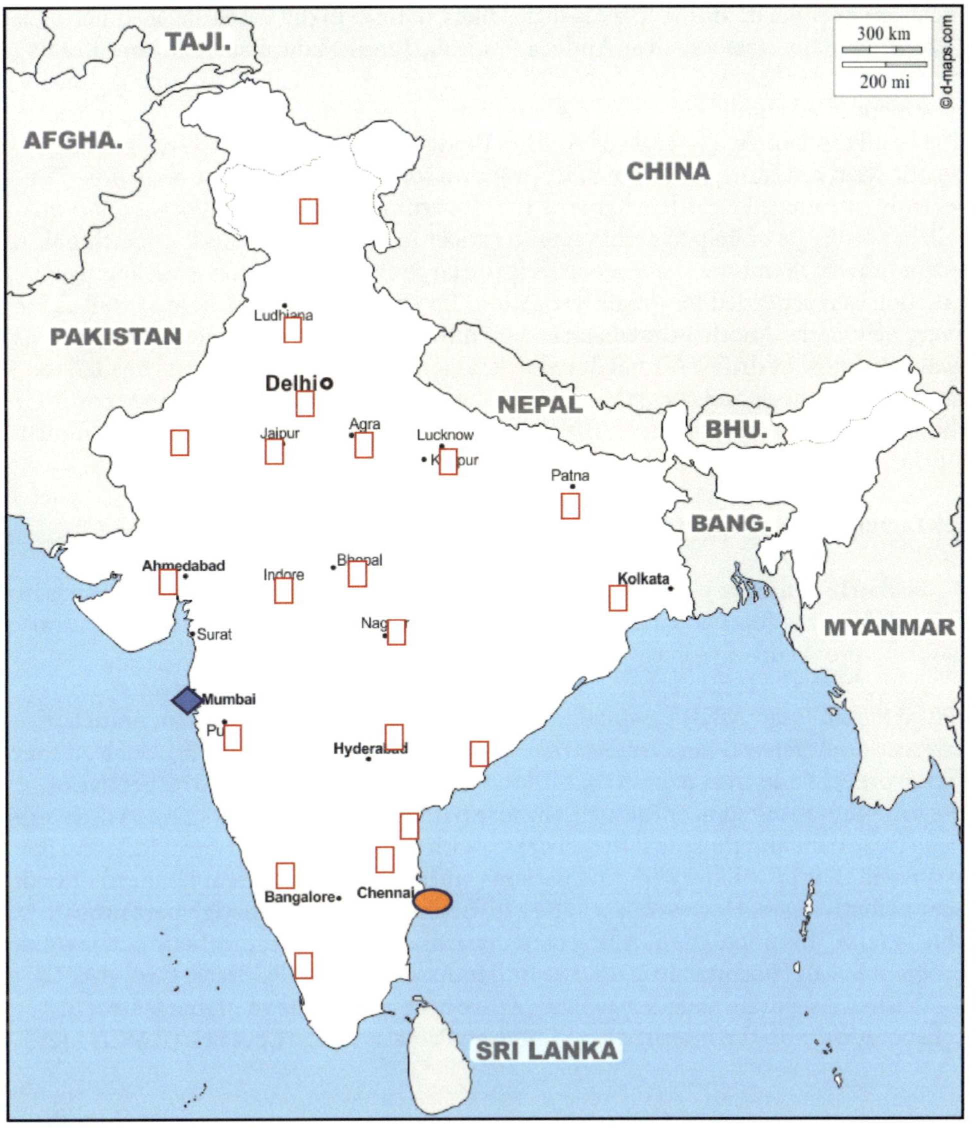


**Figure 1.**

*Pediatric oncology centers in India in various decades.* *First pediatric cancer center in India 1970's: Chennai;* *Second pediatric cancer Center in India 1990's: Mumbai;* *Pediatric oncology services currently available in India.*

government schemes providing funds for treatment of childhood cancers. However, this is just a beginning and there is a long way to go to build patient centric care for children with cancer, spread of heath literacy among the public and developing centers with skilled staff where patient and family are treated with dignity.

India, which is the fastest growing nation among developing countries in terms of human resources, development and cancer incidence in children should lead by example by improving quality of care and accessibility to Cancer care to children, in particular. Finally, it is especially important to remember that pediatric oncology departments as standalone units cannot serve and deliver comprehensive care required by a child. Collaboration between pediatricians, radiologists, surgeons, anesthetists, neurosurgeons, urologists, psychiatrists and other subspecialties would help in achieving the quality of care.

## 4. Common Childhood cancer in India and their characteristics

There is severe paucity in the data of exact incidence, prevalence, morbidity, mortality, and survivorship data of pediatric cancers in India. However, based on the available registry data, both population based and hospital based, the most common malignancies diagnosed in India in children are Leukemias, Lymphomas, CNS tumors, Retinoblastoma and Malignant Bone Tumors (**Figure 1**).

## Conflict of interest

The authors declare no conflict of interest.

## Author details

Raghunadharao Digumarti* and Venkata Pradeepbabu Koyyala
Homi Bhaba Cancer Hospital and Research Centre, Visakhapatnam, India

*Address all correspondence to: rdigumarti@gmail.com

## References

[1] Ribeiro RC, Steliarova-Foucher E, Magrath I, Lemerle J, Eden T, Forget C, et al. Baseline status of pediatric oncology care in 10 low income or mid-income countries receiving My Child Matters support: a descriptive study. Lancet 2008;9:721-729.

[2] Stiller CA, Parkin DM. Geographic and ethnic variations in the incidence of childhood cancer. Br Med Bull 1996;52:682-703.

[3] Parkin DM, Stiller CA, Draper GJ, Bieber CA. The international incidence of childhood cancer. Int J Cancer 1988;42:511-20.

[4] Barr R, Riberio R, Agarwal B, Masera G, Hesseling P, Magrath I. Pediatric Oncology in Countries with Limited Resources. In: Pizzo PA, Poplack DG, eds. Principles and Practice of Pediatric Oncology, 5 th ed. Philadelphia: Lippincott Williams and Wilkins; 2006. p. 1605-17

[5] Yadav SP, Rastogi N, Kharya G, Misra R, Ramzan M et.al. Barriers to cure for children with cancer in India and strategies to improve outcomes: a report by the Indian Pediatric Hematology Oncology Group. Pediatric Hematology and Oncology. 2014 Apr 1;31(3):217-24.

[6] Chaudhry K, Luthra UK. Cancer registration in India. WWW page. URL: www. mohfw. nic. in/WriteReadData/ l892s/Cancer% 20Registration% 20In% 20India. pdf. Last accessed February. 2021;01:2021.

[7] Sahoo SS, Verma M, Parija PP. An overview of cancer registration in India: Present status and future challenges. Oncology Journal of India. 2018 Oct 1;2(4):86.

[8] Arora RS, Eden T, Pizer B. The problem of treatment abandonment in children from developing countries with cancer. Pediatr Blood Cancer 2007;49:941-6.

[9] R. Arora, B. Arora, Acute leukemia in children: a review of the current Indian data, South Asian J. Cancer 5 (2016) 155, https://doi.org/10.4103/2278-330X.187591

[10] A.Bajel, B. George, V. Mathews, A. Viswabandya, M.L. Kavitha, A. Srivastava, M. Chandy, Treatment of children with acute lymphoblastic leukemia in India using a BFM protocol, Pediatr. Blood Cancer 51 (2008) 621-625, https://doi.org/ 10.1002/pbc.21671.

[11] Magrath, V. Shanta, S. Advani, M. Adde, L.S. Arya, S. Banavali, M. Bhargava, K. Bhatia, M. Guti'errez, D. Liewehr, S. Pai, T.G. Sagar, D. Venzon, V. Raina, Treatment of acute lymphoblastic leukaemia in countries with limited resources; lessons from use of a single protocol in India over a twenty year period [corrected], Eur. J. Cancer Oxf. Engl. 1990 (41) (2005) 1570-1583, https://doi.org/10.1016/j.ejca.2004.11.004.

[12] L.S. Arya, V. Dinand, V. Thavaraj, S. Bakhshi, R. Dawar, G.K. Rath, R. Singh, T. S. Vats, Hodgkin's disease in Indian children: outcome with chemotherapy alone, Pediatr. Blood Cancer 46 (2006) 26-34, https://doi.org/10.1002/pbc.20157.

[13] V. Radhakrishnan, M. Dhanushkodi, T.S. Ganesan, P. Ganesan, S. Sundersingh, G. Selvaluxmy, R. Swaminathan, R. Rama, T.G. Sagar, Pediatric Hodgkin lymphoma treated at Cancer institute, Chennai, India: long-term outcome, J. Glob. Oncol. 3 (2017) 545-554, https://doi.org/10.1200/JGO.2016.005314.

[14] V. Radhakrishnan, P. Shoufeej, S. Totadri, P. Ganesan, T. Ganesan,

T. Sagar, Pediatric nonblastic non-hodgkin's lymphoma: a perspective from India, Indian J. Med. Paediatr. Oncol. 39 (2018) 13, https://doi.org/10.4103/ijmpo.ijmpo_42_16.

[15] S. Suresh, A. Srinivasan, J. Scott, S. Rao, B. Chidambaram, S. Chandrasekar, Profile and outcome of pediatric brain tumors – experience from a tertiary care pediatric oncology unit in South India, J. Pediatr. Neurosci. 12 (2017) 237, https://doi.org/ 10.4103/jpn.JPN_31_17.

[16] S. Kaliki, A. Patel, S. Iram, G. Ramappa, A. Mohamed, V.A.R. Palkonda, RETINOBLASTOMA IN INDIA: clinical presentation and outcome in 1,457 patients (2,074 eyes), Retina 39 (2019) 379-391, https://doi.org/10.1097/ IAE.0000000000001962.

[17] S. Agarwala, A. Mandelia, S. Bakhshi, M. Srinivas, M. Bajpai, A.K. Gupta, D. K. Gupta, V. Bhatnagar, Neuroblastoma: Outcome over a 14 year period from a tertiary care referral centre in India, J. Pediatr. Surg. 49 (2014) 1280-1285, https://doi.org/10.1016/j.jpedsurg.2014.03.017.

[18] D. Gupta, S. Sharma, S. Agarwala, R. Carachi, Saga of Wilms' tumor: lessons learnt from the past, J. Indian Assoc. Pediatr. Surg. 10 (2005) 217, https://doi.org/ 10.4103/0971-9261.19271.

[19] Arora B, Banavali SD. Pediatric oncology in India: Past, present and future. Indian journal of medical and paediatric oncology: official journal of Indian Society of Medical & Paediatric Oncology. 2009 Oct;30(4):121.

[20] Magrath I, Santa V, Advani S, Adde M, Arya LS, Banavali S, *et al* . Treatment of acute lymphoblastic leukaemia in countries with limited resources: Lessons from use of a single protocol in India over a twenty year period. Eur J Cancer 2005; 41:1570-83.

[21] Yadav SP, Ramzan M, LallM, Sachdeva A. Childhood acute lymphoblastic leukemia outcome in India: progress on all fronts. *J Pediatr Hematol Oncol*. 2012;34(4):324.

[22] Arora B, Kanwar V. Childhood cancers in India: burden, barriers, and breakthroughs. *Indian J Cancer*. 2009;46(4):257-259.

[23] Denburg A, Arora B, Arora RS, Auste C, Bagai P, Barr R, Challinor J, Eden T, Grynzspancholc E, Hoffman R, Link M. Access to essential medicines for children with cancer: a joint SIOP-CCI position statement. The Lancet Oncology. 2017 Jan 1;18(1):20-2.

[24] Human Rights Watch. 'Please do not make us suffer any more...': access to pain treatment as a human right. 2009. Available from http://www.hrw.org/sites/default/files/reports/health0309web_1.pdf

[25] Barr R, Riberio R, Agarwal B, Masera G, Hesseling P, Magrath I. Pediatric oncology in countries with limited resources. In: Pizzo PA, Poplack DG, editors. Principles and practice of pediatric oncology, 5 th ed. Philadelphia: Lippincott Williams and Wilkins; 2006. p. 1605-17.

[26] Arora RS, Eden TO, Kapoor G. Epidemiology of childhood cancer in India. Indian J Cancer. 2009 Oct-Dec;46(4):264-73.

Section 3

# Surgical Management of CNS Tumors

Chapter 4

# Multimodal Neuronavigation for Brain Tumor Surgery

*Roberto Garcia-Navarrete, Constantino Contreras-Vázquez, Ericka León-Alvárez, Natael Olvera González, Alfonso Marhx-Bracho, Javier Terrazo-Lluch, José Luis Pérez-Gómez, Jorge Alberto Ocon Rodríguez, Judy Castañeda Goyes and Juan Alberto Díaz Ponce Medrano*

## Abstract

The current neuronavigation techniques increase safety and surgeon confidence during neurosurgical procedure performance. However, its real usefulness remains in integrating multimodal information from advanced magnetic resonance imaging, as tractography (DTI), functional studies that evaluate motor and sensitive language, motor function (BOLD techniques with different paradigms), and nuclear medicine. At the operating room, the fusion of sonographic information acquired in real-time with the predefined plan increase the chance to achieve gross-total resection of primary brain tumors. Combining these different image modalities with brain mapping and motor stimulation information in selected cases is possible, increasing surgery safety. In this review, we present our experience with multimodal neuronavigation to treat brain tumors in pediatric patients.

**Keywords:** Neuronavigation, fMRI, BOLD, PET/CT, Brain tumor, Cancer

## 1. Introduction

Gliomas are primary tumors of the central nervous system. They are derived from glial cells. They are the most common cause of solid tumors in the intracranial space in children [1]. Nearly 70,000 new cases of malignant primary and benign brain tumors of the central nervous system (CNS) are diagnosed in the United States each year. Of these, approximately 28% are gliomas, and 36% are meningiomas. Gliomas represent 80% of the primary malignant brain tumors. The incidence rates of brain tumors have increased in the last three decades. For all CNS tumors, of which brain tumors account for approximately 88%, the average annual incidence rate adjusted for age (2006 to 2010) for women (22.8 per 100,000) is higher than for men (19.1 per 100,000) [1, 2].

According to the World Health Organization (WHO) classification of brain tumors, they are divided into gliomas of the low and high degree of malignancy. Low-grade gliomas - I and II, are represented by pilocytic astrocytoma, diffuse glioma, and gemistocytic astrocytoma. They have a benign clinical course with a long survival time. High-grade gliomas, anaplastic astrocytoma (grade III) and glioblastoma multiforme (grade IV), are characterized by a rapid growth rate,

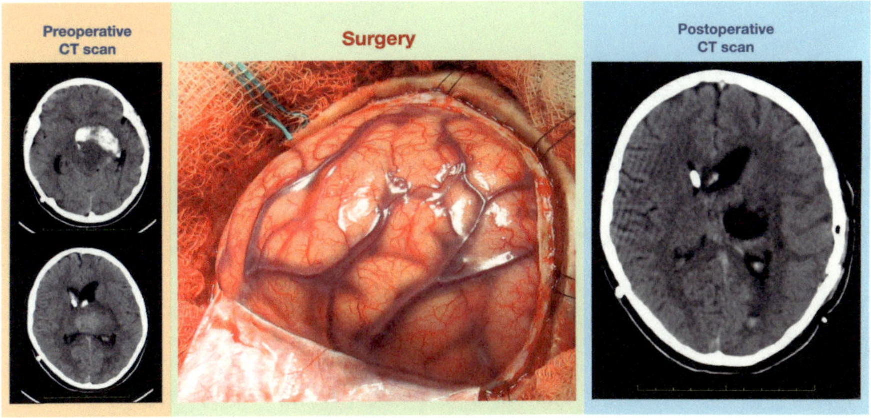


**Figure 1.**
*Intraoperative cerebral edema during emergency surgery in a patient with neurological deterioration secondary to a brain tumor bleeding.*

extensive white matter infiltration, and poor short-term prognosis [3, 4]. Therefore, the histopathological diagnosis and its proper classification are crucial for treating patients. Diffuse astrocytoma (WHO grade II) is characterized by slow growth and infiltration of neighboring brain structures **Figure 1** [5–7].

In pediatric patients, the central nervous system's tumors represent the second cause of cancer mortality after leukemia. The magnetic resonance imaging technique renders the integration of different structural images (FLAIR, diffusion, perfusion, SPGR, TRUFFI), functional aspects (DTI, BOLD), and metabolic profile (spectroscopy). They evaluated peritumoral edema by diffusion and perfusion sequences [8, 9]. The use of sequences that provide functional information allows the early identification of the risks associated with neurosurgical treatment and each case's functional prognosis [10]. Some reports show a characteristic uptake pattern for the degree of malignancy of different neoplasms. In the case of primary tumors of the CNS, significant alterations can be observed in the uptake of glucose, methionine, and tyrosine. One of the technological resources that have changed the treatment of patients with CNS neoplasms is neuronavigation.

## 2. Characteristics of Magnetic Resonance Imaging Studies for Neuronavigation

The radiological evaluation of brain tumors makes it possible to identify the structural, functional, and metabolic characteristics of neoplastic lesions and, for prognostic purposes, their relationship with healthy brain tissue by combining diverse image acquisition techniques.

The MRI imaging modalities currently used in presurgical planning for brain tumor resection are functional magnetic resonance imaging (fMRI), diffusion tensioner (DTI) imaging, diffusion tension tractography, and BOLD [2].

### 2.1 Diffusion Tensor Images (DTI)

The diffusion tensor images allow the visualization and characterization of white matter tracts [11–13]. DTI images have been used to study the architecture of white matter and the integrity of normal and diseased brains. This magnetic resonance technique is based on the general principle that the anatomical microstructure directs water diffusion, being an echo-planar technique that maps the diffusion

speed [14]. In brain tissue, diffusion rates are slower due to the typical parenchyma components that impede water movement. In specific pathological processes, water diffusion is restricted, which reduces the apparent diffusion coefficient (ADC), as in acute infarcts secondary to cytotoxic edema, abscess, lymphoma [12, 15]. Fiber tracking is the only non-invasive method to visualize the course, displacement, or interruption of white matter's main tracts according to the DTI technique. Multiple studies have shown that fiber tracking can reconstruct white matter's major fiber structures in the brain. Identifying the tracts is done by defining a rectangular interest volume (VOI) in the registered standard T1 anatomical datasets. A fast acquisition gradient echo sequence prepared with 3D magnetization weighted in T1 is used to acquire the images. T2-weighted images are acquired, inversion recovery images attenuated by T2 fluid, and 3D images weighted in T1 postcontrast are scanned. Intraoperative examinations are performed immediately when the operator considers that the lesion has been resected or intraoperative exploration was necessary to correct the cerebral displacement. For DTI, applies a sequence of echo-planar images weighted by spin-echo diffusion of a single shot (echo time, 147 milliseconds, repetition time, 9400 milliseconds, matrix size, 128 × 128, the field of view, 251 × 251 mm, the thickness of cut, 3 mm, bandwidth, 1502 Hz per pixel, diffusion encoding gradients in 12 directions with b values of 0 and 1000 s/mm$^2$, and voxel size, 1.9 × 1.9 × 3 mm) [12, 13, 16]. The 3D segmental reconstruction of the tumor is performed based on the high-resolution 3D postcontrast anatomical data set.

In the case of tumors with high uptake of contrast medium - glioblastoma multiforme, metastasis, the edge of the outermost lesion that enhances post-contrast, for example, glioblastoma, and the edge of hyperintensity or mixed hypointensity in the lesion, such as the non-malignant entity, cavernoma, represented the limit of segmentation. In non-enhancing lesions such as low-grade glioma, the T2-weighted image is used to determine the tumor's edge. For this reason, most tumors that do not have post-contrast enhancement have optimal visibility in this sequence. The existence of significant edema, which cannot be clearly distinguished from the low-grade glioma, was ruled out based on the findings of inversion recovery images with T2 fluid. The segmentation of the tumor is performed by cutting in a mode of 3D anatomical data. After profiling all the sections that contained the lesion, the three-dimensional reconstruction of the lesion was performed [13].

The techniques of DTI and tractography have overcome this obstacle and are now widely used to study the white matter in vivo. Diffusion images calculate the local direction of white matter from water diffusion measurements. Tractography takes this a step further to evaluate the functional connection between several different areas inside the same or contralateral hemisphere. The identification of water molecule's movement in all directions is known as isotropic diffusion. In the central nervous system, anisotropic diffusion is used to define water's movement in a parallel sense in the withe matter tracts defined by axons' groups. Thus, creating maps of movement of water that define the structure and orientation of with matter tracts [2, 3].

Three-dimensional visualization of white substance fibers, such as the corticospinal (pyramidal) tract, corpus callosum, cerebellar peduncles, optical radiation, and arcuate fascicle, is of great value at the preoperative evaluation and intraoperative navigation **Figure 2** [4].

### 2.2 Perfusion

There are three main techniques for perfusion imaging: T2 * enhanced dynamic magnetic susceptibility enhanced perfusion in T1-enhanced dynamic contrast, and arterial spin marking techniques, involving repetitive serial images through the tumor during blood passage been marked with contrast material.

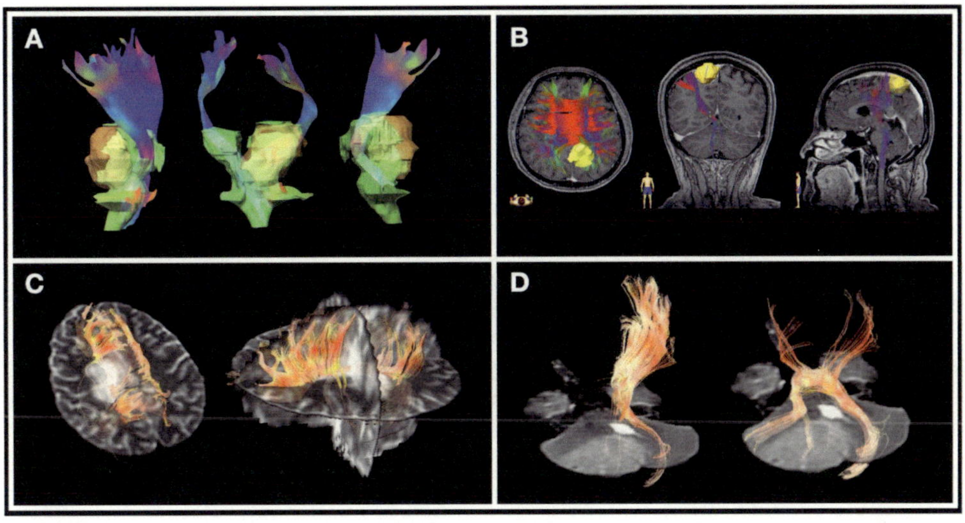


**Figure 2.**
*3D reconstructions for white matter tracts with DTI-MRI technique. (A) Thalamic high-grade glioma and his relationship with the pyramidal tract. (B) Parasagittal meningioma and its relationship with corpus callosum and pyramidal tract. (C) Supratentorial Ependymoma and its relations with Corpus callosum. (D) Fourth ventricle tumor and middle cerebellar peduncle displacement.*

Theoretically, the degree of a signal drop is proportional to the concentration of gadolinium in the tissue, obtaining relative curves of concentration - time. Dynamic contrast images weighted in T1, where the main focus is estimating tumor permeability, allow the contrast to filter into the extravascular space and reach equilibrium during multiple contrast bolus passes through the tumor bed. An arterial spin is a form of perfusion without the use of intravenous contrast; a powerful magnetic gradient is applied to the blood inlet to reverse the magnetization, effectively labeling the blood that flows upward, have impeded its application for long periods of imaging and decrease in spatial resolution compared to gadolinium [16]. Different types of tumors and grades differ in their perfusion characteristics. For example, there is a strong correlation between the degree of astrocytoma and the relative measurements of cerebral blood volume (CBV) [17]. However, low-grade astrocytomas tend to have a high cerebral blood volume, associated with the process of angiogenesis and dense capillary networks that characterize these tumors.

### 2.3 Magnetic resonance spectroscopy

It provides an analysis of the different metabolites in a delimited area within the brain and may be useful in the initial diagnosis of brain tumors. It can be done with a single voxel technique, in which a single spectrum is produced for a tissue volume, or a multivoxel technique, in which a greater volume of tissue is evaluated [18]. The primary metabolites evaluated include N-acetyl aspartate (NAA) (typical neuronal marker), choline (cell membrane marker), creatine (energy marker), lactate (metabolic acidosis), and lipids (tissue breakdown and cell death). The spectral patterns of intracranial neoplasms vary significantly due to differences in tumor types and grades. However, most CNS tumors manifest with elevated choline-creatine and co-NAA ratios caused by increases in cellularity (choline elevation) and a relative decrease in normal neurons (reduction of NAA).

### 2.4 Functional MRI Images

Functional MRI (fMRI) mapping of eloquent language cortex in patients with brain tumors after surgery is feasible and may serve as a useful reference assessment for preoperative neurosurgical planning [19].

Functional magnetic resonance imaging (MR) is an advanced tool for studying brain functions in healthy subjects and neuropsychiatric patients, identifying and locating specific metabolism and neural activity phenomena [20].

BOLD is a measure of changes in oxygenated and deoxygenated blood proportion during a particular paradigm's execution. The most commonly mapped functions during functional MRI studies include motor, auditory, somatosensory, visual perception, and language production and comprehension. When evaluating motor centers, typical tasks include tapping with fingers, pouting with lips, and flexing and extending toes [21]. Patients with mild to severe motor paresis of the hand may clench their fists instead of tapping with their fingers.

Several reports mention that a silent area around a brain tumor could recover his eloquence after the surgical resection of malignant tissue [22]. There is a latency of several seconds in the signal change observed in BOLD images, making the temporal resolution of functional MRI poor compared to other techniques such as DES or electroencephalography [23]. Because of the "delay of hemodynamic response" given the time required for the production and diffusion of vascular signal

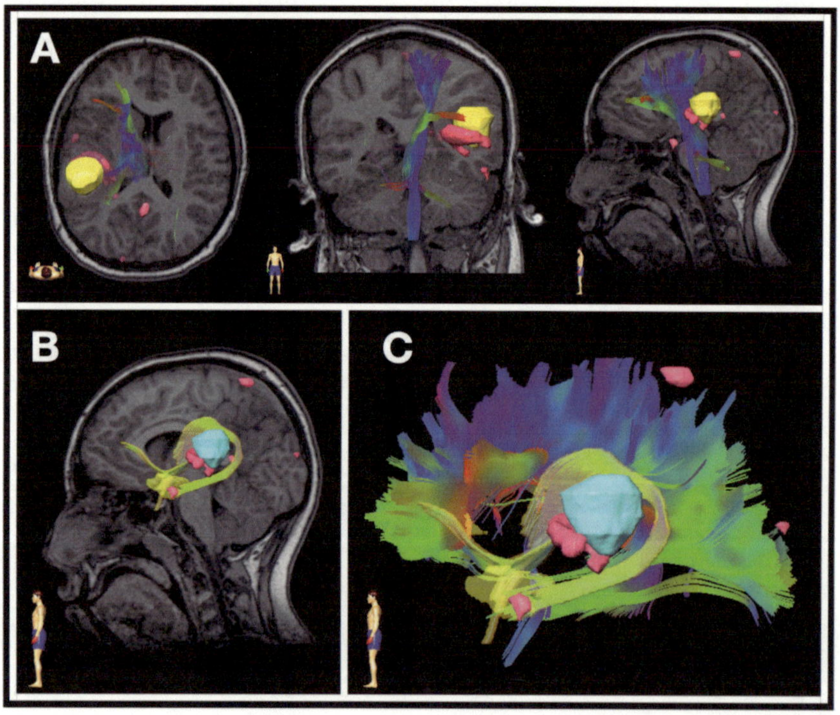


**Figure 3.**
*The utility of fMRI and tractography for surgical planning. An 8-years-old boy presents at the emergency unit with a history of intermittent language disturbances and right-hemiparesis. fMRI (language paradigm) and DTI (Pyramidal tract, Corpus callous, Arcuate fascicle) images were performed. A 3D reconstruction at the Brainlab neuronavigation station was performed. (A) Pyramidal tract reconstruction and his relationship with a neoplastic lesion (Yellow) and language areas visualized with fMRI (Red). (B) Arcuate fascicle reconstruction and language areas and their relation to the neoplastic lesion. (C) 3D reconstruction of arcuate fascicle (Yellow), language areas (Red), and neoplastic lesion (Cyan).*

substances to dilate the vascular bed and cause a deoxygenated hemoglobin wash. Another consideration is that BOLD fMRI does not directly measure neural activity but changes in the region's hemodynamic properties. So, the variability between functional localization among subjects may result from physiological differences in the BOLD signal without differences in neuronal activity per se. It has been found that several pharmacological agents may influence the BOLD signal [24].

### 2.5 The utility of fMRI and DTI in presurgical planning

The use of fMRI in conjunction with DTI for presurgical planning is currently the most established clinical application of these neuroimaging techniques. The aim is to provide the surgeon with functional information about the tumor's area and its connections to adjacent areas. The regions of interest can be defined anatomically. However, the advance of functional imaging techniques allows us to define white matter tracts more precisely. Some reports mention that it is reliable in healthy ones but maybe inaccurate in those who harbor brain injuries **Figure 3** [21].

## 3. Nuclear medicine for imaging brain tumors

In Mexico, PET positron emission tomography equipment began with opening the PET-Cyclotron Unit of the National Autonomous University of Mexico in 2002. We use nuclear medicine to determine the degree of malignancy of the lesions, evaluate the response to treatment, identify early recurrence, and radiotherapy planning.

By obtaining functional information of cellular and biological processes like glucose metabolism, protein synthesis, the PET with 18 fluoro-deoxy-glucose (FDG) PET was initially used to detect and distinguish tumors of a low and high degree of malignancy. 18 Fluoro-ethyl-tyrosine (18 F FET) evaluates the metabolism of amino acids. It provides well-contrasted images in both high and low-grade tumors. It is beneficial to take biopsies guided by image to establish a primary brain tumor diagnosis in the planning of radiotherapy treatments and distinguish between tumor recurrence or radionecrosis after initial therapy **Figure 4** [4].

It has a sensitivity of 94% and specificity of 88% for the diagnosis of brain tumors. Although the 18-FDG and 18-FET quantitative parameters allow the

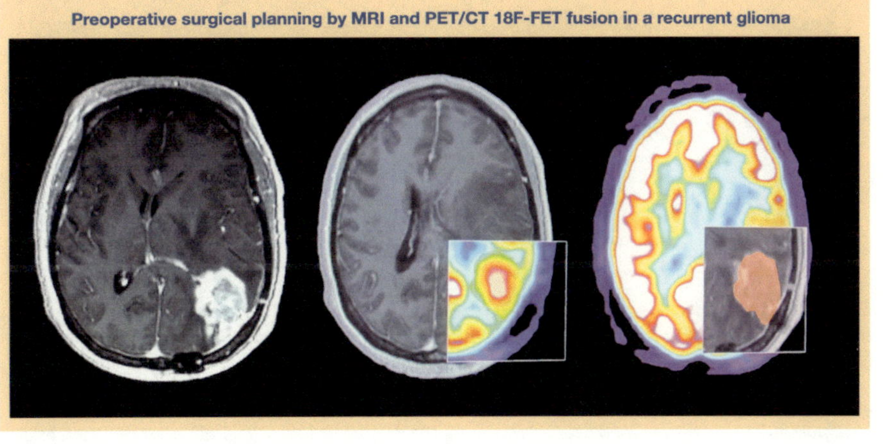


**Figure 4.**
*MRI and PET/CT 18F -FET fusion for brain tumor recurrence resection.*

distinction between low and high-grade tumors, only the 18-F FET values can distinguish between tumor and non-tumor lesions, confirming the superiority of 18-F FET over 18 FDG for the characterization of brain lesions. Since 18-FDG is unreliable for predicting the neoplastic nature due to absorption by inflammatory lesions, amino acid tracers such as FET have been developed in recent decades to increase specificity. However, to date, only a few studies limited to small population of patients compared the diagnostic value of 18-FDG and 18-FET. Goldman and Pirotte thoroughly reviewed the clinical management, images, and PET role [25].

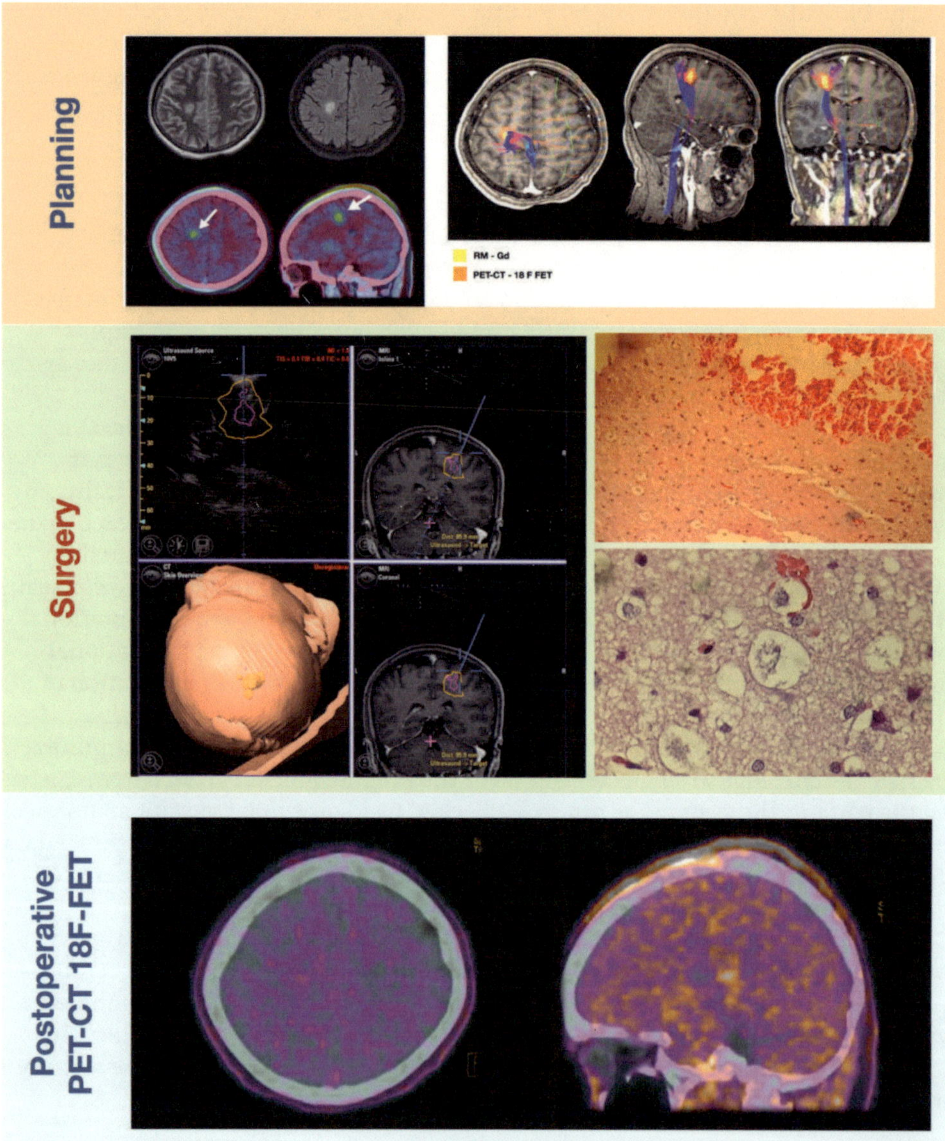


**Figure 5.**
*The utility of Multimodal Neuronavigation for brain tumor resection. A 15-years-old girl was received with a history of left hemiparesis and tonic–clonic seizures. MRI was performed, and a low-grade glioma was suspected. DTI sequences were obtained. A PET-CT 18F-FET was obtained, and fusion with structural and DTI images was performed at the Brainlab workstation. (A) Structural MRI, 18F-FET PET-CT, and DTI for pyramidal tract were fused during neuronavigation planning. (B) Right, Transoperative 3D ultrasonographic images were obtained and fused with the previous neuronavigational plan. Left, Histopathological analysis reveals a diffuse glioma. (C) At 48 months of follow-up, a new 18F-FET PET-CT was performed, no metabolic activity was detected.*

On average, glioblastoma multiforme and medulloblastoma had a uniform and intense uptake throughout the tumor, while brainstem gliomas had a low uptake in less than 50% of the tumor and ependymoma had a low uptake throughout the tumor. When more than 50% of the tumor had uptake, the apparent diffusion coefficient was lower, which agrees with the increase in cellularity. In refractory/recurrent brain gliomas, the low correlation between uptake and enhancement is associated with decreased patient survival. It may reflect concurrent tissue degradation in the disease sites that received treatment and the development of new malignancy sites characterized by increased uptake of 18-F-FDG [26, 27].

The PET/MRI fusion tool in evaluating postoperative and radiooncological treatments provides information for tumor response, progression, and necrosis by radiation, affording the patients' oncological and functional prognosis **Figure 5**.

## 4. Neuronavigation principles

Neuronavigation systems provide intraoperative guidance to the surgeon. Nevertheless, its real advantage is also to help them plan a proper surgical approach to avoid injury and incorporates functional data provided by preoperative images of magnetic resonance imaging, nuclear medicine, intraoperative sonographic studies, and in some places, magnetoencephalography (MEG) to prevent damage to eloquent areas during brain surgery [1].

Image-guided neuronavigation uses the principle of stereotaxy. The brain is considered a geometric entity divided into three imaginary spatial planes that intersect, orthogonal to each other (axial, coronal, and sagittal). Theoretically, any point within the brain is designated by a specific series of coordinates in each plane.

Neuronavigation platforms provide the unique opportunity to translate the two-dimensional information obtained from several imaging techniques – CT scan, MRI, fMRI, PET-CT, into 3D information in the patient's brain of a computational interface at the operating room [16]. The predefined targets on the navigational plan increase the chance to perform a safe and functional gross total resection of malignant primary brain tumors.

Its main objective is to facilitate the extensive resection of the lesion, minimize the risk of neurological sequelae, and favor the prognosis of survival. After registering the patient, the system's accuracy is checked by identifying constant anatomical references or craniometric points. The contour of the lesion and the functional data are fused on the reference structures. In some cases, it is possible to transfer the images to the surgical microscope's eyepieces during surgery.

The intraoperative accuracy of neuronavigation can be affected by changes in intracranial volume caused by tumor resection, brain inflammation, and cerebrospinal fluid flow **Figure 1**. Nevertheless, transoperative images can be combined with ultrasound, tomography, or magnetic resonance images. The intraoperative images offer the possibility of evaluating the residual tumor volume as the surgery progresses **Figure 6**.

### 4.1 DTI and fMRI in functional neuronavigation

Neuronavigation is currently applied in brain surgery, and it is a regular technological resource to increase safety in most neurosurgical procedures (27).

The functional navigation was described as a technological tool for brain tumor resection. It results from the merging of structural, DTI, and BOLD information concerning a malignant tumor's localization. It allows us to know the precise location of functional areas in the human brain [28].

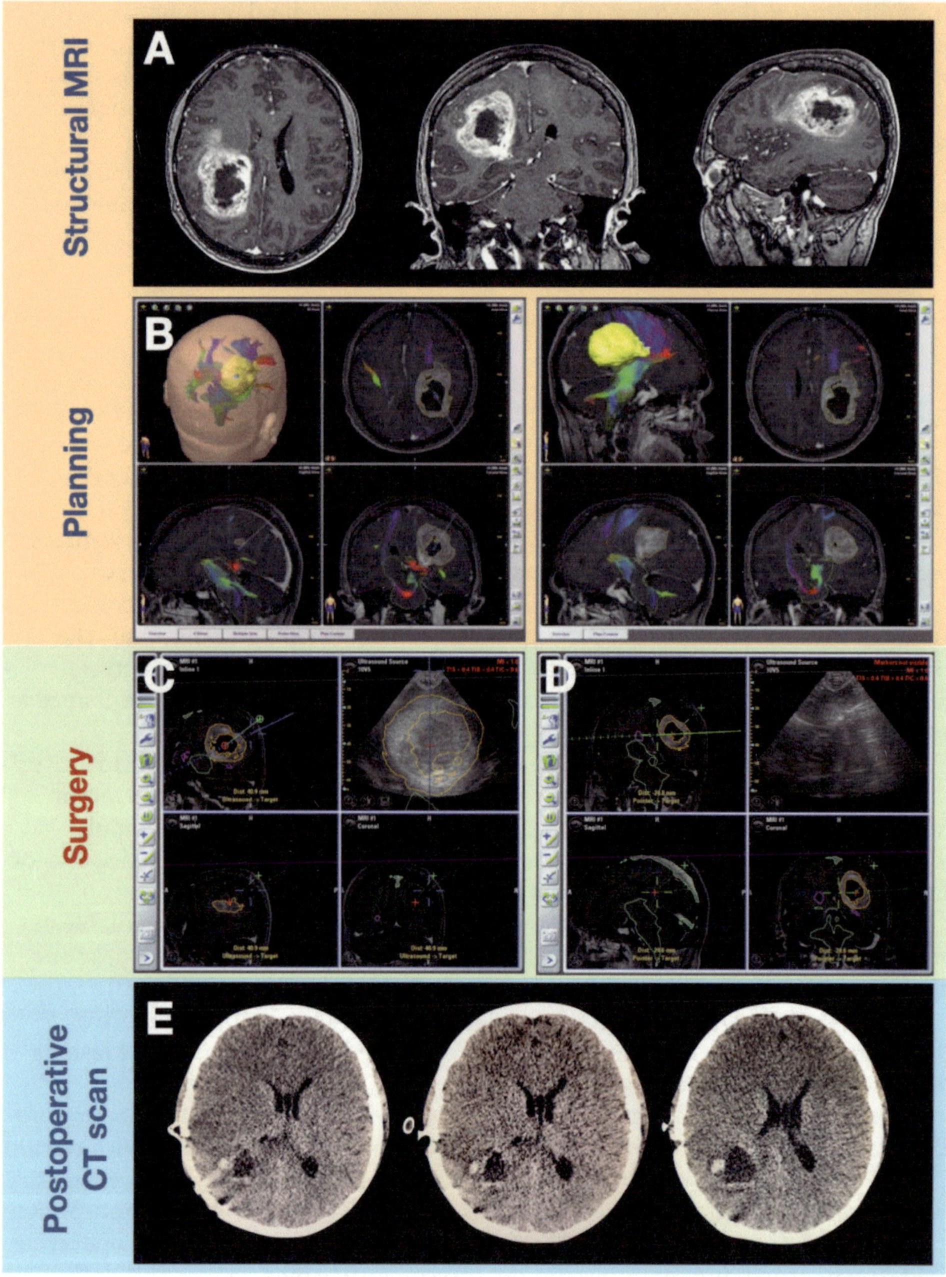


**Figure 6.**
*3D intraoperative ultrasonographic reconstruction increases the usefulness of multimodal neuronavigation for brain tumor resection. A 17-years-old boy with a history of neurofibromatosis type 1 arrives at the emergency department with a headache and left hemiparesis. On an MRI study, a glioblastoma multiforme was suspected. **(A)** MRI T1-enhanced Gd images acquired for surgery planning at **(B)** Brainlab workstation. **(C)** 3D ultrasonographic acquisition to fusion with predefined neuronavigation's plan to achieve a gross total resection. **(D)** Immediate postoperative CT Scan.*

Clinical articles have suggested that the brain shift observed after the opening of the dura and cerebrospinal fluid depletion is the main disadvantage for neuronavigation precision. Nevertheless, several reports suggest that intraoperative MRI use can solve this consequence of brain displacement satisfactorily [29]. In our country, these facilities are not available. To solve it, we correct the brain shit with

three-dimensional ultrasound (3D-US) scans before the dural opening, after the dural opening, and at the end of the resective surgery. Taking advantage of merging this new 3D-US information with previously developed navigation plans with information on the different modalities of structural, functional, and metabolic information tumor and the neighboring tissue. In order to preserve and restore the functional status of each patient. Some limitations to consider for applying these techniques are the biological variability among individuals, the displacement of deep brain structures, and the previously mentioned brain-shift.

## 5. Neuronavigation and intraoperative electrical stimulation

Prof. Hugues Duffau considers the brain as an entirely eloquent organ; every millimeter of the cerebral cortex represents, sometimes a well-recognized function, and others the association area for several complex functions as language and his diverse characteristics that sometimes define a person, visuospatial perception, auditive integration, and so forth.

In the pediatric patient, the patient's age determines a more complex scenario because the stage of neurodevelopment at the time of brain tumor surgery determines the functions' profile to evaluate. Some functions depend on the correct integration of cortical and subcortical areas in the developing brain. Thus, the extensive evaluation and integration in neuronavigation devices of structural, functional, and metabolic imaging techniques are essential to reduce the chance to produce functional sequels.

Undoubtedly, DTI has contributed substantially to the intraoperative identification of withe matter tracts. Perhaps the most studied are those related to motor function. It has been widely described that subcortical continuous monopolar stimulation can help identify the pyramidal pathway with a comprehensive concordance with its counterpart visualized by DTI.

Transoperative electrical stimulation is one more of the resources available to promote extensive glioma resection. The purpose is to preserve the patient's functionality while attempting to dry out as much of the injury as possible [30].

In our experience, the integration of neuronavigation with intraoperative electrical stimulation and brain mapping considerably reduces the risk of lesions secondary to brain tumor resection.

Monopolar continuous stimulation seems to be the most useful and reproducible procedure for the pyramidal tract's subcortical characterization. With the aid of DTI, it is possible to identify the modifications preoperatively in the trajectory, density, and resultant distortion secondary to a CNS malignancy. The neuronavigation plan defines precisely the location of the pyramidal tract. In the operative field, the neuronavigation tools and the intraoperative monopolar stimulation can effectively identify its location at subcortical, thalamic, and peduncular regions.

Recently advances suggest that intraoperative acquisition of DTI images can reduce the risk of sequelae.

## 6. Conclusions

The current neuronavigational technologies allow us to reach deep regions inside the human brain without an increased risk of disability.

The interrelation of different radiological information modalities – structural, functional, and metabolic, in the planning phase of the case and during the surgical procedure permit us to increase the gross-total resection rate for brain tumor resection.

The integration of neurophysiological information into the neuronavigational platform during the neurosurgical procedure reduces complications by monitoring and stimulating withe matter tracts related to language and motor functions.

All multidisciplinary effort is directed to increase surgical techniques' safety to benefit the quality of life of children who suffer from brain tumor disease.

## Acknowledgements

Many people have changed my life, mom, sister, wife, son, and teachers. We acknowledge the incredible patient's confidence; thank you for touching my life, by improving yours.

This work is dedicated to respect and honor relatives and all medical staff members who fell during the COVID-19 pandemic.

## Conflict of interest

"The authors declare no conflict of interest."

## Author details

Roberto Garcia-Navarrete[1,2,3]*, Constantino Contreras-Vázquez[4], Ericka León-Alvárez[5], Natael Olvera González[6], Alfonso Marhx-Bracho[2], Javier Terrazo-Lluch[2,3], José Luis Pérez-Gómez[2], Jorge Alberto Ocon Rodríguez[2], Judy Castañeda Goyes[2] and Juan Alberto Díaz Ponce Medrano[7]

1 Neurosurgery Department, Centro Medico Naval, Secretaria de Marina, Mexico

2 Neurosurgery Department, Instituto Nacional de Pediatria, Mexico

3 Neurosurgery Department, Centro Medico ABC, Mexico

4 Radiology Department, Centro Medico Naval, Secretaria de Marina, Mexico

5 Anesthesiology Department, Instituto Nacional de Pediatria, Mexico

6 Anesthesiology Department, Centro Medico Naval, Secretaria de Marina, Mexico

7 Centro Medico Naval, Secretaria de Marina, Mexico

*Address all correspondence to: roberto.gns@gmail.com

## References

[1] Ganslandt O, Behari S, Gralla J, Fahlbusch R, Nimsky C. Neuronavigation: concept, techniques and applications. Neurol India. 2002 Sep;50(3):244-255. PMID: 12391447.

[2] Kyle M. Walsh, Epidemiology of Brain Tumors. Neurological Surgery. 2017; 118: p. 856-863

[3] Floeth, F.W., Pauleit, D., Wittsack, H.J., et al. 2005. Multimodal metabolic imaging of cerebral gliomas: positron emission tomography with [18F] fluoroethyl-L- tyrosine and magnetic resonance spectroscopy. Journal Neurosurgery., 102 p. 318-327

[4] Dunet, V., Rossier, C., Buck, A., et al. 2012. Performance of 18F-fluoro-ethyl-tyrosine (18F-FET) PET for the differential diagnosis of primary brain tumor: a systematic review and metaanalysis. Journal of Nuclear Medicine. 53 p. 207-214

[5] Concha Enrique, Pelayo Besa, Gutiérrez Jorge. Astrocitic and Oligodendroglial Brain Tumors Management. Clinica las Condes. 2017; 28: p. 392-400

[6] Consejo de Salubridad General. Guia práctica Clínica. Evidencia y recomendaciones. CENETEC. 2010. Tratamiento de Astrocitoma y Medulo-blastoma, en niños y adolescentes.

[7] Filss, C.P., Galldiks, N., Stoffels, G., et al. 2014. Comparison of 18F-FET PET and perfusion-weighted MR imaging: a PET/MR imaging hybrid study in patients with brain tumors. Journal of Nuclear Medicine., 55: p. 540-545.

[8] Lily L. Wang, MBBS, MPH, James L. Leach, John C. Breneman, Cristopher M. Mc. Pherson Critical Role of Imaging in the Neurosurgical and Radiotherapeutic Management of Brain Tumors, Radiographics. 2014; 34:p. 702-721.

[9] Lundemann M, Cardoso Costa J, Law I, Aage S, Mujic A. Patterns of failure for patients with glioblastoma following O-(2-[18F]fluoroethyl)-L-tyrosine PET- and MRI-guided radiotherapy. Elsevier Radiotherapy and Oncology. 2017; 122 p: 380-386

[10] Tyler, J Fraum, MD, Kathryn J. Fowler, MD, Jonathan Mc Conathy, MD, PhD. PET/MRI Emerging Clinical al Applications in Oncology. Academic Radiology. Vol 23; Febrero 2016 p. 220-236. Vincent Dunet, Anastasia Pomoni, Andreas Hottinger, Marie Nicod-Lalonde and John O. Prior. Performance of 18F-FET versus 18F-FDG-PET for the diagnosis and grading of brain tumors: systematic review and meta-analysis. Neuro oncology. March 2016; 18: p. 426-344.

[11] Schonberg T, Pianka P, Hendler T, Pasternak O, Assaf Y (2006) Characterization of white matter displaced by brain tumors using combined DTI and fMRI. NeuroImage 30: 1100-1111.

[12] Lily L. Wang, MBBS, MPH, James L. Leach, John C. Breneman, Cristopher M. Mc. Pherson Critical Role of Imaging in the Neurosurgical and Radiotherapeutic Management of Brain Tumors, Radiographics. 2014; 34:p. 702-721

[13] Guo –Chen Sun, Xiao-lei Che, Yan Zhao, Fei Wang, Bao. Intraoperative High-Field Magnetic Resonance Imaging Combined With Fiber Tract Neuronavigation-Guided Resection of Cerebral Lesions Involving Optic Radiation. Neurosurgery. Research human clinical studies Neurosurg. Noviembre 2011; 69: p. 1070-1084

[14] Jenkinson, M.D., Du Plessis, D.G., Walker, C., Smith, T.S. 2007. Advanced MRI in the management of adult gliomas. British Journal of Neurosurgery, 21: p. 550 -561

[15] Yamasaki, F., Kirusu, K., Satoh, K., et al. 2005. Apparent diffusion coefficient of human brain tumors at MR imaging. Radiological Society of North America. 235: p. 985-991

[16] Borogovac Ajna, Asllani Iris. Arterial spin labeling (ASL), fMRI: advantages theoretical constrains, and experimental challenges in neurosciences. International Journal of Biomedical Imaging 2012: p. 1-13

[17] Thompson, G., Mills, S.J., Stivarios, S.M., Jackson, A. 2010. Imaging of brain tumors: perfusión/permeability. Neuroimaging Clinics of North America. 20(3):337-353.

[18] Bendszus, M., Warmuth- Metz, M., Klein, R., et al 2000. MR sprectoscopy in gliomatosis cerebri. American Journal of Neuroradiology. 21 (2): 375-380.

[19] Peck KK, Bradbury M, Petrovich N, Hou BL, Ishill N, Brennan C, Tabar V, Holodny AI. Presurgical evaluation of language using functional magnetic resonance imaging in brain tumor patients with previous surgery. Neurosurgery. 2009 Apr;64(4):644-652; discussion 652-3. doi: 10.1227/01. NEU.0000339122.01957.0A. PMID: 19197223.

[20] Labbé Atenas, T; Ciampi Díaz, E; Cruz Quiroga, JP; Uribe Arancibia, S; Cárcamo Rodríguez, C. Resonancia magnética funcional: principios básicos y aplicaciones en neurociencias. Radiología, ISSN: 0033-8338, Vol: 60, Edición: 5, Página: 368-377.

[21] Schonberg T, Pianka P, Hendler T, Pasternak O, Assaf Y (2006) Characterization of white matter displaced by brain tumors using combined DTI and fMRI. NeuroImage 30: 1100-1111.

[22] Roux F.E., Boulanouar K., Ibarrola D., et al: Functional MRI and intraoperative brain mapping to evaluate brain plasticity in patients with brain tumours and hemiparesis. J Neurol Neurosurg Psychiatry 2000; 69: pp. 453-463.

[23] Okada T, Nishida N, Taki J, Enatsu R, Ikeda A, Miki Y, Hanakawa T et al (2007) Comparación entre el registro de potenciales evocados motores y el seguimiento de fibras para estimar los tractos piramidales cerca de tumores cerebrales. J Neurosurg 106 (1): 128-133.

[24] Stadlbauer A, Nimsky C, Buslei R, Salomonowitz E, Hammen T, Buchfelder M, Moser E, Ernst-Stecken A, Ganslandt O (2007) Diffusion tensor imaging and optimized fiber tracking in patients with glioma: histopathological evaluation of the white matter with invasive tumor structures. NeuroImage 34 (3): 949-956

[25] Goldman, S., Pirotte, B.J. 2011. Brain tumors. Methods in Molecular Biology, Springer., 727: p. 291-315

[26] Zukotyrski, K. Fahey, F., Kocak, M., et al. 2014. 18-FDG PET and MR imaging associations across spectrum of pediatric brain tumors. A report from the pediatric brain tumor consortium, Journal of Nuclear Medicine., 55:1473-148

[27] Sunaert S (2006) Presurgical planning for tumor resection. J Magn Reson Im 23: 887-905

[28] Rasmussen IA Jr, Lindeth F, Rygh O, Berntsen E, Selbekk T, Xu J, Hernes TN, Harg E, Haberg A, Unsgaard G (2007) Functional neuronavigation combined with intraoperative 3D ultrasound: initial experiences during surgical resections close to brain areas eloquent and future directions in automatic compensation for cerebral displacement of preoperative data. Acta Neurochir (Vienna) 149: 365-378.

[29] Kleiser R, Staempfli P, Valvanis A, Boesiger P, Kollias S (2010) Impact of

advanced fMRI-guided DTI fiber tracking techniques on their clinical applications in patients with brain tumors. Neuroradiology 52: 37-46.

[30] Nossek, E., Korn, A., Shahar, T., Kanner, A. A., Yaffe, H., Marcovici, D., Ben-Harosh, C., Ben Ami, H., Weinstein, M., Shapira-Lichter, I., Constantini, S., Hendler, T., & Ram, Z. (2011). Intraoperative mapping and monitoring of the corticospinal tracts with neurophysiological assessment and 3-dimensional ultrasonography-based navigation, Journal of Neurosurgery JNS, *114*(3), 738-746.

Chapter 5

# Awake Craniotomy and Brain Mapping for Brain Tumor Resection in Pediatric Patients

*Roberto Garcia-Navarrete, Javier Terrazo-Lluch, Alfonso Marhx-Bracho, Ericka León Alvárez, Natael Olvera González, Beatriz Alvárez-Mora, Rosario Aguilar Silva, Cointa Arroyo, Vianey Maceda Morales, Luz María Cordero, Daniel Magos Rodríguez, Sandra Luz Lizarraga-Lopez, Ana Niembro Zúñiga and Juan Alberto Díaz Ponce Medrano*

## Abstract

Brain tumor resection in pediatric patients constitutes a real challenge. In order to improve survival and to preserve neurological function, we will further on describe our experience with awake craniotomy and functional mapping for brain tumor resection in pediatric patients. Although our experience with this technique was relatively short, we did not observe complications, and a gross total resection was successfully achieved in all cases. In the postoperative period we did not find any new deficiency in our patients. We observed functional recovery - motor and sensitive aphasia, motor strength improvement in hemiplegic patients, and recovery of neurodevelopmental milestones during follow-up. In our experience, the use of awake craniotomy and brain mapping for brain tumor resection in pediatric patients is truly safe and reliable.

**Keywords:** Awake craniotomy, Brain mapping, Brain tumor, Cancer

## 1. Introduction

The last year, the *Instituto Nacional de Pediatría* at Mexico is commemorating the 50th anniversary of its foundation. Throughout the years, the Pediatric Neurosurgery Department has consolidated itself as an emblematic service in our hospital among the civilian population and has become the reference center in Mexico to treat brain tumors and complex neurosurgical diseases.

The *Centro Médico Naval* is the referral center for the treatment of complex neurosurgical diseases in the health services of the *Secretaría de Marina* of Mexico. We serve military personnel and their families, as well as civilian population under certain public health circumstances, as COVID-19 pandemic. The Neurosurgery Department is equipped with the ultimate technological devices for brain tumor

treatment, such as neuronavigational systems (Brainlab and Medtronic Systems), intraoperative imaging devices (O-arm), neurophysiological equipment for brain mapping and subcortical stimulation.

This review describes our protocol in both centers for **Awake craniotomy and brain mapping for brain tumor resection in pediatric patients.**

In recent years, the collaborative work performed by an experienced group of neuroscientific specialties - Neuroanesthesiologist (LAE, NOG), Neuropsychologist (BAM, RAS, CA), Neurophysiologist (LMC/DMR), and a specialist from the Intensive care unit (SLL) and pediatric oncologist (AN); allows us to treat brain tumors located in eloquent areas in young brains.

## 2. Neuropsychological evaluation

Most neurological diseases have variable expressiveness; the severity of symptoms that define the disorder varies between individuals. The variability of symptom expression should be identified, and the expected effects of treatment defined. The neurological pathology is complex and comprises a set of unique conditions, therefore it is required a multidisciplinary team of professionals and specialists in pediatric neurosurgery and neuropsychology.

Neuropsychological pediatric evaluation faces certain peculiarities. The brain's functional systems are in development. Thus, certain functions are not able to be properly evaluated. The neuropsychological evaluation tries to obtain a capacity profile which contains weak and strong points. When certain neuropsychological abilities (behavioral and cognitive) are selectively impaired, they may be compatible with the neurological alteration detected. The purpose of an evaluation depends mainly on the reference reason, and this, in turn, depends on the patient's age, academic grade and cognitive development. Neuropsychological tests are essential for establishing a cognitive disorder; in a patient with a brain tumor, it is crucial to have several chronologically ordered evaluations. All improvements can also be monitored by repeating a series of tests, and changes in symptomatology can be detected early. Furthermore, the intervention's effectiveness can be documented, and neuropsychological rehabilitation interventions can be scheduled.

Concerning tumors, the tumor growth site does often relate to neuropsychological deficits (e.g., left hemisphere tumors often affect language). However, due to compression and displacement effects, more widespread damage and overall neuropsychological impairment may occur [1].

It is essential to mention that neuropsychological functions result from a complex functional system that cannot be located in restricted areas of the cerebral cortex or isolated cells. With the use of such specific MRI techniques as blood oxygenation level dependent imaging (BOLD), we know that those functions must be organized into systems of areas that work harmoniously, each of which plays its part within the complex functional system, being located in entirely different areas often very distant from each other in the brain.

Neuropsychological functioning is related to tumor malignancy and behavior; neuropsychological performance assessment may be more sensitive in predicting early tumor recurrence than imaging techniques [1].

In recent years, there has been an increase in the need for neuropsychological evaluations in people who have suffered from known organic diseases and psychiatric pathologies where brain dysfunction is suspected. Interestingly, in most western countries, there has been a crescent incorporation of neuropsychologists into hospital services.

The neuropsychological assessment's primary objective is to identify a possible alteration of functions which are regulated by the cerebral cortex and powerful neuropsychological interventions during sequelae early identification and treatment [2].

When someone faces the need to perform a neuropsychological evaluation, they deal with people who retain a very diverse set of skills depending on their personality characteristics, disease topography, brain edema. These conditions prevent the talk of a rigid evaluation protocol and a set of tests established in advance; they require, on the other hand, a certain level of knowledge to determine in each case the most appropriate evaluation tests [2].

The neuropsychological evaluation has been used during surgeries such as epilepsy and deep brain stimulation to identify adverse outcome risks. The results of this evaluation represent the starting point for neuropsychological treatment and rehabilitation [3].

In a pediatric patient with a brain tumor, the neuropsychological evaluation is performed to determine the patient's overall cognitive status, specifying the skills preserved in contrast with those affected by brain edema and destruction of tissue secondary to the tumor [4, 5].

To set up the overall cognitive status of the patient before surgery, it requires the application of specific instruments, including standardized batteries, or a set of tests which adapt to the specific problems and needs of each patient; allowing to establish:

a. Preserved and altered cognitive functions, i.e., a baseline against which to evaluate postoperative function.

b. The ability of patients to cooperate with transoperative and postoperative needs.

The role of the Neuropsychologist in CNS surgery is divided into different stages. The preoperative evaluation aims to locate, if possible, the focus by associating cognitive deficits in a particular brain region. Set a baseline for measuring changes. Predict cognitive risks after surgery and, in conjunction with the neurosurgeon and family members, assess the procedure's risks/benefits in their quality of life. It is useful as a guide to the neurosurgeon to decide which areas of the brain are at risk and adjust, from there, educational and cognitive rehabilitation programs. Finally, the evaluation can help diagnose psychiatric disorders and their potential impact on cooperation in the operating room. Several reports note that much of the success of awake patient surgery is due to the patient's active participation in the intraoperative process. During functional testing, patient cooperation allows the team to make real-time surgical decisions to achieve maximum tumor resection with minimal functional deterioration to ensure a better quality of life.

There is no protocolized structure for neuropsychological exploration and monitoring that these patients need; there is not enough information about candidates' psychological profiles and eligibility criteria. The transoperative evaluation is based on the literature on the Wada test's use, mainly evaluating language and memory in the dominant hemisphere.

The evaluation depends on the patient's cooperation and what can be applied; if possible, it should include the functions of speech and language:

- Verbal fluency
- Denomination
- Verbal understanding

- Repetition of sentences
- Oral reading (if possible)

Memory evaluation should include:

- Guidance
- Sequencing
- Image remembrance/recovery
- Repetition of digits
- Calculation

Already standardized test subtests measure these areas such as Wechsler Scales, Luria test, Woodkock test, a word list with a letter. These tests are appropriate for the child's age and the evaluation context.

Postoperative evaluation allows monitoring of its evolution, possible sequelae, and the creation of stimulation programs to achieve its full potential.

It has been estimated that there are transient changes in cognitive functioning within the first three months of post-surgical recovery, which are relatively permanent within the following six months after the intervention. However, the most significant changes can occur up to one year after the intervention.

## 3. Neuroanesthesiological evaluation

Several anesthetic considerations for awake craniotomy should be granted to avoid injuries in brain surgery. The primary goal is to carry out the lesion's resection with maximum preservation of neurological functions [6, 7]. This type of management in pediatric patients is limited by anxiety and insufficient understanding, limiting their cooperation during the procedure [8].

The awake craniotomy technique had been developing since the second half of the 19th century when local anesthetics (LA) became widely available. With proper local analgesia, Prof. Horace Horsley was able to perform a craniotomy in awake patients. The benefits were not recognized until 1951, when Prof. Wilder Penfield published LA value for craniotomy in patients with epilepsy to facilitate the resection of epileptogenic focuses [9].

Prof. Penfield argumented that patients with functional neurological pathology should be operated on awake modality and at the same time performing complex and motor activities.

It was initially designed for patients undergoing functional neurological surgery. It is currently offered in pathologies that involve eloquent or motor areas, where real-time monitoring of superior or motor functions is required during tumor resection [10].

The anesthesiologist should know the problems faced during the brain tumor resection in the awake patient, should be aware that at any time, surgery can be switched to a classic craniotomy under total endovenous anesthesia [11].

Scenarios that may be confronted during both phases, asleep or awake, are seizures or movements typical of the patient, result of the suboptimal neuromuscular blockage, or movements in the presence of anxiety or insufficient analgesia. These

symptoms can result in severe damage, from lacerations to the scalp, skull fractures, including cervical spine injuries [9]. This technique aims to provide the neurosurgeon tools to perform the lesion's resection with maximum preservation of eloquent or motor anatomical areas, preserve the patient's integrity, minimize neurological damage and not to increase the deficit already installed [7, 8]. This technique involves inducing general anesthesia and maintaining airway control with a supraglottic device, it also includes invasive monitoring (catheter placement and urinary catheter), administration of scalp blockage, patient positioning, including fixing the skull to Mayfield's head clamp to opening the dura mater [9, 10].

The technique consists of awakening the patient, ousting the supraglottic device, and performing cortical mapping or delimitation of the lesion and resection. At the end of the resection, general anesthesia is again continued, the supraglottic device is reinserted, and the dura mater, skull, and skin are closed.

The main objective of anesthetic management is to ensure adequate patient cooperation, maintain comfort throughout the procedure concerning the chosen position for surgery, prevent and treat nausea, vomiting, seizures, and maintain systemic and neurological homeostasis to provide adequate ventilation, hemodynamic stability, and brain relaxation [11].

Optimal tumor resection is maximum mass removal without significant neurological deficits, such as damage to motor or language function. Therefore, it is now considered the treatment of choice for brain tumor surgery in eloquent areas. Compared to craniotomy under general anesthesia, an awake craniotomy may provide a higher degree of tumor removal without postoperative neurological deficits and better survival rates in these patients [12].

The pediatric patient represents a tremendous challenge for the awake craniotomy technique's success. The cognitive level and emotional maturity will determine their cooperation during the procedure. It is well known that the patient under the age of 16 does not yet have an adult's maturity, and therefore requires more significant psychological support. In the literature, few patients from 8 to 15 years of age have demonstrated this procedure's feasibility [11]. Patients under the age of 10, chosen for this procedure, must demonstrate a rigorous level of maturity and motivation, so the child's degree of development will determine the possibility of exercising this technique [10].

Multidisciplinary assessment (Pediatric neurosurgeon, Neuroanesthesiologist, Neuropsychologist, and Neurophysiologist) is indispensable to mitigate the patient's stress. Some authors prepare the patient psychologically using videos and teaching material to explain the procedure. The previous visit to the operating theater can be an excellent option to gain the child's trust and confidence [12, 13].

The Neuroanesthesiologist should know the surgical and neurophysiological needs required for this procedure. We have a wide variety of anesthetics that can be useful but should be individualized to each patient. Propofol, remifentanil, dexmedetomidine, and scalp nerve blockage provide the right conditions for intraoperative brain mapping. Proper patient selection, adequate perioperative psychological support, and correct anesthetic management at each stage of surgery are all crucial for the safety, satisfaction, and success of the procedure. All of them must allow analgesia and a required sedation level according to the surgical moment [10]. It should be emphasized that certain anesthetics may affect the neurophysiological evaluation [12].

The neuroanesthesiologist should describe the procedure to follow, including position, scalp nerve blockage, possible discomfort, motor, and language testing. It would help to relieve the patient's anxiety and discomfort and to ensure the surgery's success [13, 14].

There are different craniotomy techniques in an awake patient, but Sleep-Awake-Sleep (SAS) is the most convenient in pediatric patients for its cognitive

characteristics. Regardless of the technique chosen, the Neuroanesthesiologist or the person designated for the case must always maintain visual and verbal communication throughout the procedure. The communication at each stage should be clear, and according to the patient's age, questions and tasks should be planned to consider, explain what the sensation may be, explain the noises of the room and maintain an adequate distraction of the patient to avoid anxiety. Heavy traffic within the room should also be avoided, limit staff access, and minimize room noises that confuse the patient which may cause anxiety. (4) Cooperation will depend on the total absence of pain, leading to an outstanding surgical experience; this is based on the anesthetics offered during the procedure, including efficient regional anesthesia with scalp blockage [15].

The premedication should be personalized according to each patient's needs; short-lived anxiolytics such as midazolam is preferred. It does not affect neurocognitive functions and limits confusion or delirium during the procedure. Minimum doses (100-200mcg/kg) are beneficial for controlling anxiety in young patients with normal preoperative neurological functions. However, in the case of mapping and resection of epileptogenic lesions, any suppressive medication of epileptiform and anticonvulsant activity, including benzodiazepines and barbiturates, should be avoided [16].

Analgesia during awake craniotomy is achieved by blocking nerves in the scalp with local anesthetics. Therefore, the patient's hemodynamic and physiological state may be more stable in awake craniotomy than in general anesthesia [13].

The first phase of surgery may be performed with total intravenous anesthesia and a supraglottic device. There are current reports of possible adverse effects of general anesthetic agents, including inhaled agents and opioids, on cancer prognosis, such as increased recurrence or metastasis after surgery [14].

Anesthesiologists should provide sufficient sedation and analgesia during the initial craniotomy; a combination of remifentanil and propofol has been considered the standard protocol for sedation of the first stage of awake craniotomy due to ease of use and reliability. The state of drowsiness but with a quick response, is considered the optimal level of sedation in awake craniotomy. Schneider's model is recommended for propofol's controlled infusion into awake craniotomy to maintain patients' spontaneous ventilation [17].

Dexmedetomidine, an alpha-2 agonist, is a propofol alternative for sedation in such procedures, minimally interferes with neurophysiological monitoring, and it also has a minimal respiratory depressant effect. Concomitant dexmedetomidine with scalp blockage provides sufficient conditions for performing awake craniotomy, compared to the propofol-remifentanil combination and the increased risk of respiratory depression [13].

Complications of awake craniotomy include seizures (3–30%), respiratory depression or airway obstruction (7–16%), hypertension (17–24%), nausea and vomiting (0–9%), cerebral edema (7–14%) [18, 19]. In expert hands, the failure of awake craniotomy occurs in less than 2% of cases, regardless of the proper anesthetic technique carried out [18, 20].

Monitored anesthesia care involves keeping the patient awake under spontaneous breathing with low doses of sedative to resection the lesion by avoiding an acute transition from sleep to wakefulness, leading to hypoactive or hyperactive delirium and decrease mapping reliability [19]. The team's skill and experience are required to achieve optimal sedation, maintaining spontaneous breathing with the patient drowsy but easily reactive [21, 22].

**Advantages:** Lower requirements for anesthetic agents, lower opioid use, better cooperation during intraoperative testing, shorter surgery duration, and shorter hospital stay.

**Disadvantages:** Oversedation leading to airway obstruction with respiratory depression, carbon dioxide ($CO_2$) retention, and consequent cerebral edema; or sub-optimal sedation that leads to the patient's likelihood of anxiety and movements [21].

The SAS technique is preferred in cases of requiring more profound sedation during the craniotomy until before the resection of the tumor, and its objectives are to provide comfort for the patient and the surgical team during the pre-awakening phase, protection of painful sensations, to avoid ventilation distress, and to dismiss postoperative memories about the awake phase throughout the surgery [19].

**Advantages:** Provides the opportunity to control brain edema through hyperventilation, to avoid intraoperative movements of the patient, to lower frequency of seizures and agitation. Used during the implementation of this technique in new hospitals or during the surgical team's learning curve [8].

**Disadvantages:** In high-risk patients with comorbidities, difficult airway predictors, or a high risk of bleeding; the SAS technique is controversial [21].

### 3.1 Anesthetic depth monitoring in awake craniotomy

Researchers compared the Patient State Index, Masimo's PSi, an electroencephalogram (EEG) parameter obtained from SedLine's brain function monitoring system® with Medtronic's Bispectral Index (BIS™) for anesthetic depth monitoring, found that PSi 1.0 was less affected by monopolar Bovie device [23].

Both can be used to monitor anesthetic depth trends in the Sleep-Awake-Sleep phase, to achieve an early and gentle awakening of total intravenous anesthesia [24]. The use of processed electroencephalography indices improves anesthetic titration in the intraoperative period. Processed EEG monitors deliver raw stroke data, numerical anesthesia/sedation depth index, and 2D spectrogram. Deep sedation is associated with poor short- and long-term outcomes in critical patients; cognitive and psychological complications, increased hospital stay and mortality [25].

The use of processed EEG systems as an objective guide to sedative dosing, may decrease medical complications of excessive sedation, such as depressed cardiac contractility and hypotension. BIS's use provides a decrease in the use of sedation, analgesia, decreased agitation, and fewer failures in extubation.

Processed electroencephalogram can help optimize drug doses in individuals with different pharmacogenomics and sedative clearance; global knowledge of the technology and processed EEG traces is required to avoid misinterpretations, significantly when muscle activity interferes with the processing algorithm [26].

Some pathological states, such as seizures or altered EEG states (Suppression of iatrogenic bursts or seizure coma), may be revealed by processed EEG and thus a complete EEG may be requested [27].

PSi values can range from 0 to 100; higher values indicate a lower degree of sedation as follows: 0–24 outbreak suppression with varying degrees of suppression, 25–49 general anesthesia, and > 50 mild sedation [23]. The algorithm uses specific frequency band performance power combined with symmetry and synchronization changes in multiple cortical regions [24]. Without a doubt, processed EEG systems are an excellent tool to optimize sedation and plan proper awakening in awake craniotomy.

## 4. Electrocorticography and brain stimulation for brain tumor resection in the awake pediatric patient

Neurophysiological brain cortical mapping is a valuable tool for brain tumor resection by optimizing the extent of resection and minimizing or avoiding a neurological deficit. In the context of resection of supratentorial malignancies,

the gross-total resection improves survival, and by the usage of brain mapping, the functional outcome and quality of life are safeguarded in the postoperative period [28].

### 4.1 Principles

Stimulation can be bipolar or monopolar. In bipolar stimulation, the cathode and anode are at the level of the selected tissue. It is made using a grid of electrodes, deep electrodes, or an intraoperative manual stimulator (**Figure 1**).

The electric field produced is confined to a small area, usually half the distance between the electrodes, having a low risk of distal activation. Stimulation does not occur unless the electrodes are set directly over the tract, activating the axon's initial part and its Ranvier nodes, where the most sodium channels are contained. Bipolar stimulation in cortical mapping and the technique described by Penfield and Ojemann, are the most commonly used [29, 30].

The standard stimulation paradigm for cortical stimulation described by Penfield, is based on applying a rectangular two-phase pulse with a frequency of 50 Hz on trains lasting 3 to 5 seconds. Pulse duration remains constant at 0.3 ms, starting with an intensity of 1 mA, which increases from 1 mA waiting for a response to stimulation, to a maximum of 15 mA. When using the depth electrodes, the pulse intensity is diminished to a range of 0.5–2.5 mA. In contrast, in monopolar stimulation, a single electrode administers the stimulus, and another reference electrode, usually inserted into the temporal muscle, receives it. The stimulus field is diffuse, and the volume of brain tissue is more significant, with the possibility of activating numerous axons in the motor pathways at a distance of 20 to 25 mm from the stimulation point. It is generally used for subcortical tracks and is known as the High-Frequency Train Technique or Taniguchi Technique [31].

This technique can be used for subcortical functional monitoring in patients under the effect of general anesthesia. A five-pulse monopolar train is typically administered at frequencies between 300 and 500 Hz, with a repetitive frequency

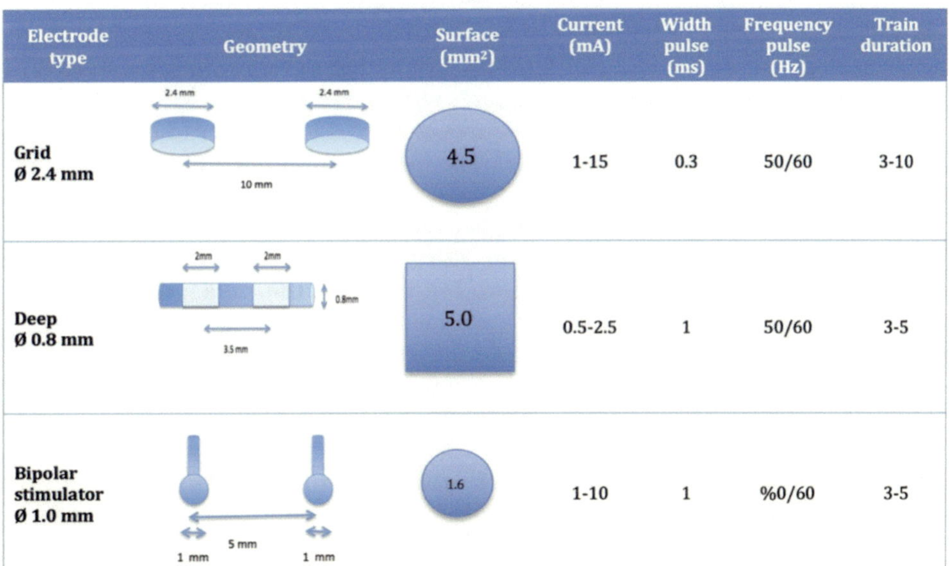


**Figure 1.**
*Principal characteristics of electrodes for brain mapping and bipolar stimulation.*

of 1 to 3 Hz, including a pulse duration of 0.5 milliseconds and a range between stimuli of 2 to 4 milliseconds (**Figure 2**). This method is used to assess motor pathways and can also produce motor responses at lower intensities. It is not affected by the preoperative motor state, and the possibility of post-stimulation discharges is low.

The register is carried out through the potential evoked motor with electrodes placed in the contralateral limb muscles, such as the abductor pollicis brevis, the flexor, and forearm extender, which are usually good options for the upper extremity. In contrast, the abductor hallucis brevis is the best muscle in the case of the lower limb. For facial muscles, we have as options the orbicularis of the mouth and eyes, and the genius, which allow us to register the language articulation.

### 4.2 Indications

The intraoperative functional mapping in awake patients is directed to those with neoplastic or epileptogenic diseases located adjacent to the motor, visual, somatosensory, or language areas. We require patient cooperation to detect the change or deficit of their cognitive functions by stimulation during the procedure. Monitoring cortical and subcortical regions, allows us to resect brain tumors near eloquent cortical and white matter tracts, respectively, at the same surgical event. The limitation is that we have little time to perform the cognitive tasks necessary for transoperative assessment. It could represent an anesthesiological challenge because of the technical difficulty of performing a craniotomy in the awake patient and the high risk of transoperative seizures.

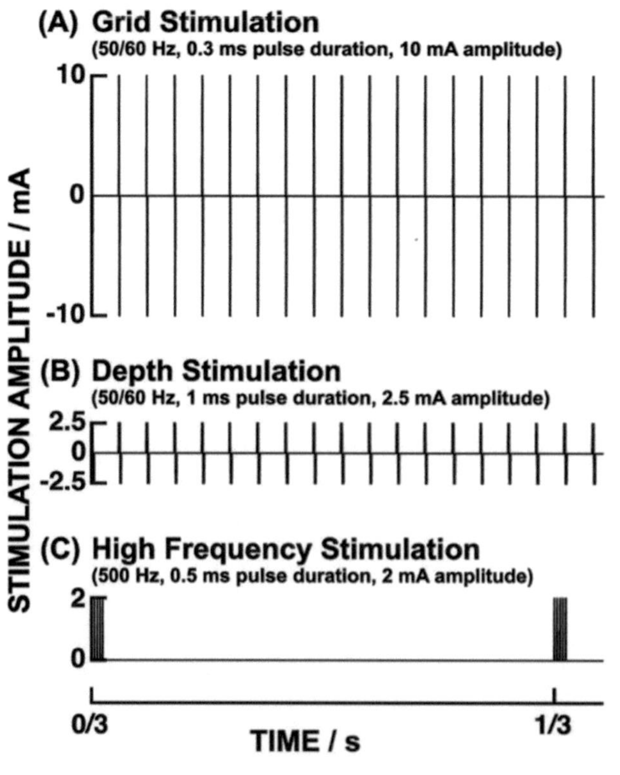


**Figure 2.**
*Stimulation techniques.*

## 4.3 Procedure

General Considerations. Patients are premedicated with midazolam. The surgeon performs local anesthesia with a mixture of 1:1 bupivacaine at 0.5% and lidocaine at 1%; 1:100000 epinephrine for infiltration upon placement of the Mayfield's head clamp. Sedation is performed by means of propofol (above 100 ug/kg/min) and remifentanil (0.05–2 ug/kg/min). Once the craniotomy is completed, the dura mater and the muscle are infiltrated with lidocaine, and no sedation is offered. At all times of the mapping, propofol and icy ringer solution should be ready to use to suppress post-stimulation discharges. Once the mapping is finished, sedation is carried out with dexmedetomidine (1 ug/kg/min) and remifentanil (0.05 ug/kg/min) [32].

In the case of monitoring asleep patients, the purpose of mapping is exclusively to monitor motor response, so that short-acting opioids, such as remifentanil, supplemented with propofol or dexmedetomidine, are used. Almost all agents inhaled at high doses suppress motor responses, so it is suggested to use at low doses (less than 0.25 MAC), with nitrous oxide being the least suppressive. Propofol, commonly used for mapping, can suppress the motor response between 30 and 60% at levels of 1 to 2 mg/ml, so it is suggested at 1ug/ml doses. Other agents, such as ketamine, opioids, benzodiazepines, have minimal effect on motor responses. The most commonly used scheme is a short-acting opioid with propofol or dexmedetomidine.

Other factors to consider in surgery include temperature, blood pressure, oxygen saturation, and $CO_2$. Hypothermia (less than 35 degrees) or hyperthermia (greater than 38 degrees) can increase the motor response latency, decrease amplitude or suppress it altogether. Hypercapnia (greater than 70 mmHg) and hypocapnia (13 to 30 mmHg) can alter mapping and promote cerebral edema.

Due to late myelinization, larger intensities of 15 mA and a longer stimulus duration of 500 ms are recommended in pediatric patients. It is suggested that the minimum age for evaluating language should be ten years old and for motor evaluation a minimum of 5 years. In case the patient does not cooperate and needs to remain under general anesthesia, the monopolar subcortical stimulation technique is recommended, where a stimulus is administered with a train of five monopolar pulses at frequencies typically between 300 and 500 Hz, with a repeat frequency of 1 to 3 Hz including a pulse duration of 0.5 milliseconds, and an interval of 2 to 4 milliseconds between stimuli.

## 4.4 Functional mapping

Once the craniotomy is performed and exposed to the cerebral cortex to map, the bipolar stimulation already described is carried out:

| Pulse | Biphasic |
|---|---|
| Frequency | 50 Hz |
| Pulse duration | 0.2–03. ms |
| Stimulus duration | 3–5 s |
| Language | 5 s<br>Negative almost 10 s |
| Current intensity | Increase 0.5–1 mA |
| Maximal current intensity | 10–15 mA |

| Brain function | Anatomic stimulation | Clinical response |
|---|---|---|
| **Motor** | Primary motor cortex (Brodmann 4): precentral gyrus, 10 mm anterior to the central sulcus and posterior region of central sulcus. | Contralateral muscle contraction. |
| | Supplementary sensitive-motor area: dorsal region of the superior frontal gyrus. | Limb movements vocalization and contralateral cephalic movements. |
| | Silent primary motor cortex: inferior or medial frontal gyrus.<br>Supplementary motor cortex: mesial surface of the superior frontal gyrus, paracentacral lobule and cingulum gyrus. | The negative response inhibits the motor response in the awake patient. |
| **Sensitive** | Sensitive primary cortex (Brodmann 3,1,2): poscentral gyrus. | Contralateral paresthesias o dysesthesias. |
| **Language** | Expressive language (Broca's area): posterior region of the inferior frontal gyrus in dominant hemishere.<br>Posterior region of medial frontal gyrus, and anterior region of superior temporal gyrus in dominant hemisphere. | Negative response or language disturbances when the patient is asked to read, count numbers, or repeat sentences. |
| | Sensitive language (Wernicke's area): posterior temporoparietal area or temporal basal area of language (Inferior temporal gyrus, fusiform or hippocampal gyrus). | Negative response; alterations in understanding. Visual confrontation and nomination pictures. |
| **Visual** | Primary visual cortex (Brodmann 17): occipital cortex. | Contralateral phosphenes and disturbances in perception of shapes, colors, or lines. |
| | Secondary visual cortex (Broadmann 18) and secondary association cortex (Brodmman 19). | Visual illusions. |
| **Hearing** | Primary auditive cortex (Brodmann 22)<br>Posterior peri-Syilvian region. | Hearing distortion.<br>Complex listening experiences. |

**Table 1.**
*Cortical areas to stimulate during functional mapping.*

The stimulus should be applied at least three times; it is considered positive when at least 2 out of three times an answer is found. Responses can be either positive (regional movements, dysesthesias, phosphenes) or negative (motor inhibition, language alteration, anomia) (**Table 1**).

Language tasks such as nomination, articulation, reading, counting, and comprehension are evaluated. It is stimulated with a pulse duration of 0.25 ms on trains from 4 to 60hz, usually used from 1.5 mA and increased to 6. The stimulation is applied from one to two seconds during the completion of the task. The point is stimulated at least three times. A positive point is considered when a 66% language error is observed, such as the absence of language, anomia, and paraphasia. Some authors [30, 33, 34] have established the 10–20 mm concept as a safe margin, i.e., the distance from the resection edge to the mapped language site, in order to determine the risk of language deficits during the postoperative period. Usually, if this distance is greater than 1, the risk of language deficit in the frontal lobe is low.

## 4.5 Functional mapping considerations

The limitation of the technique is associated with several factors:

a. **Patient's condition.** Previous deficit. These include a pre-existing deficit; usually the most accurate responses are obtained in patients with preserved motor and language functions. Any significant variation in sensation, motor paresis, or alterations of language or anomia, will not allow an appropriate check-in in those areas. Patient's age. Reduced myelination in pediatric patients, so motor responses are typically more challenging to activate than the standard parameters used in adults. Due to incomplete functional maturation, the motor and language areas can be identified with confidence after 5 and 10 years old, respectively. Some suggested strategies to improve motor monitoring include pulse duration as large as 500 microseconds and increasing load intensity (more than 25 mA); this has been observed in children between 5 and 7 years old, but as they grow and enter adolescence, they get thresholds similar to adulthood. One option for pediatric patients who cannot perform awake functional mapping, is to use other techniques such as primary motor cortex localization using the reserve phase technique, which indirectly allows us to locate the motor area (**Figure 3**).

b. **Effect of different types of brain injuries.** Pre-existing injuries, i.e., brain edema, hemorrhage, herniation syndromes, can increase stimulation thresholds. The restoration of local homeostasis improves the stimulation threshold. Moreover, modification in the functional expressiveness of cortical areas due to the mass effect secondary to neoplasms. In patients with cortical malformations such as dysplasia, an abnormal somatotopic organization is observed and induces several secondary mechanisms, leading to a compensatory reorganization known as neural plasticity [35].

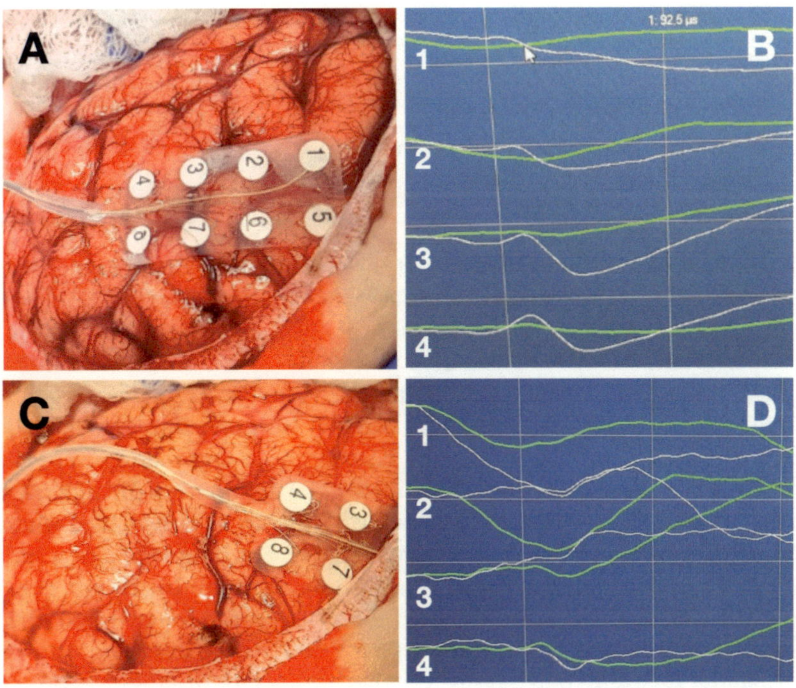


**Figure 3.**
*Reverse-phase. An electrode grid is applied to identify the motor and somatosensory primary cortex. A) Parietal lobule exploration. B) Neurophysiological typical response for somatosensory cortex stimulation. C) Electrode-grid relocation to identify primary motor cortex. D) Reverse-phase demonstration.*

## 4.6 Technical limitations

### *4.6.1 Lack of standardization*

Negative mapping does not protect and creates a questionable problem concerning the reliability of the stimulation. There is a lack of consensus on stimulation paradigms and techniques. Significant variations were observed, not only in stimulation environments, but also in proven functions and protective margins preserved in resection. An example is deficit in language functions after functional mapping. In the survey, several centers where the functional mapping is practiced, only half responded that they regularly tested the four commonly checkable functions (speech production, comprehension, denomination, reading), creating the possibility of false-negative results related to unproven function. It may explain why 41% of centers reported persistent postoperative language deficiencies despite the preservation of language areas, and 56% of this group mentioned the failure to identify crucial language sites [28]. Variability in mapping thresholds has been observed not only at the population level but also in individual patients. One maneuver to facilitate the response in eloquent areas could be to increase the current at each cortical site, regardless of the adjacent post-estimate discharge threshold, instead of mapping the entire exposed cortex into a single current level. Besides, their findings highlighted the need for ECoG during electrocortical stimulation mapping, both to identify when post-stimulation discharges occur and to verify stimulation by recording stimulation artifacts [36].

### *4.6.2 Post-stimulation*

Post-stimulation discharges can evolve into seizures during the surgical procedure, which is why the anesthesiologist should always be ready with propofol as well as the surgeon with an icy ringer solution. These stimuli thresholds are not significantly higher than those used to stimulate sensory, motor, or linguistic responses. However, post-stimulation discharges have been reported during awake craniotomy at 12% [37, 38].

### *4.6.3 Anesthesiologic challenge*

From an anesthetic perspective, cortical functional mapping with an awake patient imposes essential demands on the anesthesiologist ability to facilitate sleep-awake-sleeping procedures and avoid inadequate or excessive sedation. Pain, emesis, and emotional intolerance to the technique are rarely observed, and, of course, seizures can occur. Failure of the functional cortical mapping technique leads to a lower macroscopic total resection incidence and increased postoperative morbidity.

## 4.7 Intraoperative electrocorticography

### *4.7.1 Objectives and limitations of intraoperative electrocorticography*

Epilepsy surgery involves complete resection of the epileptogenic area (the alleged site generating epileptic seizures, removal or disconnection is necessary in order to prevent further seizures) with minimal postoperative deficits. Electrocorticography (ECoG) allows the epileptogenic zone to be delimited using flexible electrodes placed before and after resection, and to use the electrodes to stimulate and delimit the eloquent area. However, sampling is limited by reduced registration time during surgery [39].

So ECoG is not sufficient to define the epileptogenic zone; many preoperative studies are required, such as video-EEG, functional and structural MRI including PET, SPECT, and sometimes invasive recording with grid placement. The ECoG intraoperative utility as a single element for defining the epileptogenic zone in a reliable way, is based on the assumption that interictal discharges are trustworthy markers of the epileptogenic zone. This assumption has proven unreliable in many cases. One of the most significant transoperative electrocorticography limitations is that primary epileptiform discharges may not be identified from secondary ones by propagating to a distant area. More importantly, ECoG's in patients with refractory epilepsy to medical treatment has shown interictal multifocal activity, making focus identification a difficult task.

Interictal activity may be affected by anesthetic agents use, as some of those agents decrease activity while others increase them. It is said that the log is reliable when a pattern of awake interictal poly points is observed with a tip frequency exceeding one per minute. Some activation maneuvers, such as hyperventilation or some intravenous anesthetics such as methohexital, etomidate, propofol, and thiopental, have been used.

Unfortunately, the activation induced by these agents could be expanded to previously silent areas. Opioids, such as remifentanil and alfentanil, increase the activity in the epileptogenic zone. Remifentanil has been reported to suppress tips in the normal brain.

Other attempts have been made to locate the epileptogenic area using repetitive cortical electrical stimulation and evaluate its susceptibility to start a discharge and reproduce the patient's usual seizure. Although early researchers expected post-stimulation discharges originating in the epileptogenic area to have distinctive characteristics (lower post-discharge thresholds and longer durations), this is not true. The use of electrical stimulation to induce the patient's usual seizures has also shown not to be useful.

Three types of electrodes are used to register intraoperatively, often in combination:

The first type consists of silver wires insulated with a carbon ball or a distal silver ball/silver chloride located on the cortical surface. These electrodes are arranged in an electrode clamping device mounted on the skull at the edge of the craniotomy and attached to the recording device inputs. Although flexible and precise electrode placement, particularly along the resection cavities, is an excellent resource of this type of electrode; the exact distance between electrodes can be problematic, limiting the ability to engrave in a bipolar assembly. Therefore, recording in a reference montage is preferred. Also, electrode placement is limited only to the cortex areas, so it is impossible to register from the lower and medial surfaces. These electrodes can be sterilized and reused.

The second type of electrode is disposable and consists of silver stainless steel, or platinum disc electrodes embedded in silicone sheets. These blades are arranged in advance as strips containing 4 to 8 electrodes, with a separation of 10 to 15 mm, or larger grids containing 64 electrodes or more. These electrodes can be placed on the exposed cortical surface and allow the flexibility to slide under the craniotomy margins to cover the cortex uncovered surfaces. Because the distances between electrodes are standardized, it is possible to make recordings in both bipolar and referencing assemblies. However, due to the potential for cancelation of common-mode activity under two adjacent electrodes in a bipolar recording, referencing assembly remains preferred and universally accepted as being more reliable. Functional stimulation can also be performed through band and grid electrodes.

Finally, a four-contact depth electrode can also be used to be inserted into the brain's deeper structures. It is not uncommon for these various electrodes to be used

simultaneously, with ball electrodes used to register over the lateral cortex or along the resection margins, while electrode strips are placed in the cortical areas. The recording electrodes can be referenced to several locations, including the mastoid, cervical, and bone flap region.

The ECoG can be registered using digital or analog instruments, although digital has become more used. As the activity recorded on the cortical surface is significantly higher than the one recorded on the skin surface, the recording parameters must be adjusted. Sensitivities between 10 and 50 mV/mm are the most commonly used. Other recommended recording parameters include a 0.5 Hz low-frequency filter and a 70 Hz high-frequency filter.

The usefulness of electrocorticography in anteromedial temporal lobectomy allows delimiting the degree of resection of the hippocampus. The most significant cause of seizure recurrence after temporal lobectomy is the incomplete resection of the affected hippocampus. Therefore, the resection of the hippocampus guided by electrocorticography has been the only procedure with a predictive value. Its usefulness has also been seen in patients with refractory epilepsy to extratemporary location medical treatment, where the need for all patients to require an invasive chronic record is controversial.

In patients with a high concordance between neuroimaging (MRI, PET, and SPECT) and the clinic of seizures, although EEG may not be conclusive in identifying the ictal area, it is indicated to perform the resection of the epileptogenic focus in a single surgical time guided by electrocorticography.

Electrocorticography is very useful in the resection of structural lesions that generate seizures, such as low-grade astrocytomas or malformations, and the surrounding epileptogenous cortex. Patients who had only the lesion resection, have a probability of being free of crisis by 50% and increasing to 87% when electrocorticography is offered.

Electrocorticographography has been very useful in cortical dysplasia resection, where sometimes the image is not very clear, especially in type I cortical focal dysplasias, and where electrocorticography helps define the edges of the margins of the resection.

Finally, ECoG should be used during functional mapping to detect post-stimulus discharges that can occur over a wide threshold range (2 to 15 mA), usually lasting seconds, but some downloads last more than 90 seconds. Post-stimulus discharges have been present in 12% of patients undergoing cortical functional mapping; 65% of these discharges involve more than one electrode, and 10% become epileptic electrographic activity.

## 5. Clinical experience

Since 2017, we have performed awake craniotomies and brain mapping for brain tumor resection in 8 and 5 cases, respectively. The average age of patients was 12.2 years old with a range of 10–15 years old. No gender predominance was observed (Male/Female ratio 1). The neuropsychological evaluation was performed in all cases. A series of neuropsychological tests were applied to meet the maturity and neurological performance in all cases. Before considering each case as a candidate for an awake craniotomy, an assay was conducted by the neurosurgeon and the neuroanesthesiologist to gain the patient's confidence. In all cases, the technique was completed. In some cases, conversion to total-endovenous anesthesia was necessary. Intraoperative seizures were not observed during brain mapping or stimulation of eloquent areas in the neighborship of brain tumors.

In order of frequency, the most common histopathological diagnosis was diffuse glioma (n = 3), supratentorial glioblastoma multiforme (n = 2), dysembryoplastic tumor (n = 2), and Primitive Neuroectodermal Tumor (PNET) (n = 1). In all cases, gross total resection was achieved. In malignant gliomas, the overall survival was 32 months. In this group, all patients received adjuvant chemotherapy and radiotherapy. In the cases of diffuse glioma, we have not observed fatalities so far. Currently, the overall survival is 38 months. In the case of PNET, adjuvant therapy and radiotherapy with a linear accelerator were indicated. The free of disease period was 18 months, a new surgical treatment was indicated to improve survival, but in the postoperative period, the patient's family declined the second-line chemotherapy, and the patient died after 28 months— **Case 1** VIDEO.

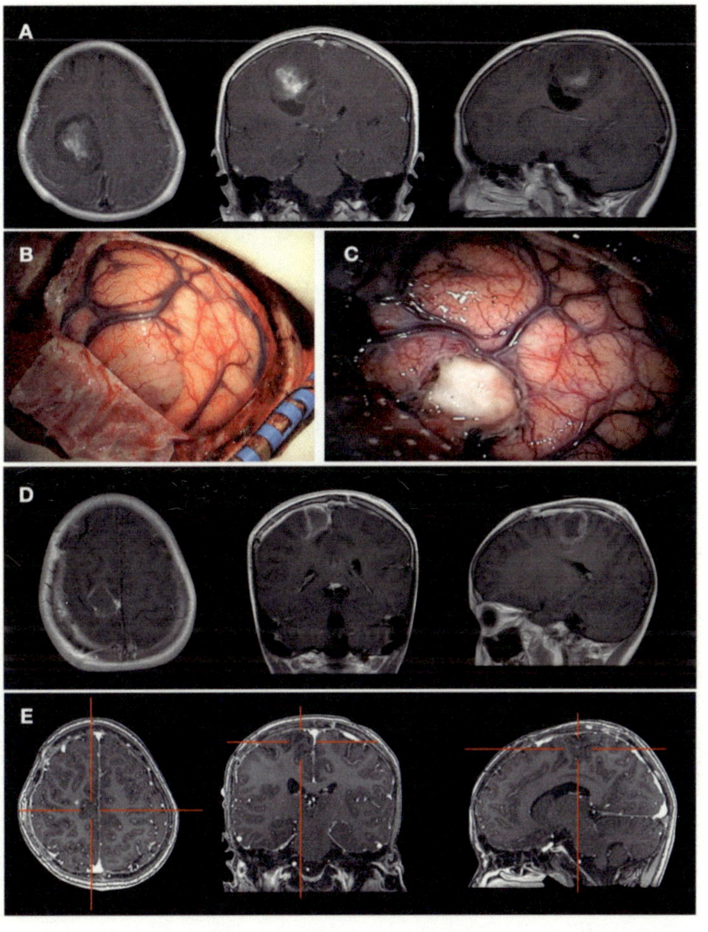


In all cases, during follow-up, we observed a clinical improvement of neurological deficits. In the two cases of epilepsy secondary to brain tumor activity – dysembryoplastic tumor, the cortical mapping and brain stimulation in eloquent areas improved the seizure control and functional recovery in the postoperative period. In one of these cases, after the tumor's gross-total resection, a new ECoG helped us identify epileptic activity isolated from the brain tumor. Histopathological analysis revealed cortical dysplasia. After removing the epileptic foci by corticectomy, the new ECoG register showed regular electrocorticographic activity — **Case 2** Currently, the two patients with dysembryoplastic tumors are seizure-free (Engel's class Ia).

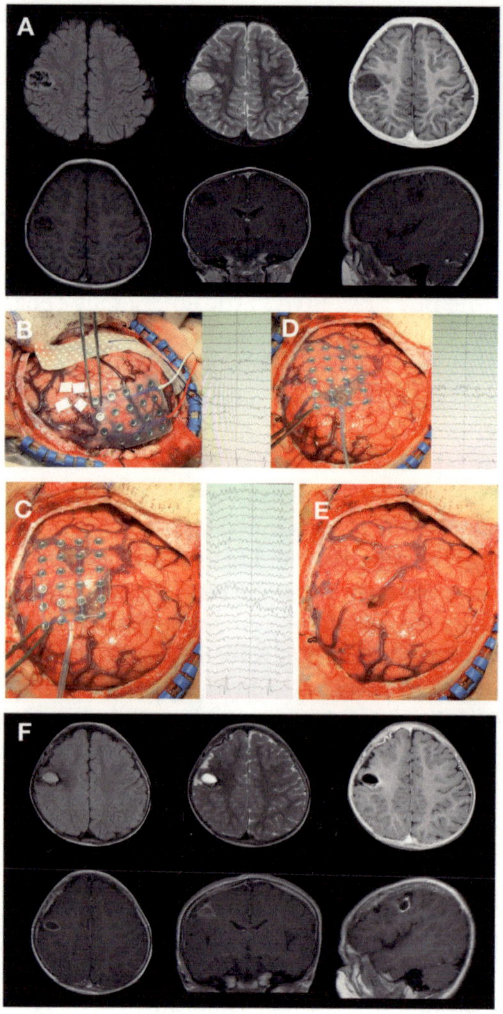


## 6. Conclusions

The SAS technique is a reproducible, safe, and probably the most convenient technique for awake craniotomy in pediatric patients with brain tumors. It is imperative to maintain good communication with the patient from pre-anesthetic assessment, explaining the most confident procedure. SAS will provide the most outstanding comfort before awakening and during neuropsychological and motor tests, recognizing that the neurological evaluation during and after the surgical procedure will be the best indicator of the patient's condition and success.

Cortical functional mapping allows us to delimit lesions that require resection, such as an epileptogenic zone or a tumor from eloquent regions. For this purpose, with a mature and cooperative patient, surgery may be performed with an awake patient. This technique is reserved for patients without severe neurological deficits in order to preserve the language, somatosensory, or motor functions. If the patient does not cooperate, as are pediatric patients below eight years old, the cortical functional mapping for motor functions could be performed with general anesthesia.

Electrocorticography is widely used in epilepsy and brain tumor surgery. Its usefulness has also been seen in patients undergoing temporary mesial lobectomy

to determine the hippocampus degree of resection. Another utility is in resective surgery for structural lesions that cause seizures (tumors, cortical, vascular malformations), in order to delimit the surrounding epileptogenic zone and expand it.

Finally, electrocorticography must be accompanied by the mapping procedure to identify post-stimulation discharges.

## 7. Clinical cases

**Case 1.** An 8-year-old boy presented at the emergency department with a two-month history of headache, left-sided weakness (1/5), and generalized seizures. MRI study shows a premotor right brain tumor (A). An awake craniotomy was performed, and gross total resection was achieved. VIDEO. (https://bit.ly/3vXzr2S) (C). The pathology service reports a Primitive Neuroectodermic tumor. The patient receives chemotherapy (Iphosphamide - Carboplatine - Etoposide) and radiotherapy 54 Gy (Lineal-accelerator). During follow-up, a recurrence was suspected (D), and a new surgical treatment was performed (E).

**Case 2.** A 4-year-old female presented to the neurosurgery department with a history of symptomatic epilepsy since she was 3 years old. A few months later, autism disorder was detected. Partial motor seizures with hand-forearm-shoulder involving and secondary generalization were observed. An MRI study was performed, and a neoplastic lesion in the primary motor cortex was identified. A comprehensive case review was performed. Because of the history of autism disorder, the patient was dismissed as a candidate for awake craniotomy. However, she was considered a candidate for surgical treatment by total endovenous anesthesia. The primary motor cortex was identified with the reverse-phase technique in the operating room, and transoperative electrocorticography was performed. The gross-total resection was achieved for the brain tumor, and a subpial resection was completed after the identification of epileptic foci identified by a new ECoG. A) Preoperative MRI. B) ECoG to define the epileptic activity. C) ECoG after brain tumor resection. D) ECoG identifies epileptic activity in the rostral region of pars triangularis. E) After subpial resection of epileptic foci. F) Follow-up MRI.

## Acknowledgements

We acknowledge the intense work, dedication, and commitment of Pediatry and Pediatric Specialties residents, to the great nurse's team and social workers at the Instituto Nacional de Pediatría and at the Centro Médico Naval of México.

This work is dedicated to respect and honor relatives and worldwide medical staff members who fell during the COVID-19 pandemic.

## Conflict of interest

"The authors declare no conflict of interest."

## Author details

Roberto Garcia-Navarrete[1,2,3*], Javier Terrazo-Lluch[1,3], Alfonso Marhx-Bracho[1], Ericka León Alvárez[4], Natael Olvera González[5], Beatriz Alvárez-Mora[6], Rosario Aguilar Silva[7], Cointa Arroyo[7], Vianey Maceda Morales[6], Luz María Cordero[8], Daniel Magos Rodríguez[8], Sandra Luz Lizarraga-Lopez[9], Ana Niembro Zúñiga[10] and Juan Alberto Díaz Ponce Medrano[11]

1 Neurosurgery Department, Instituto Nacional de Pediatria, Mexico City, Mexico

2 Neurosurgery Department, Centro Medico Naval (Secretaria de Marina Armada de Mexico), Mexico City, Mexico

3 Neurosurgery Department, Centro Medico ABC, Mexico City, Mexico

4 Anesthesiology Department, Instituto Nacional de Pediatria, Mexico City, Mexico

5 Anesthesiology Department, Centro Medico Naval, Secretaria de Marina Armada de Mexico, Mexico City, Mexico

6 Psychology Department, Centro Medico Naval, Secretaria de Marina Armada de Mexico, Mexico City, Mexico

7 Mental Health Department, Instituto Nacional de Pediatria, Mexico City, Mexico

8 Neurophysiology Department, Instituto Nacional de Pediatria, Mexico City, Mexico

9 Intensive Care Unit, Instituto Nacional de Pediatria, Mexico City, Mexico

10 Oncology Department, Instituto Nacional de Pediatria, Mexico City, Mexico

11 Centro Medico Naval, Secretaria de Marina Armada de Mexico, Mexico City, Mexico

*Address all correspondence to: roberto.gns@gmail.com; rgarcianavarretes@pediatria.gob.mx

IntechOpen

## References

[1] Ownsworth T, Chambers S, Walker D.G., and Shum D. Neuropsychological Assessment of Individuals with Brain Tumor: Comparison of Approaches Used in the Classification of Impairment. Front Oncol. 2015; 5: 56.

[2] Rausch, R. Psychological evaluation. In: Surgical treatment of epilepsies. New York. Raven Press. 2001.

[3] Tröster A. Some Clinically Useful Information that Neuropsychology Provides Patients, Carepartners, Neurologists, and Neurosurgeons About Deep Brain Stimulation for Parkinson's Disease. Arch Clin Neuropsychol. 2017 Nov; 32(7): 810-828

[4] Kaplan, E. F., Goodglass, H., & Weintraub, S. The Boston naming test. Philadelphia: Lippincott Williams & Wilkins, 1983-2001

[5] Peña-Casanova J. Integrated neuropsychological exploration program-Barcelona test revised. Barcelona: Masson; 2005

[6] Luria, A.R. El cerebro en acción. Barcelona; Martinez Roca; 1984

[7] Everett LL, Van Rooyen IF, Warner MH, Shurtleff HA, Saneto RP, Ojemann JG. Use of dexmedetomidine in awake craniotomy in adolescents: Report of two cases. Paediatric Anaesthesia 2006; 16 (3): 338-342.

[8] Ramírez-Segura EH. Anestesia para craneotomía con el paciente despierto: Técnica dormido-despierto-dormido. Revista Mexicana de Anestesiología 2014; 37(1): 42-46.

[9] Chui J. Anestesia para craneotomía en el paciente despierto: una actualización. Revista Colombiana de Anestesiología 2015; 43: 22-28.

[10] McClain CD, Landrigan-Ossar M. Challenges in Pediatric Neuroanesthesia. Awake Craniotomy, Intraoperative Magnetic Resonance Imaging, and Interventional Neuroradiology. Anesthesiology Clinics 2014; 32(1): 83-100.

[11] Solera RI, Uña OR, Valero I, Laroche F. Awake craniotomy. Considerations in special situations. Revista Española de Anestesiología y Reanimación 2013; 60(7): 392-398.

[12] Meng L, McDonagh DL, Berger MS, Gelb AW. Anesthesia for awake craniotomy: a how-to guide for the occasional practi- tioner. Can J Anaesth 2017; 64: 517-529.

[13] Gerritsen JKW, Arends L, Klimek M, Dirven CMF, Vincent AJE. Impact of intraoperative stimulation mapping on high-grade glioma surgery outcome: a meta-analysis. Acta Neurochir (Wien) 2019; 161: 99-107.

[14] Richardson AM, McCarthy DJ, Sandhu J, Mayrand R, Guerrero C, Rosenberg C, et al. Predictors of successful discharge of pa- tients on postoperative day 1 after craniotomy for brain tumor. World Neurosurg 2019; 126: e869–e877.

[15] Delion M, Terminassian A, Lehousse T, Aubin G, Malka J, N'Guyen S, Menei P. Specificities of awake craniotomy and brain mapping in children for resection of supratentorial tumors in the language area. World Neurosurgery 2015; 84(6): 1645-1652.

[16] Zhang K, Gelb AW, Francisco FS. Awake craniotomy: indications, benefits, and techniques. Colombian Journal of Anesthesiology 2018; 46: 49-55.

[17] Soehle M, Wolf CF, Priston MJ, Neuloh G, Bien CG, Hoeft A, et al. Propofol pharmacodynamics and bispectral index during key moments of awake craniotomy. J Neurosurg Anesthesiol 2018; 30: 32-38.

[18] Spena G, Roca E, Guerrini F, Panciani PP, Stanzani L, Salmaggi A, et al. Risk factors for intraoperative stimulation-related sei- zures during awake surgery: an analysis of 109 consecutive pa- tients. J Neurooncol 2019; 145: 295-300.

[19] Eseonu CI, ReFaey K, Garcia O, et al. Awake craniotomy anesthesia: a comparison of the monitored anesthesia care and asleep-awake-asleep techniques. World Neurosurg 2017; 104:679-686.

[20] Flexman AM, Wang T, Meng L. Neuroanesthesia and outcomes: evidence, opinions, and speculations on clinically relevant topics. Curr Opin Anaesthesiol. 2019 Oct;32(5):539-545.

[21] Kulikov A, Lubnin A. Anesthesia for awake craniotomy. Current Opinion in Anaesthesiology 2018; 31(5): 506-510.

[22] Sewell D, Smith M. Awake craniotomy: Anesthetic considerations based on outcome evidence. Current Opinion in Anaesthesiology 2019; 32(5): 546-552.

[23] Bloom, J., Wyler, D., Torjman, M. C., Trinh, T., Li, L., Mehta, A., ... Romo, V. (2020). High Incidence of Burst Suppression during Propofol Sedation for Outpatient Colonoscopy: Lessons Learned from Neuromonitoring. Anesthesiology Research and Practice, 2020, 1-6.

[24] Castellanos Peñaranda, C., Casas Arroyave, F. D., Gómez, F. J., Pinzón Corredor, P. A., Fernández, J. M., Velez Botero, M., ... Marulanda Toro, C. (2020). Technical and clinical evaluation of a closed loop TIVA system with SEDLineTM spectral density monitoring: Multicentric prospective cohort study. Perioperative Medicine, 9(1). doi:10.1186/s13741-019-0130-2

[25] Wang ZH, Chen H, Yang YL, et al. Bispectral index can reliably detect deep sedation in mechanically ventilated patients: a prospective multicenter validation study. Anesth Analg. 2017;125:176-183

[26] Wang ZH, Chen H, Yang YL, et al. Bispectral index can reliably detect deep sedation in mechanically ventilated patients: a prospective multicenter validation study. Anesth Analg. 2017; 125:176-183.

[27] Devlin JW, Skrobik Y, Gélinas C, et al. Clinical Practice Guidelines for the Prevention and Management of Pain, Agitation/Sedation, Delirium, Immobility, and Sleep Disruption in Adult Patients in the ICU. Crit Care Med. 2018;46:e825–e827

[28] Ritaccio AL, Brunner P, Schalk G. Electrical stimulation maping of the brain: Basic Pinciples and emergin alternatives J Clin Neurophysiol, 2018 Marzo (2): 86-97.

[29] Penfield W, Boldrey E. Somatic Motor and sensory representation in the cerebral cortex of man as studied by electrical stimulation. Brain 1937; 60:389-443

[30] Ojemann G, Ojemann J, Lettich E, Berger M. Cortical language localization in left, dominant hemnisphere. An Electrical stimulation mapping investigation in 117 patiens. J Neurosurg 1989;71:316-326

[31] Taniguchi M, Cedzich C, Schramm J. Modification of cortical stimulation for motor evoked potentials under general anestesia: technical description. N ueursurgey, 1993, 91 379-385

[32] Wang DD, Rolston JD Berger M. Cortical stimulation and Mapping. Cataltepe O, Jallo GI. Pediatric Epilepsy Surgery. Thieme 2ª ed 2020, 277-283

[33] Haglund MM, Berger MS, Shamseldin M, Lettich E, Ojemann GA. Cortical localization of temporal lobe

language sites in patients with gliomas. Neurosurgery. 1994; 34:567-576. discussion 576.

[34] Berger MS, Kincaid J, Ojemann GA, Lettich E. Brain mapping techniques to maximize resection, safety, and seizure control in children with brain tumors. Neurosurgery. 1989; 25:786-792.

[35] Tuxhorn I, Extra- and Intraoperative electrocortical stimulation. Cataltepe O, Jallo GI. Pediatric Epilepsy Surgery. Thieme 2ª ed 2020,134-142

[36] Galletine WB, Mikati MA Intraoperative Electrocorticography and cortical stimulation in children. Journal of Clinical Neurophysiology 2009;26(2): 95-108

[37] Bank AM, Schevonb CA, Hamberger MJ. Characteristics and clinical impact of stimulation-evoked seizures during extraoperative cortical mapping. Epilepsy & Behavior. 2014; 34:6-8

[38] Nossek E, Matot I, Shahar T. Barzilia O, Rapopolrt Y, Gonene T, et al. Intraoperative seizures during awake craniotomy: incidence and consequiences: analisys of 4677 patients. Neurosurgery 2013; 73 135-140

[39] Pouratian N, Cannestra AF, Bookheimer SY, et al. Variability of intraoperative electrocortical stimulation mapping parameters across and within individuals. J Neurosurg. 2004;101: 458-466.

Section 4

# Molecular Classification of CNS Tumors

Chapter 6

# The Distribution and Significance of *IDH* Mutations in Gliomas

*Nu Thien Nhat Tran*


## Abstract

In 2009, the discovery of isocitrate dehydrogenase (IDH) mutations in gliomas is a powerful example of understanding of the relationship between tumor genetics and human diseases. IDHs, catalyze the oxidative decarboxylation of isocitrate to α-ketoglutarate with production of NADH/NADPH, is the key enzymes in the Krebs cycle. IDH mutations, which occur early in gliomagenesis, change the function of the enzymes, causing them to produce 2–hydroxyglutarate, and to not create NADPH. Gliomas with mutated IDH have improved prediction of patient outcomes compared to its with wild-type IDH. Thus, the WHO Classification of Tumors of the Central Nervous System was revised in 2016 to incorporate molecular biomarkers (including the IDH mutations) – together with classic histological features – in an integrated diagnosis, in order to define distinct glioma entities as precisely as possible. The aim of this chapter is to review the findings on the epidemiology and significance of IDH mutations in human gliomas, from discovery to the current knowledge about their molecular pathogenesis.


**Keywords:** *IDH* mutation, gliomas, Isocitrate dehydrogenase, significance, therapies

## 1. Introduction

Isocitrate dehydrogenase (IDH) is a key enzyme in the Krebs cycle and plays an important role in energy metabolism. This enzyme is involved in a number of cellular processes, such as mitochondrial oxidative phosphorylation, regulation of cellular redox status, glutamine metabolism as well as lipogenesis or glucose sensing.

In 2008, Parsons et al. discovered a link between *IDH* mutations and gliomas. After that, further studies showed that *IDH* mutations are not only common but also closely related to the diagnosis, treatment and prognosis of gliomas. Therefore, the WHO classification of Tumors of the Central Nervous System of 2016, gliomas are subdivided based on combined classical histological with molecular markers (including the *IDH* mutations). This reclassification is expected to guide treatment decisions and improve outcome prediction.

The aim of this chapter is to review the findings on the epidemiology and significance of *IDH* mutations, from current knowledge about molecular pathogenesis to the value these mutations in gliomas.



IntechOpen

## 2. IDH enzymes

### 2.1 Normal enzymes

#### *2.1.1 Genetics and classification enzymes*

IDH is a small molecule protein which is mainly distributed in the liver, heart muscle and skeletal muscle. In humans, there are three isozymes of IDH, which differ in subcellular localization, structural organization, allosteric regulation, catalytic mechanism and cofactor requirement. These are IDH1, IDH2 and IDH3.

These isozymes are encoded by five separate genes. IDH1, encoded by *IDH1* gene on 2q33.3, is configured as a homodimer with two enzymatically active sites and most of its activity is detected in the cytosol and in peroxysomes, Main function of IDH1 is believed to be the synthesis of NADPH, required for reducing reactions and for lipid synthesis [1–3].

IDH2, which is found in mitochondrial, encoded by the *IDH2* gene on 15q26.1, in [4]. Similar to IDH1, this enzyme is structured as a homodimer. Recent findings show that the IDH2 may be the main catalyst for the oxidation of isocitrate (ICT) to α-ketoglutarate (α-KG) in the citric acid cycle (TCA) in [5]. IDH3 is composed of three subunits encoded by *IDH3A* (subunit alpha), on 15q25.1-q25.2, *IDH3B* (subunit beta) on 20p13 and *IDH3G* (subunit gamma), on Xq28 [6–8].

IDH3 is a multi-tetrameric enzyme (2α1β1γ) with α – subunits being catalytic and the β- and γ- subunits being believed to be regulatory [9, 10]. Since *IDH3* mutations do not occur with a significant frequency in glioma [11] this chapter focuses on the roles of IDH1 and IDH2 in glioma biology and uses IDH to refer to both IDH1 and IDH2 but not IDH3 (**Figure 1**).

#### *2.1.2 Mechanism and function of IDH enzymes*

IDH exists in NADP-dependent forms [2]. Both IDH1 and IDH2 exist as homodimers, share considerable sequence similarity (70% identity humans). IDH1 is highly expressed in the mammalian liver (IDH1 provides NADPH for peroxisomal fat and cholesterol synthesis) with only moderate to absent expression in other tissues, whereas IDH2 is highly expressed in heart, muscle, and activated lymphocytes [13].

The main function of IDH is to catalyze the oxidative decarboxylation of ICT to α-KG. This reaction also produces a molecule called NADPH, which is necessary for

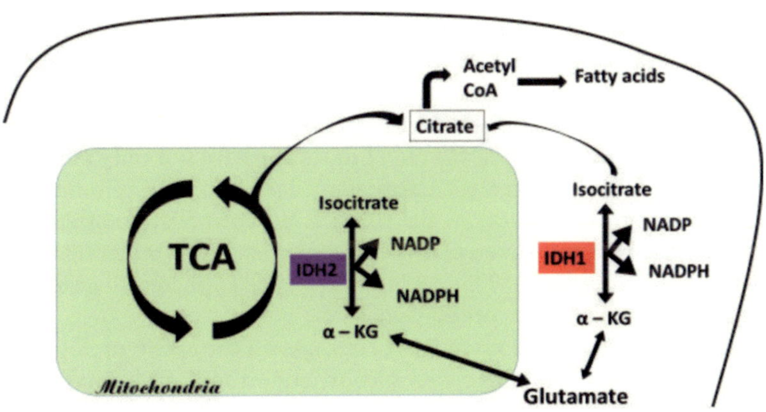


**Figure 1.**
*IDH1 is localized in the cytoplasm and peroxisomes, whereas IDH2 is founded within the mitochondrial matrix [12].*

multiple cellular processes. The NADPH is involved in the breakdown of lipids for energy, and also protects cells from potentially harmful molecules called reactive oxygen species.

By providing mitochondrial NADPH for NADPH-dependent antioxidant enzymes, IDH maintains a pool of reduced glutathione and peroxiredoxin [14]. These molecules protect mitochondria from ROS-mediated oxidative damage, ensuing lipid peroxidation and DNA damage, and from stress induced by heat shock, cadmium, excess fructose, or tumor necrosis factor-α (TNF-α) [13, 14]. These data suggest that IDH is important for cell stress responses, mitochondrial bioenergetics, and macromolecular synthesis to support cell survival and growth.

### 2.2 Molecular pathogenesis of IDH mutations

*IDH1* mutations almost occur at Arginine 132 resulting in amino acid exchange, including R132H (most common, 88%), R132C, R132L, R132S, and R132G. *IDH2* mutations typically occur at R140 or R172. Of *IDH2* mutations, R172K is most common. *IDH1* and *IDH2* mutations are mutually exclusive [15].

#### *2.2.1 Enzymatic properties of mutant IDHs*

Mutations in *IDH* are neomorphic gain-of-function mutations, which affect cofactor binding affinity and conformation of the enzymes' active center. When mutated, the enzymes' binding affinity to ICT decreases, while affinity to NADPH increases. Mutations result in a dominant gain-of-function that catalyzes the NADPH-dependent reduction of α -KG to D-2-hydroxyglutarate (D-2HG or R-2HG) but not further carboxylated [16]. D-2HG is a competitive inhibitor of multiple α -KG-dependent dioxygenases, including histone demethylase. As a result, D-2HG makes histone methylation and blocks cell differentiation. Therefore, D-2HG is called oncometabolite.

All *IDH* mutant enzymes produce D-2HG; their allelic frequency, enzymatic property, and association with overall prognosis, however, are markedly different. For example, while the IDH2Arg140 mutation is exclusively found in myeloid malignancies [17], the IDH1Arg132 and IDH2Arg172 mutations are common in gliomas.

In addition, due to essential roles of IDHs in producing cytoplasmic and mitochondrial NADPH, tumor cell survival may also be dependent on basal IDH activities to maintain cytoplasmic and mitochondrial redox homeostasis.

#### *2.2.2 Mutant IDH enzymes control cellular growth*

A large body of evidence indicates that IDH mutation inhibits cell proliferation [18–20]. Theoretically, D-2HG inhibits ATP synthase, resulting in decreased mTOR (mammalian target of rapamycin) signaling and cell growth. Moreover, by inhibiting the FTO (fat mass and obesity-associated) demethylase activity, D-2HG promotes cell-cycle arrest, thereby increasing N6-methyladenosine modification of MYC/CEBPA (CCAAT/enhancer binding protein alpha) transcripts for destabilization and, thus, decreasing proliferative signaling [20].

There is a study in mice indicating that IDH1R132H homozygous expression in neural progenitor cells (NPCs) results in extensive cerebral hemorrhage and perinatal lethality [21]. On molecular levels, high-level accumulation of D-2HG inhibits prolyl-hydroxylation and subsequent maturation of collagen. Immature collagens accumulate, resulting in an aberrantly formed basement membrane and the initiation of an endoplasmic reticulum (ER) stress response. As a result, mice developed hydrocephalus and grossly dilated lateral ventricles.

Collectively, these studies provide strong evidence that IDH mutation targets various signaling pathways to inhibit glial cell proliferation.

### 2.3 IDH mutation involvement human cancers

Mutations in *IDH1* and *IDH2* have recently been discovered in CNS cancers like gliomas, and a number of types of leukemia, including acute myeloid leukemia. This discovery has been extended to prostate cancer, intrahepatic cholangiocarcinoma, colon cancer, and thyroid cancer as well since 2009.

Mutations targeting IDH in different types of tumors share four distinct biochemical features. First of all, *IDH* mutations are almost somatic and rarely germline. In addition, predominantly all reported cases have been frameshifts or deletions, whereas nonsense mutations have not been observed in cancer.

Second, the vast majority of *IDH* mutations (Mut) are heterozygous with a wild-type (Wt) allele [22, 23]. The existence of wild type-mutant (Wt-Mut) and mutant-mutant (Mut-Mut) dimers in addition to wild type-wild type (Wt-Wt) dimer in a cell heterozygous for *IDH* mutation has been reported [24]. An illustration of the three dimer types allele is provided in **Figure 2**.

From what has been mentioned so far, the most likely model is as follows: substitution of two arginine residues on both monomers inactivates both forward oxidative decarboxylation and reverse reductive carboxylation reactions while the presence of one arginine fully inhibits the forward oxidative decarboxylation reaction but changes the product of the reverse reductive carboxylation reaction to be D-2HG instead of ICT.

It is conceivable that the Mut-Mut dimer is totally, while the Wt-Mut dimer increases the production of D-2HG from 2KG through the reverse reaction and does not interconvert ICT and 2KG. Since D-2HG is thought to inactivate 2KG utilizing enzymes, it is possible that it also inhibits the Wt-Wt dimer form and that might explain the dominant negative effect of heterozygous arginine substitution (**Figure 3**) [24, 25].

Third, nearly all *IDH* mutations cause a single amino acid replacement, Arg132 in *IDH1* (into one of six amino acid residues -His, Cys, Leu, Ile, Ser, Gly

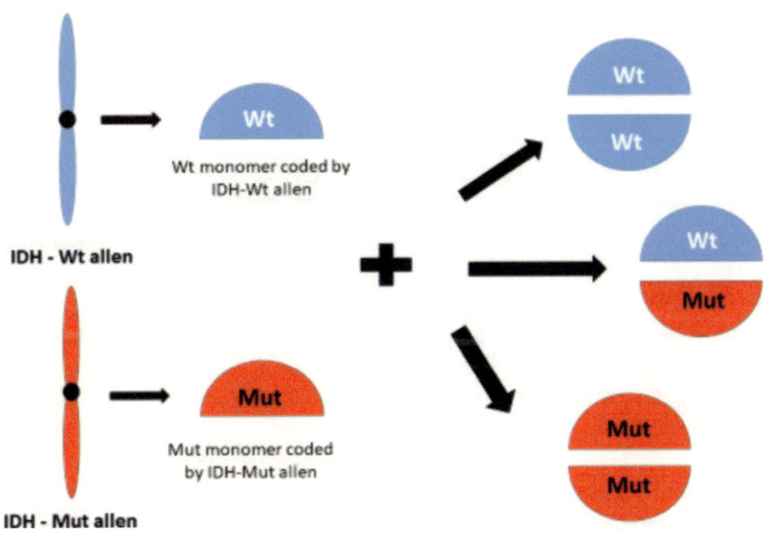


**Figure 2.**
*The three dimer types formed in a cancer cell heterozygous for IDH mutation.*

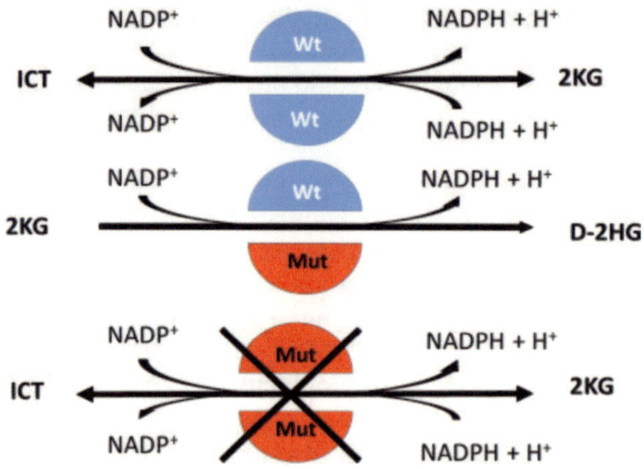


**Figure 3.**
*The model gains of function and dominant negative effect exerted by heterozygous IDH mutation. (D)-2HG (d) 2-hydroxyglutarate, ICT: isocitrate, Mut: mutant, Wt: wildtype.*

and Val), as well as Arg172 in *IDH2* (into one of four other residues -Lys, Met, Gly and Trp), and Arg140 in *IDH2* to either Gln or Trp. Rarely *IDH1* mutations also are reported, including R100A in adult glioma, G97D in colon cancer cells and a pediatric glioblastoma. The synthesis of cancer-associated *IDH* mutations in the functional region of the enzyme suggested that these mutations might give the mutant protein with a new and possibly oncogenic enzymatic activity.

Lastly, the mutual exclusivity seen in mutant *IDH1* and *IDH2* alleles in most cases. Obviously, in a cancerous cell transformed by one of these mutant alleles, the forward oxidative decarboxylation reaction catalyzed by the remaining wild-type isoform would still be important for that cell to be able to produce NADPH. In other words, cancerous cells that have mutant IDH2, would still need the wild type IDH1 isoform to catalyze the forward oxidative decarboxylation reaction to produce NADPH. Only rarely, individual tumors have been found to sustain mutations in both the *IDH1* and *IDH2* genes [26].

*IDH* mutations also exhibit three distinct clinical features. First, they exist in a highly restricted tumor spectrum. For example, they occur frequently in low-grade gliomas and secondary glioblastomas (GBM), but rarely in primary GBM. Likewise, they are often found in genetically normal AML. Second, the *IDH* mutations occur at an early stage in tumor formation, and occur the earliest known mutation in glioma. Finally, in glioma, AML and intrahepatic cholangiocarcinoma, *IDH* mutations alone or in combination with other genetic mutations (in the case of AML) are associated with better prognosis.

### 2.4 *IDH* mutations in human gliomas

Glioma stem cells are small numbers of tumor cells that act as stem cells in glial cells. According to the "seed and soil" theory put forward by Paget, if the tumor microenvironment is soil, then glioma stem cells are seeds.

The IDH mutations enhance function in glial tumor cells, leading to the accumulation and secretion of large amounts of the oncometabolite, D-2HG, which ultimately inhibits the catalytic activity of α-KG-dependent dioxygenase, damaging the key steps in angiogenesis, hypoxic stress, and mature differentiation of cells. These processes are closely related to the occurrence and development of tumors. However, researches showed that D-2HG is a weak competitive inhibitor

of α-KG. Thus, it can only be observed to inhibit the differentiation of glioma stem cells when the accumulation of D-2HG is high. Therefore, the formation of gliomas requires not only seeds (glioma stem cells) but also soil (tumor microenvironment).

It was found that the *IDH* mutations could promote tumorigenesis microenvironment by increasing the expression of VEGF and making it suitable for glioma stem cell growth.

Interestingly, VEGF is initiated transcription by HIF-1α, and hypoxia can cause an increase in VEGF. IDH mutants can modulate VEGF to promote tumor microchip formation by inhibiting HIF-1α degradation. Moreover, quick growth of tumors will rapidly consume the surrounding energy and nutrients. Thus, HIF-1α is a stably expressed surrounding tumor. *IDH* mutations make tumor microenvironments easier to form.

With the appropriate soil, glioma tumor stem cells grow rapidly and continue to invade the surrounding tissues, ultimately accelerating the growth of gliomas.

*IDH* mutations occur in about 80% of all grade II/III gliomas (low-grade gliomas - LGG) and secondary glioblastomas, which progress from the less malignant grade 2 diffuse astrocytomas or grade 3 anaplastic astrocytomas. In contrast, IDH mutations accounted for less than 5% of primary glioblastomas, which arise de novo [27, 28] and approximately 10% of pediatric glioblastomas [26, 29]. This suggests that LGG and secondary GBM are minimally overlapping disease subtypes.

In contrast to diffuse gliomas, *IDH* mutations are rare in many of WHO grade I gliomas, for example gangliogliomas, subependymal giant cell tumors, pilocytic astrocytomas, ependymomas and pleomorphic xanthoastrocytoma.

Aggregate data from multiple preclinical and clinical studies have shown that *IDH* mutations alone are not enough to turn malignant. *IDH* mutations occur early in gliomas formation and often have secondary genetic abnormalities such as mutations in *TP53*, chromosomal region 1p/19q co-deletion or loss of nuclear ATRX reactivity.

These changes relate to the histological classification of the disease. For example, diffuse astrocytomas, mutant *IDH*, often contain *TP53* mutations and lose ATRX. In contrast, almost histologically confirmed IDH mutant oligodendrogliomas have 1p/19q co-delection. In particular, the majority of glioma patients with IDH mutation and 1p/19q co-deletion also had a mutation in the promoter regions of

| **Type of IDH** | **IDH1/2** | **IDH1/2** | **IDH1** | **IDH1/2** | **IDH1** |
|---|---|---|---|---|---|
| **Author** | **Yan et al [29]** | **Hartmann et al [26]** | **Ichimura et al [33]** | **Park et al [34]** | **Watanabe et al [35]** |
| Pilocytic astrocytoma | 0% | | 0% | 0% | 10% |
| Diffuse astrocytoma | 90% | 74% | 59% | >80% | 88% |
| Anaplastic astrocytoma | 73% | 65% | 52% | | 78% |
| Secondary glioblastoma | 85% | | 50% | >95% | 82% |
| Primary glioblastoma | 5% | | 3% | | 5% |
| Oligodendroglioma | 84% | 87% | 68% | 100% | 79% |
| Anaplastic oligodendroglioma | 94% | 75% | 60% | | 75% |
| Oligoastrocytoma | 100% | 83% | 50% | | 94% |
| Anaplastic oligoastrocytoma | 100% | 72% | 78% | | 71% |

**Table 1.**
*Frequency of IDH mutations in different types of gliomas.*

| | **Author** | **Yan et al [29]** | **Hartmann et al [26]** | **Sanson et al [36]** | **Pusch et al [37]** |
|---|---|---|---|---|---|
| **Gene** | **Amino acid change** | | | | |
| *IDH1* | R132H | 83.5% | 89.4% | 89% | 91.5% |
| | R132C | 4.1% | 3.9% | 3.2% | 4.3% |
| | R132S | 2.4% | 1.5% | 1.9% | 1.6% |
| | R132G | 0.6% | 1.3% | 4.5% | 1.9% |
| | R132L | 4.1% | 0.3% | 1.3% | 0.6% |
| *IDH2* | R172K | 2.4% | 2.7% | | |
| | R172M | 1.8% | 0.8% | | |
| | R172W | | 0.7% | | |
| | R172G | 1.2% | | | |

**Table 2.**
*Frequency of specific IDH mutations in gliomas.*

the telomerase reverse transcriptase (*TERT*). These mutations are thought to be mutually exclusive [30–32], thus aiding in distinguishing diffuse astrocytomas from oligodendrogliomas (**Tables 1** and **2**) [38].

## 3. Clinical indications involving the discovery of IDH-mutated glioma

### 3.1 Diagnosis

The latest WHO classification of CNS tumors using the integrated phenotypic and molecular parameters (including the *IDH* mutation) have re-established the CNS tumors classification. This classification includes glioblastoma, *IDH*-wildtype, *IDH*-mutant or NOS; diffuse astrocytoma, *IDH*-wildtype, *IDH*-mutant or NOS; anaplastic astrocytoma, *IDH*-wildtype, *IDH*-mutant or NOS; oligodendroglioma, *IDH*-mutant and 1p/19q-codeleted or NOS; oligodendroglioma, *IDH*-mutant and 1p/19q-codeleted or NOS; anaplastic oligodendroglioma, *IDH*-mutant and 1p/19q-codeleted or NOS.

There are wo features make *IDH* mutations easily detectable, reliable as biomarkers. First, nearly all tumors carry *IDH* mutations located at specific residues, such as Arg132 in *IDH1* or Arg140 and Arg172 in *IDH2*, which are located in a single exon 4 and can be simply identified through PCR-based amplification and sequencing. Second, antibodies specifically recognizing mutant IDH1R132H protein have been developed, thus it may be identified through conventional immunohistochemistry (IHC). Based on these hypotheses, to determine *IDH* mutations, currently, different methods are available to diagnose this status. They analyze either the nucleotide sequence of the gene (as the direct method) or the altered structure of the protein (as the indirect method).

Practical guidelines are available for detection of *IDH* mutations with molecular genetics techniques. In this regard, crucial aspects are the availability of tumor tissue, the tumor cell content and the quality of the respective genomic DNA (gDNA). Among them, conventional Sanger sequencing is a relatively inexpensive method and therefore is widely used in laboratories. As a consequence, it becomes the "gold standard" for the detection of *IDH* mutations. Beside, alternative methods to assess

the *IDH* mutation status exist. They include derived cleaved amplified polymorphic sequence (dCAPS), PCR-based restriction length polymorphism assays, cold PCR high resolution melting (HRM), post-PCR fluorescence melting curve analysis (FMCA) and SNaPshot assays. These are new methods and unapproved for clinical use in determining IDH status.

As the indirect method to confirm *IDH* status, immunohistochemistry of the *IDH1* mutant proteins is used. IHC using IDH1 R132H mutation-specific antibody detects *IDH1* mutation. However, this method can miss about 10% of gliomas carrying an *IDH1* mutation and all gliomas with an *IDH2* mutation [39]. It is conceivable that, when the IHC is negative for IDH1 R132H, the tumor can carry the IDH1 mutation in another location or the IDH2 mutation. In this case, subsequent genetic analysis is recommended.

All of the above methods have in common the need for tissue samples. Thus, surgery or biopsy of the tumor is necessary. This is a diagnostic difficulty. Therefore, recently, studies on non-invasive methods are being carried out, in which diagnosis by magnetic resonance spectroscopy (MRS) and amide proton transfer-weighted (APTw) have been shown to be promising [40–42]. In IDH mutant gliomas, D-2HG accumulates to sufficient levels as a brain metabolite, which renders its visibility on MRS. Therefore, this may provide crucial longitudinal data for the determination of disease progression and therapy response.

Identification of *IDH* status allows differential diagnosis between gliomas and non-neoplastic CNS lesions (astrocytoma or therapy-induced changes), between gliomas and non-glial CNS tumors, and within glioma subtypes. As discussed above, *IDH* status may be used to differentiate primary from secondary glioblastomas. In addition, IDH status associated with 1p/19q co-deletion became the key in the diagnosis of oligodendroglioma.

### 3.2 Prognostic

Generally, *IDH* mutations are associated with a better outcome than other types of mutations [43–45]. In 2008, Parsons et al. reported that mutations in IDH1 occurred in most secondary GBM, and were related with better overall survival (OS) [46]. Similar trends were reported in variety studies using different datasets [29]. For example, in a prospective translational cohort study of the German Glioma Network, patients with anaplastic astrocytoma carry *IDH1* wild-type exhibited a worse overall survival rate than patients with glioblastomas with *IDH1* mutation [47] *IDH*-mutated astrocytomas harboring ATRX mutation also were shown to form a subgroup of astrocytomas with a favorable prognosis [48].

Furthermore, in the SongTao study, *IDH* mutations were associated with prolonged PFS together with MGMT promoter methylation and 1p/19q codeletion and a higher rate of objective response to temozolomide in secondary glioblastomas [43]. Even in primary glioblastomas, *IDH1*/2 mutations define a subgroup of tumors of long-term survival patients [49].

In 2009, using a large clinical dataset, Yan et al. reported that GBM patients with *IDH* mutations tended to prolonged median OS compared with patients carrying *IDH* wild-type GBM. Similar findings were also observed in patients with anaplastic astrocytoma.

The median OS was 65 months for gliomas patients with *IDH* mutant, compared with 20 months for those with IDH wild-type. Furthermore, the progression-free survival (PFS) was also improved among GBM patients with IDH mutations compared with other patients [29].

Extensive meta-analysis (2,190 cases) confirmed *IDH* mutation as a prognostic biomarker of gliomas [44]. Many other studies have shown that *IDH* mutations are an independent prognostic marker for improved PFS and OS in patients with grade III gliomas [47, 50–52].

Several studies have explained that the favorable prognosis of IDH mutant gliomas is due to their increased sensitivity to chemotherapy and radiotherapy [47, 53]. IDH mutant gliomas likely harbour defects in multiple DNA repair pathways, which render them vulnerable to radiotherapy- or chemotherapy-induced DNA damage [54, 55]. These findings indicate that IDH mutation could serve as an important predictive factor for treatment response among glioma patients.

#### *3.2.1 Novel therapies*

Glioma is the most frequent brain tumor and has a notably high mortality and disability rate. For its complex pathogenesis, the surgical and drug-assisted treatments do not seem to be effective. Therefore, it is of great significance to find new targets for diagnosis and treatment. The detection of IDH mutations in gliomas offers bases to research new therapies.

Some studies indicated that IDH-mutated gliomas maintain the IDH-mutated allele even after acquiring oncogenic driver mutations [56, 57]. This may show that IDH-mutated gliomas may remain vulnerable to the targeted therapies developed specifically for IDH mutations even at progression or after malignant transformation to higher grade glioma. The therapeutic effects may be further enhanced by combining different targeted therapies or with traditional chemotherapeutics or radiation.

#### *3.2.2 IDH-mutated inhibitors*

Since the neomorphic activity of IDH mutants is correlated with malignant transformation, direct targeting of the mutant enzymes becomes a heavily pursued strategy.

Over the past decade, several attempts have been made to find and develop small molecular compounds that directly inhibit the IDH-mutated enzymes. Some synthetic inhibitors reported as AGI-5198, ivosidenib (AG-120) and vorasidenib (AG-881), demonstrated effective and safe in treating IDH-mutated myeloid malignancies and solid tumors, including glioma [58–60]. BAY1436032, another IDH-mutant inhibitor, had shown tumor-suppressing effects as experimental therapeutics for the treatment of AML and astrocytoma in animal models [61, 62]. Recently, ivosidenib and vorasidenib have been approved by the Food and Drug Administration as a therapeutic option for IDH-mutated AML.

Despite the promising success of the IDH-mutated inhibitors, a number of studies have indicated the potential limitations of their application. As discussed above, IDH-mutated enzymes enhance sensitivity to chemotherapy and radiotherapy. So that, using these inhibitors reduces D-2HG production and relieves the burden on the multiple DNA repair pathways, resulting in chemoresistance. For example, AGI-5198 might increase their resistance to genotoxic therapies, such as radiation and chemo agents [63, 64].

Overall, targeting IDH-mutated activity is a straightforward strategy and has shown efficacy gliomas in humans. However, whether inhibition of mutant IDH and subsequent reduction in D-2HG production are sufficient to halt tumor growth in gliomas and other solid tumors remains unclear. In addition, whether these drugs will cross the blood brain barrier for admission to IDH mutant glioma cells is a question that requires further studies.

### *3.2.3 Targeting redox homoeostasis*

Redox homeostasis has been reported to be greatly affected by IDH mutations, notably elevated levels of oxidative stress. Targeting redox homeostasis may be effective in gliomas with IDH mutations. In fact, in IDH-mutated gliomas, the synthesis of NAD is largely compromised. As a result, tumor cells rely on a path of salvation to create NAD. Consequently, the IDH-mutated gliomas cells can be extremely sensitive to the blockade of the salvage pathway.

In addition, one study demonstrated that levels of glutamate, glutamine and glutathione decreased in tumor regions in patients with IDH-mutated glioma, compared with levels in contralateral regions. Furthermore, the glutathione level negatively correlates with the level of D-2HG, suggesting that glutathione is required for IDH-mutated cells to maintain redox homoeostasis [65]. An animal preclinical study has shown that inhibiting glutamine metabolism using the glutaminase inhibitor CB-839 leads to impaired redox homoeostasis and makes IDH-mutated glioma sensitivity to radiotherapy [66].

Since the disruption of redox homoeostasis results in potent cytotoxicity accompanied by tumor suppression, current therapeutic compounds are mostly at the preclinical stage and show considerable systemic toxicity. Nevertheless, developing the next generation of therapeutic compounds with both potency and selectivity will be of great help for targeting redox imbalance in IDH-mutated malignancies.

### *3.2.4 Immunotherapies*

With evidence that IDH mutation is an early event in tumorigenesis and is present homogenously in all glioma tumor cells at specific codons. These mutations are ideal immunotherapy targets.

In fact, there are increasing evidences that the IDH mutation might play critical roles in altering the immunological microenvironment of the tumor, as shown by an inhibition of tumor-infiltrating lymphocytes, cytotoxic T cells and natural killer cells [67, 68]. Additionally, the presence of IDH mutation correlates with a decrease in the expression of PD-L1 (Programmed Death-Ligand 1). Decreased expression of PD-L1 in IDH-mutated gliomas implies a stronger T cell activation, because PD-L1 is a cellular surface protein that modulates the immune system and promotes self-tolerance through inhibition T cell activity [69].

The combination with the IDH-mutated inhibitors shows an improvement in the efficacy of PD-1-resistant derived immunotherapy, which induces intracellular CD4 + T-cell proliferation. The result is a reduction in tumor size and a prolonged survival. Further studies are currently under investigation, promising to bring positive results.

### *3.2.5 Vaccines*

Vaccination is the most effective measure of disease prevention and control. In many low-grade glioma patients, the spontaneous immune response to IDH1 mutation has been found [70]. The use of the self-immune response to tumor treatment has also been a heavily researched subject in recent years and provides evidences that is worth the wait. For example, in animal experiments, it was found that the vaccine not only was able to prevent from IDH1 mutant cells growing in the brain, but also did not destroy the normal physiological function of the IDH1 enzyme [70].

Specifically, a phase 1 clinical trial is ongoing to confirm the safety and therapeutic efficacy of the IDH1 R132H mutant peptide vaccine (NOA-16)

in newly diagnosed grade III and IV gliomas with IDH1 mutation. The first reported results demonstrated the safety and immunogenicity of NOA-16, with 80% of patients having mutation-specific T cell immune responses, and 87% of the patients displaying humoral immune responses; no deaths have been reported [71].

It is difficult to completely remove gliomas by surgery and drugs, so they often recur. Moreover, the recurrent gliomas after clearance generally tend to be more resistant and invasive. Vaccines can play a maintenance role in these cases. So finding a suitable vaccine will greatly benefit patients and help them escape the magic spell of glioma recurrence.

### *3.2.6 Other therapies*

In addition to the treatments outlined above, there are other methods base on vulnerability of IDH-mutant cells to NAD+ depletion, hypoxia-inducible factor-1? (HIF-1?) pathway of IDH mutation or mammalian target of rapamycin (mTOR) signaling pathway. These are all new methods, are preclinical models and promise to bring about a change in treatment for gliomas with IDH mutations.

It is generally known that trials of IDH mutant inhibitors, vaccines, immunotherapies and so on in IDH mutant gliomas and recurrent gliomas have been conducted. Meanwhile, old drugs for other tumors have also been developed to treat gliomas with IDH mutations, such as azacitidine, nivolumab, and temozolomide.

In summary, targeting the distinctive vulnerabilities of IDH-mutated glioma has been shown to be successful, as cancer cells are less likely to compensate for the loss of essential biological pathways. However, development of further studies is needed for more convincing evidence to apply these novel therapies to treatment.

## 4. Conclusion

The discovery of the IDH mutation not only adds to the landscape of glioma genetics but also supports diagnosis and prognosis. For IDH-mutated gliomas, numerous attempts have been made to define selective and effective therapeutics that target the biological signatures, with the aim of improving standard treatments.

From the above mentioned biological bases, IDH mutation is an important target for the prevention and treatment of gliomas. However, due to the short and uncertain clinical trial duration, most clinical trials of vaccines, IDH inhibitors or other methods are still underway. Much research still needs to be completed. However, we believe that the great potential of these new treatments offers hope in patients with gliomas.

Finally, a major obstacle in IDH-mutated glioma is that the critical oncogenic drivers of this disease remain controversial. One of the main questions remains the molecular pathogenesis of WHO grade II and III gliomas without IDH mutations, which often do not show changes in genes typically associated with gliomas. In-depth investigation of critical molecular pathways will be of great importance to develop highly potent and selectivity treatment.

## Author details

Nu Thien Nhat Tran
Thu Duc City Hospital, Ho Chi Minh City, Viet Nam

*Address all correspondence to: nhat24.10@gmail.com

## References

[1] Narahara K, Kimura S, Kikkawa K, et al. Probable assignment of soluble isocitrate dehydrogenase (IDH 1) to 2q33. 3. Human genetics. 1985;71:37-40. DOI: 10.1007/BF00295665.

[2] Geisbrecht BV, Gould SJ. The human PICD gene encodes a cytoplasmic and peroxisomal NADP+-dependent isocitrate dehydrogenase. Journal of Biological Chemistry. 1999;274:30527-33. DOI: 10.1074/jbc.274.43.30527.

[3] Shechter I, Dai P, Huo L, et al. IDH1 gene transcription is sterol regulated and activated by SREBP-1a and SREBP-2 in human hepatoma HepG2 cells: evidence that IDH1 may regulate lipogenesis in hepatic cells. Journal of lipid research. 2003;44:2169-80. DOI: 10.1194/jlr.M300285-JLR200.

[4] Grzeschik K-H. Assignment of a gene for human mitochondrial isocitrate dehydrogenase (ICD-M, EC 1. 1. 1. 41) to chromosome 15. Human genetics. 1976;34:23-8. DOI: 10.1007/BF00284430.

[5] Hartong DT, Dange M, McGee TL, et al. Insights from retinitis pigmentosa into the roles of isocitrate dehydrogenases in the Krebs cycle. Nature genetics. 2008;40:1230-4. DOI: 10.1038/ng.223.

[6] Kim Y, Park S, Kang Y, et al. Assignment of mitochondrial NAD+-specific isocitrate dehydrogenase (Beta subunit) gene (IDH3B) to human chromosome band 20p13 by in situ hybridization and radiation hybrid mapping. Cytogenetic and Genome Research. 1999;86:240. DOI: 10.1159/000015348.

[7] Brenner V, Nyakatura G, Rosenthal A, et al. Genomic Organization of Two Novel Genes on Human Xq28: Compact Head to Head Arrangement ofIDH? andTRAP? Is Conserved in Rat and Mouse. Genomics. 1997;44:8-14. DOI: 10.1006/geno.1997.4822.

[8] Huh TL KY, Oh IU, et al. Assignment of the human mitochondrial NAD+ -specific isocitrate dehydrogenase alpha subunit (IDH3A) gene to 15q25.1-->q25.2by in situ hybridization. Genomics. 1996;32:6. DOI.

[9] Ramachandran N, Colman RF. Chemical characterization of distinct subunits of pig heart DPN-specific isocitrate dehydrogenase. Journal of Biological Chemistry. 1980;255: 8859-64. DOI.

[10] Weiss C, Zeng Y, Huang J, et al. Bovine NAD+-dependent isocitrate dehydrogenase: alternative splicing and tissue-dependent expression of subunit 1. Biochemistry. 2000;39:1807-16. DOI: 10.1021/bi991691i.

[11] Krell D, Assoku M, Galloway M, et al. Screen for IDH1, IDH2, IDH3, D2HGDH and L2HGDH mutations in glioblastoma. PloS one. 2011;6:e19868. DOI: 10.1371/journal.pone.0019868.

[12] Cairns RA, Mak TW. Oncogenic isocitrate dehydrogenase mutations: mechanisms, models, and clinical opportunities. Cancer discovery. 2013;3:730-41. DOI: 10.1158/2159-8290.CD-13-0083.

[13] Smolková K, Ježek P. The role of mitochondrial NADPH-dependent isocitrate dehydrogenase in cancer cells. International journal of cell biology. 2012;2012. DOI: 10.1155/2012/273947.

[14] Jo S-H, Son M-K, Koh H-J, et al. Control of mitochondrial redox balance and cellular defense against oxidative damage by mitochondrial NADP+-dependent isocitrate dehydrogenase. Journal of Biological Chemistry. 2001; 276:16168-76. DOI: 10.1074/jbc.M010120200.

[15] Han CH, Batchelor TT. Isocitrate dehydrogenase mutation as a therapeutic

target in gliomas. Chin Clin Oncol. 2017;6:33. DOI: 10.21037/cco.2017.06.11.

[16] Dang L, White DW, Gross S, et al. Cancer-associated IDH1 mutations produce 2-hydroxyglutarate. Nature. 2009;462:739-44. DOI: 10.1038/nature 08617.

[17] DiNardo CD, Ravandi F, Agresta S, et al. Characteristics, clinical outcome, and prognostic significance of IDH mutations in AML. American journal of hematology. 2015;90:732-6. DOI: 10.1002/ajh.24072.

[18] Bralten LB, Kloosterhof NK, Balvers R, et al. IDH1 R132H decreases proliferation of glioma cell lines in vitro and in vivo. Annals of neurology. 2011;69:455-63. DOI: 10.1002/ana.22390.

[19] Chittaranjan S, Chan S, Yang C, et al. Mutations in CIC and IDH1 cooperatively regulate 2-hydroxyglutarate levels and cell clonogenicity. Oncotarget. 2014;5:7960. DOI: 10.18632/oncotarget.2401.

[20] Su R, Dong L, Li C, et al. R-2HG exhibits anti-tumor activity by targeting FTO/m6A/MYC/CEBPA signaling. Cell. 2018;172:90-105. e23. DOI: 10.1016/j.cell.2017.11.031.

[21] Sasaki M, Knobbe CB, Itsumi M, et al. D-2-hydroxyglutarate produced by mutant IDH1 perturbs collagen maturation and basement membrane function. Genes & development. 2012; 26:2038-49. DOI: 10.1101/gad. 198200.112.

[22] Dang L, Jin S, Su SM. IDH mutations in glioma and acute myeloid leukemia. Trends in molecular medicine. 2010;16:387-97. DOI: 10.1016/j.molmed.2010.07.002.

[23] Bleeker FE, Lamba S, Leenstra S, et al. IDH1 mutations at residue p. R132 (IDH1R132) occur frequently in high? grade gliomas but not in other solid tumors. Human mutation. 2009;30:7-11. DOI: 10.1002/humu.20937.

[24] Zhao S, Lin Y, Xu W, et al. Glioma-derived mutations in IDH1 dominantly inhibit IDH1 catalytic activity and induce HIF-1?. Science. 2009;324:261-5. DOI: 10.1126/science.1170944.

[25] Al-Khallaf H. Isocitrate dehydrogenases in physiology and cancer: biochemical and molecular insight. Cell & bioscience. 2017;7:1-18. DOI: 10.1186/s13578-017-0165-3.

[26] Hartmann C, Meyer J, Balss J, et al. Type and frequency of IDH1 and IDH2 mutations are related to astrocytic and oligodendroglial differentiation and age: a study of 1,010 diffuse gliomas. Acta neuropathologica. 2009;118:469-74. DOI: 10.1007/s00401-009-0561-9.

[27] Balss J, Meyer J, Mueller W, et al. Analysis of the IDH1 codon 132 mutation in brain tumors. Acta neuropathologica. 2008;116:597-602. DOI: 10.1007/s00401-008-0455-2.

[28] Bleeker FE, Atai NA, Lamba S, et al. The prognostic IDH1 R132 mutation is associated with reduced NADP+-dependent IDH activity in glioblastoma. Acta neuropathologica. 2010;119:487-94. DOI: 10.1007/s00401-010-0645-6.

[29] Yan H, Parsons DW, Jin G, et al. IDH1 and IDH2 mutations in gliomas. New England journal of medicine. 2009;360:765-73. DOI: 10.1056/NEJM oa0808710.

[30] Network CGAR. Comprehensive, integrative genomic analysis of diffuse lower-grade gliomas. New England Journal of Medicine. 2015;372:2481-98. DOI: 10.1056/NEJMoa1402121.

[31] Leeper HE, Caron AA, Decker PA, et al. IDH mutation, 1p19q codeletion and ATRX loss in WHO grade II gliomas. Oncotarget. 2015;6:30295. DOI: 10.18632/oncotarget.4497.

[32] Reuss DE, Sahm F, Schrimpf D, et al. ATRX and IDH1-R132H immunohistochemistry with subsequent copy number analysis and IDH sequencing as a basis for an "integrated" diagnostic approach for adult astrocytoma, oligodendroglioma and glioblastoma. Acta neuropathologica. 2015;129:133-46. DOI: 10.1007/s00401-014-1370-3.

[33] Ichimura K, Pearson DM, Kocialkowski S, et al. IDH1 mutations are present in the majority of common adult gliomas but rare in primary glioblastomas. Neuro-oncology. 2009;11:341-7. DOI: 10.1215/15228517-2009-025.

[34] Mukasa A, Takayanagi S, Saito K, et al. Significance of IDH mutations varies with tumor histology, grade, and genetics in Japanese glioma patients. Cancer science. 2012;103:587-92. DOI: 10.1111/j.1349-7006.2011.02175.x.

[35] Watanabe T, Nobusawa S, Kleihues P, et al. IDH1 mutations are early events in the development of astrocytomas and oligodendrogliomas. The American journal of pathology. 2009;174:1149-53. DOI: 10.2353/ajpath.2009.080958.

[36] Sanson M, Marie Y, Paris S, et al. Isocitrate dehydrogenase 1 codon 132 mutation is an important prognostic biomarker in gliomas. J Clin Oncol. 2009;27:4150-4. DOI: 10.1200/JCO.2009.21.9832.

[37] Pusch S, Schweizer L, Beck A-C, et al. D-2-Hydroxyglutarate producing neo-enzymatic activity inversely correlates with frequency of the type of isocitrate dehydrogenase 1 mutations found in glioma. Acta neuropathologica communications. 2014;2:1-10. DOI: 10.1186/2051-5960-2-19.

[38] Chen R, Ravindra VM, Cohen AL, et al. Molecular features assisting in diagnosis, surgery, and treatment decision making in low-grade gliomas. Neurosurgical focus. 2015;38:E2. DOI: 10.3171/2015.1.FOCUS14745.

[39] Liu X, Ling Z-Q. Role of isocitrate dehydrogenase 1/2 (IDH 1/2) gene mutations in human tumors. 2015. DOI: 10.14670/HH-11-643.

[40] Tietze A, Choi C, Mickey B, et al. Noninvasive assessment of isocitrate dehydrogenase mutation status in cerebral gliomas by magnetic resonance spectroscopy in a clinical setting. Journal of neurosurgery. 2017;128:391-8. DOI: 10.3171/2016.10.JNS161793.

[41] Han K, Ahn SS, Choi YS, et al. Amide proton transfer imaging might predict survival and IDH mutation status in high-grade glioma. European radiology. 2019;29:6643-52. DOI: 10.1007/s00330-019-06203-x.

[42] Jiang S, Zou T, Eberhart CG, et al. Predicting IDH mutation status in grade II gliomas using amide proton transfer? weighted (APTw) MRI. Magnetic resonance in medicine. 2017;78:1100-9. DOI: 10.1002/mrm.26820.

[43] SongTao Q, Lei Y, Si G, et al. IDH mutations predict longer survival and response to temozolomide in secondary glioblastoma. Cancer science. 2012; 103:269-73. DOI: 10.1111/j.1349-7006.2011.02134.x.

[44] Zou P, Xu H, Chen P, et al. IDH1/IDH2 mutations define the prognosis and molecular profiles of patients with gliomas: a meta-analysis. PloS one. 2013;8:e68782. DOI: 10.1371/journal.pone.0068782.

[45] Gorlia T, Delattre J-Y, Brandes AA, et al. New clinical, pathological and molecular prognostic models and calculators in patients with locally diagnosed anaplastic oligodendroglioma or oligoastrocytoma. A prognostic factor analysis of European Organisation for Research and Treatment of Cancer Brain Tumour Group Study 26951. European journal of cancer. 2013;49:3477-85. DOI: 10.1016/j.ejca.2013.06.039.

[46] Parsons DW, Jones S, Zhang X, et al. An integrated genomic analysis of human glioblastoma multiforme. science. 2008;321:1807-12. DOI: 10.1126/science.1164382.

[47] Hartmann C, Hentschel B, Wick W, et al. Patients with IDH1 wild type anaplastic astrocytomas exhibit worse prognosis than IDH1-mutated glioblastomas, and IDH1 mutation status accounts for the unfavorable prognostic effect of higher age: implications for classification of gliomas. Acta neuropathologica. 2010;120:707-18. DOI: 10.1007/s00401-010-0781-z.

[48] Wiestler B, Capper D, Holland-Letz T, et al. ATRX loss refines the classification of anaplastic gliomas and identifies a subgroup of IDH mutant astrocytic tumors with better prognosis. Acta neuropathologica. 2013;126:443-51. DOI: 10.1007/s00401-013-1156-z.

[49] Krex D, Klink B, Hartmann C, et al. Long-term survival with glioblastoma multiforme. Brain. 2007;130:2596-606. DOI: 10.1093/brain/awm204.

[50] Ichimura K. Molecular pathogenesis of IDH mutations in gliomas. Brain tumor pathology. 2012;29:131-9. DOI: 10.1007/s10014-012-0090-4.

[51] Juratli T, Kirsch M, Geiger K, et al. The prognostic value of IDH mutations and MGMT promoter status in secondary high-grade gliomas. Journal of neuro-oncology. 2012;110:325-33. DOI: 10.1007/s11060-012-0977-2.

[52] Shibahara I, Sonoda Y, Kanamori M, et al. IDH1/2 gene status defines the prognosis and molecular profiles in patients with grade III gliomas. International journal of clinical oncology. 2012;17:551-61. DOI: 10.1007/s10147-011-0323-2.

[53] Houillier C, Wang X, Kaloshi G, et al. IDH1 or IDH2 mutations predict longer survival and response to temozolomide in low-grade gliomas. Neurology. 2010;75:1560-6. DOI: 10.1212/WNL.0b013e3181f96282.

[54] Wang P, Wu J, Ma S, et al. Oncometabolite D-2-hydroxyglutarate inhibits ALKBH DNA repair enzymes and sensitizes IDH mutant cells to alkylating agents. Cell reports. 2015;13:2353-61. DOI: 10.1016/j.celrep.2015.11.029Get.

[55] Lu Y, Kwintkiewicz J, Liu Y, et al. Chemosensitivity of IDH1-mutated gliomas due to an impairment in PARP1-mediated DNA repair. Cancer research. 2017;77:1709-18. DOI.

[56] Johnson BE, Mazor T, Hong C, et al. Mutational analysis reveals the origin and therapy-driven evolution of recurrent glioma. Science. 2014;343:189-93. DOI: 10.1126/science.1239947.

[57] Wakimoto H, Tanaka S, Curry WT, et al. Targetable signaling pathway mutations are associated with malignant phenotype in IDH-mutant gliomas. Clinical cancer research. 2014;20:2898-909. DOI: 10.1158/1078-0432.CCR-13-3052.

[58] Rohle D, Popovici-Muller J, Palaskas N, et al. An inhibitor of mutant IDH1 delays growth and promotes differentiation of glioma cells. Science. 2013;340:626-30. DOI: 10.1126/science.1236062.

[59] DiNardo CD, Stein EM, de Botton S, et al. Durable remissions with ivosidenib in IDH1-mutated relapsed or refractory AML. New England Journal of Medicine. 2018;378:2386-98. DOI: 10.1056/NEJMoa1716984.

[60] Mellinghoff IK, Penas-Prado M, Peters KB, et al. Phase 1 study of AG-881, an inhibitor of mutant IDH1/IDH2, in patients with advanced IDH-mutant solid tumors, including glioma. J Clin Oncol. 2018;36:2002. DOI: 10.1200/JCO.2018.36.15_suppl.2002.

[61] Pusch S, Krausert S, Fischer V, et al. Pan-mutant IDH1 inhibitor BAY 1436032 for effective treatment of IDH1 mutant astrocytoma in vivo. Acta neuropathologica. 2017;133:629-44. DOI: 10.1007/s00401-017-1677-y.

[62] Chaturvedi A, Herbst L, Pusch S, et al. Pan-mutant-IDH1 inhibitor BAY1436032 is highly effective against human IDH1 mutant acute myeloid leukemia in vivo. Leukemia. 2017;31:2020-8. DOI: 10.1038/leu.2017.46.

[63] Sulkowski PL, Corso CD, Robinson ND, et al. 2-Hydroxyglutarate produced by neomorphic IDH mutations suppresses homologous recombination and induces PARP inhibitor sensitivity. Science translational medicine. 2017;9. DOI: 10.1126/scitranslmed.aal2463.

[64] Molenaar RJ, Botman D, Smits MA, et al. Radioprotection of IDH1-mutated cancer cells by the IDH1-mutant inhibitor AGI-5198. Cancer research. 2015;75:4790-802. DOI: 10.1158/0008-5472.CAN-14-3603.

[65] Andronesi OC, Arrillaga-Romany IC, Ly KI, et al. Pharmacodynamics of mutant-IDH1 inhibitors in glioma patients probed by in vivo 3D MRS imaging of 2-hydroxyglutarate. Nature communications. 2018;9:1-9. DOI: 10.1038/s41467-018-03905-6.

[66] McBrayer SK, Mayers JR, DiNatale GJ, et al. Transaminase inhibition by 2-hydroxyglutarate impairs glutamate biosynthesis and redox homeostasis in glioma. Cell. 2018;175:101-16. e25. DOI: 10.1016/j.cell.2018.08.038.

[67] Ren F, Zhao Q, Huang L, et al. The R132H mutation in IDH 1 promotes the recruitment of NK cells through CX 3 CL 1/CX 3 CR 1 chemotaxis and is correlated with a better prognosis in gliomas. Immunology and cell biology. 2019;97:457-69. DOI: 10.1111/imcb.12225.

[68] Bunse L, Pusch S, Bunse T, et al. Suppression of antitumor T cell immunity by the oncometabolite (R)-2-hydroxyglutarate. Nature medicine. 2018;24:1192-203. DOI: 10.1038/s41591-018-0095-6.

[69] Chen L, Han X. Anti-PD-1/PD-L1 therapy of human cancer: past, present, and future. The Journal of clinical investigation. 2015;125:3384-91. DOI: 10.1172/JCI80011.

[70] Schumacher T, Bunse L, Pusch S, et al. A vaccine targeting mutant IDH1 induces antitumour immunity. Nature. 2014;512:324-7. DOI: 10.1038/nature13387.

[71] Platten M, Schilling D, Bunse L, et al. A mutation-specific peptide vaccine targeting IDH1R132H in patients with newly diagnosed malignant astrocytomas: A first-in-man multicenter phase I clinical trial of the German Neurooncology Working Group (NOA-16). American Society of Clinical Oncology; 2018.10.1200/JCO.2018.36.15_suppl.2001

Chapter 7

# CNS High Grade Glioma

*Liam Chen*


## Abstract

Since the publication of the 2016 edition of the WHO Classification of CNS Tumors, advances in neuropathology have enhanced our understanding of the molecular underpinnings of CNS tumors, providing new elements to refine their classification and improve pathological diagnosis of these neoplasms. This chapter will review the highlights of the updated recommendations which provide guidance for how even in the absence of histopathological characteristics of the highest malignancy grade, molecular markers can be used to reach a diagnosis of glioblastoma, IDH–wild-type or astrocytoma, IDH-mutant, grade IV. These changes have important implications for the management of patients with CNS tumors in current neuro-oncology practice.


**Keywords:** astrocytoma, oligodendroglioma, glioblastoma, IDH-mutant glioma, molecular pathology

## 1. Introduction

The 2016 WHO classification divided the glial tumors into these categories: diffuse astrocytic and oligodendroglial tumors, other astrocytic tumors, ependymal tumors, and other gliomas [1]. It for the first time broke a nearly century-old tradition of classifying CNS tumors based merely on concepts of histogenesis and histological features by incorporating well-established molecular parameters into the classification of different gliomas. Further refinements of the classification were subsequently proposed by the Consortium to Inform Molecular and Practical Approaches to CNS Tumor Taxonomy — Not Officially WHO (cIMPACT- NOW) [2–8]. The chapter will review the highlights of the published cIMPACT-NOW updates and discusses their implications for the management of patients with CNS tumors in current neuro-oncology practice. We will focus on the adult high grade CNS glioma. Infant and pediatric high grade gliomas are beyond the scope of our discussion, but viewers can refer to some of a few excellent reviews [9, 10] published recently.

## 2. Grading of CNS tumors

The taxonomy and grading of neoplasms have evolved over time as clinical studies have become more sophisticated. Moreover, as the field of bioinformatics has exploded, and statistical analysis has become more powerful, pathologist, clinicians and scientists have employed these tools to better stratify nervous system tumors. In most cases, tumor classifications and grading schemes are based on

| WHO Grade | Features | Prognosis* |
|---|---|---|
| I | • Usually circumscribed<br>• Low proliferation<br>• Potential for complete resection | • Good |
| II | • Infiltrative<br>• Relatively low proliferation<br>• Increased risk of recurrence or progression to higher grade | • Fair (usually >5 years) |
| III | • Histologic evidence of malignancy<br>• Brisk mitotic activity<br>• Often require adjuvant chemo and/or radiation therapy | • Poor (usually 2-3 years) |
| IV | • Histologic malignancy, brisk mitotic activity, and necrosis<br>• Rapid pre- and post-surgical progression<br>• Prone to CSF spread | • Dismal (usually 1 year) |

**Table 1.**
*WHO grading system.*

retrospective studies of patients with a given tumor. Data from different pathologic features such as number of mitotic figures per 10 high powered fields (HPF) (400x magnification), nuclear anaplasia, presence or absence of necrosis, growth pattern, and specific histology are analyzed using complex multivariate analysis models to determine which factors represent statistically significant independent risk factors for aggressive behavior. In many cases, two or three of the most important features are used to determine different grades of a given tumor. For example, one criterion of the grading scheme of anaplastic oligodendroglioma, IDH-mutant and 1p/19q-codeleted, requires a mitotic count. Based on a series of studies, neuropathologists and physician collaborators determined that tumors with greater than 6 mitoses per 10 HPF were shown to have a worse prognosis, and were thereby designated "anaplastic" oligodendroglioma, WHO Grade 3. The current WHO grading scheme of CNS neoplasms is summarized in **Table 1**. Obviously, this is a gross oversimplification, especially considering the prognosis of tumors, given the advances in chemotherapy, radiotherapy, and diagnosis.

## 3. Astrocytoma, IDH-mutant

IDH-mutant astrocytoma is a diffusely infiltrating astrocytoma with a mutation in either *IDH1* or *IDH2* gene. This tumor most commonly affects young adults and occurs throughout the CNS, but is preferentially located in the frontal lobes. This is similar to the preferential localization of IDH-mutant and 1p/19q-codeleted oligodendroglioma and supports the hypothesis that these gliomas develop from a distinct population of precursor cells [11]. Seizures are common presenting symptom. MRI studies usually show T1-hypodensityh and T2-hyperintesnsity, with enlargement of the areas involved early in the evolution of the tumor. Gadolinium enhancement is not common in low-grade diffuse astrocytoma, but tends to appear during tumor progression as diffuse astrocytomas have an intrinsic capacity for malignant progression to IDH-mutant anaplastic astrocytoma and eventually to IDH-mutant glioblastoma.

Fibrillary astrocytoma is the classic type of diffuse astrocytoma. Another variant is the gemistocytic astrocytoma that is characterized by the presence of a conspicuous proportion of gemistocytic neoplastic astrocytes. The gemistocytes have plump, glassy, eosinophilic cell bodies and eccentric nuclei. Nevertheless, both types carry mutations in *IDH* genes. Glioma-associated IDH mutations impart a gain-of-function phenotype to the respective metabolic enzymes IDH1 and IDH2, which overproduce the oncometabolite 2-hydorxylutarate [12]. The physiological consequences of 2-hydroxyglutarate overproduction are widespread, including profound effects on cellular epigenomic states and gene regulation. Specifically, IDH mutations induce G-CIMP, by which widespread hypermethylation in gene promoter regions silences the expression of several important cellular differentiation factors. In this way, IDH mutation and C-CIMP are thought to maintain glioma cells of origin in stem cell-like physiological states inherently more prone to self-renewal and tumorigenesis. The vast majority of IDH-mutant diffuse astrocytomas also harbor loss-of-function mutations in *TP53* and *ATRX*. *ATRX* encodes an essential chromatin-binding protein, and its deficiency has been associated with epigenomic dysregulation and telomere dysfunction. In particular, *ATRX* mutations seem to induce an abnormal telomere maintenance mechanism known as alternative lengthening of telomeres. *ATRX* mutations and alternative lengthening of telomeres are mutually exclusive with activating mutations in the *TRET* gene, which encodes the catalytic component of telomerase. Interestingly, TERT mutations are found in the vast majority of oligodendrogliomas and IDH-wildtype glioblastomas [13]. ATRX deficiency has also been associated with generalized genomic instability, which can induce p53-dependent cell death. Therefore, *TP53* mutations in diffuse astrocytoma may enable tumor cell survival in the setting of ATRX loss.

Multiple studies have identified homozygous deletion of *CDKN2A/B* as a marker of poor prognosis in patients with IDH-mutant diffuse astrocytic gliomas [6]. Thus,

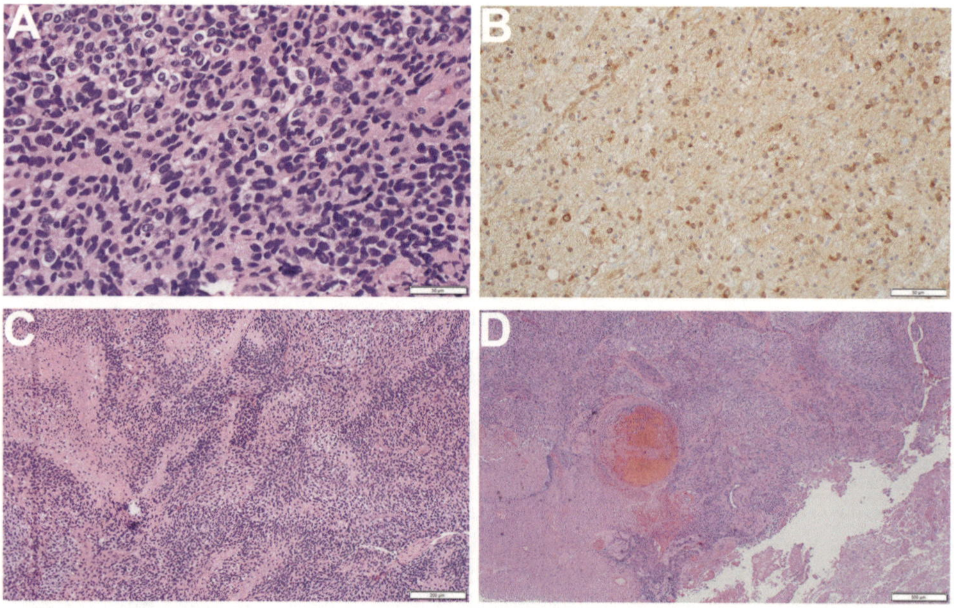


**Figure 1.**
*Neuropathological features of high grade gliomas. Hypercellularity, nuclear pleomorphism, significant proliferative activity (A) and a mutation in IDH1 R132H as detected by immunohistochemistry (B) are essential features of astrocytoma, IDH-mutant, grade 3. A hypercellular band of cells tracing the border of necrotic zones in what is known as pseudopalisading necrosis (C) and/or microvascular proliferation (D) are required histological characteristics for diagnosis of glioblastoma, grade 4.*

IDH-mutant astrocytomas that lack significant mitotic activity, histologic anaplasia, microvascular proliferation, necrosis and *CDKN2A/B* homozygous deletion are referred to as Astrocytoma, IDH-mutant, grade 2. Patients with these tumors have a median overall survival greater than 10 years. An IDH-mutant astrocytoma that contains elevated mitotic activity and histologic anaplasia, yet lacks microvascular proliferation, necrosis and *CDKN2A/B* homozygous deletion, currently fits into the designation of Astrocytoma, IDH-mutant, grade 3 (**Figure 1A-B**). Recognizing that no validated published criteria exist for mitotic count cut-off values for grading IDH-mutant astrocytomas, "significant" mitotic from grade 2 tumors. Most neuropathologists use a threshold of ≥2 mitoses within the entire specimen, or one mitosis in very small biopsies, while large specimens may require more. Lastly, IDH-mutant astrocytomas with microvascular proliferation or necrosis or CDKN2A/B homozygous deletion, or any combination of these features, correspond to WHO grade 4.

## 4. Glioblastoma, IDH-wildtype

By far, the most frequent malignant brain tumor in adults is glioblastoma, accounting for approximately 15% of all intracranial neoplasms and approximately 45-50% of all primary malignant brain tumors. The annual incidence of glioblastoma in the USA, adjusted to the United States Standard Population, is 3.19 cases per 100, 000 population. It preferentially affects older adults, with peak incidence occurring in patients aged 55-85 years. A series of environmental and genetic factors have been studies as potential causes of glioblastoma. To date, the only validated risk factor associations are an increased risk after ionizing radiation to the head and neck and a decreased risk among individuals with a history of allergies and atopic disease [14]. Glioblastoma is most often centered in the subcortical white matter of the cerebral hemispheres. Glioblastoma is particularly notorious for its rapid invasion of neighboring brain structures. Infiltration occurs most readily along white matter tracts, but can also involve cortical and deep gray structures. When infiltration extends through the corpus callosum, with subsequent growth in the contralateral hemisphere, the result can be a bilateral, symmetrical lesion (so called butterfly glioma). The symptoms depend largely on the tumor location, primarily manifesting as focal neurological deficits and edema with increase in intracranial pressure. As many as half of all patients are diagnosed after an inaugural seizure. On MRI, glioblastomas are irregularly shaped and have a ring-shaped zone of contrast enhancement around a dark, central area of necrosis.

Glioblastoma is typically a highly cellular glioma, usually composed of poorly differentiated, sometimes pleomorphic tumor cells with nuclear atypia and brisk mitotic activity. Tumor necrosis is a fundamental feature of glioblastoma. Palisading form, which consists of multiple, small, irregularly shaped band-like or serpiginous foci surrounded by radially oriented, densely packed glioma cells, is a histological hallmark of glioblastoma (**Figure 1C**). The other histological hallmark is microvascular proliferation (**Figure 1D**). Glioblastomas are among the most vascularized of all human tumors. Hypoxia is a major driving force of glioblastoma angiogenesis and leads to intracellular stabilization of the master regulator HIF1A [15]. HIF1A accumulation leads to transcriptional activation of over a hundred of hypoxia-regulated genes encoding proteins that control angiogenesis. Among them, VEGFA seems to be the most important mediator of glioma-associated vascular functions; it is primarily produced by perinecrotic palisading cells as a consequence of cellular stress such as hypoxia and hypoglycaemia. Therapeutic blocking of VEGFA by monoclonal antibodies is effective to target small, immature vessels and

lead to vascular normalization accompanied by improved perfusion and oxygenation [16]. On light microscopy, microvascular proliferation typically presents as so-called glomeruloid tufts of multilayered mitotically active endothelial cells together with smooth muscle cells/pericytes. Another less common form is hypertrophic proliferating endothelial cells within medium-sized vessels.

Multiple studies have concluded that a substantial subset of IDH-wildtype diffuse or anaplastic astrocytomas in adults has an aggressive clinical course, with overall patient survival time almost equal to the patients with IDH-mutant glioblastoma, WHO grade 4 [17, 18]. Thus, cIMPACT has reached a consensus that despite the WHO grade 2 or 3 histology, IDH-wildtype diffuse astrocytic tumors would follow an aggressive clinical course and considered as an entity equivalent to glioblastoma if they have the genotype of epidermal growth factor receptor (EGFR) amplification and/or combined whole chromosome seven gain and whole chromosome ten loss (+7/−10) and/or TERT promoter mutation. Although these tumors possess so-called "GBM genotypes", there has been a reluctance to designate the tumor as a glioblastoma in the absence of histological features including palisading necrosis and microvascular proliferation. cIMPACT has thus reached consensus on the designation of diffuse astrocytic glioma, IDH-wild type, with molecular features of glioblastoma, WHO grade 4 as the most appropriate terminology at this time, since this conveys the histologic, molecular and clinical features of glioblastoma that does not alter the long-standing histologic definition [4]. Glioblastoma is highly resistant to therapy, with only modest survival increases achieved in a minority of patients, even after aggressive surgical resection, external beam radiation therapy, and maximum tolerated doses of chemotherapy. MGMT promoter methylation is the only predictive biomarker for the efficacy of and response to alkylating and methylating chemotherapy agents in glioblastoma [19].

## 5. Oligodendroglioma

While astrocytoma represents roughly 80-90% of all gliomas, oligodendroglioma, the second most common primary CNS tumor, represents only about 5-6% of all gliomas, with peak incidence in patients aged 35-44 years [20]. Approximately two-thirds of patients present with seizures. The frontal lobe is the most common location. They are characterized by cortex and white-matter based proliferations of neoplastic cells morphologically resembling oligodendrocytes which have a characteristic "fried-egg" appearance (a delayed fixation tissue artifact seen on H&E permanent sections, and rarely observed on frozen section), delicate "chicken wire" vasculature, mucoid/cystic degeneration and microcalcifications. The current WHO classification of oligodendroglioma requires demonstration of *IDH1* or *IDH2* mutation, typically by immunohistochemistry using the mutation-specific antibody against R132H-mutant IDH1 (followed by DNA genotyping when R132H-mutant IDH1 immunostaining is negative), as well as demonstration of 1p/19q codeletion by FISH or molecular genetic testing. Mutations in the *CIC* gene on 19q13.2 and *FUBP1* gene on 1p31.1, among other genes on 1p and 19q, may contribute to the distinctive biology of 1p/19q codeletion [21]. Unlike IDH-mutant diffuse astrocytomas, oligodendroglioma usually lacks wide-spread nuclear p53 staining, a finding consistent with the mutual exclusivity of *TP53* mutation and 1p/19q deletion [22]. In addition, oligodendrogliomas lack *ATRX* mutation but virtually always carry activating mutations in the *TERT* promoter region, leading to increased expression of TERT [23]. In this manner, 1p/19q testing can be skipped if an IDH-mutant tumor appears clearly astrocytic and the ATRX/p53 immunohistochemistry results are consistent with an astrocytic genotype (*ATRX* and/or *TP53* mutations).

There is no WHO grade 1 variant of oligodendroglioma. WHO grade 2 oligodendroglioma is defined by a diffusely infiltrating, slow-growing glioma without evidence of increased mitotic activity (a few mitoses are permitted), endothelial proliferation, or necrosis. In contrast, WHO grade 3 anaplastic oligodendroglioma is defined by histological features of anaplasia. In particular, microvascular proliferation and/or increased mitotic activity (there is debate among experts, although classic studies have indicated a cutoff of ≥6 mitoses/10 HPF) have been suggested to be of important indicators of anaplasia in oligodendroglioma. Interestingly, contrast enhancement has been detected in <20% of WHO grade 2, but in >70% of grade 3 anaplastic oligodendrogliomas [24]. Thus lack of contrast enhancement does not exclude anaplastic oligodendroglioma. 1p/19q codeletion has been found to be associated with better therapeutic response and longer survival in patients treated with adjuvant radiotherapy and chemotherapy [25]. Not surprisingly, long-term follow-up data indicate higher median overall survival times (>10 years) for patients with anaplastic oligodendrogliomas who were treated with combined radiotherapy and chemotherapy.

Finally, to make matters even slight more complicated, there is a class of tumors that combines the histologic features of both astrocytomas and oligodendrogliomas. The existence of these entities is hotly contested; however, as of the 2016 iteration of the WHO classification, there is a grade II oligoastrocytoma, NOS and a grade III anaplastic oligoastrocytoma, NOS. They usually manifest in adult patients, with preferential localization in the cerebral hemispheres. Again, NOS indicates that molecular testing could not be completed or is inconclusive.

## 6. Diffuse midline glioma, H3 K27M-mutant

By definition, this entity is an infiltrative midline glioma with predominantly astrocytic differentiation and a K27M mutation in either *H3F3A* or *HIST1H3B/C* [3]. K27M mutations affecting H3.3 (encoded by *H3F3A*) are about three times as prevalent as the same mutation in histone variant H3.1 (occurring in *HIST1H3B* or *HIST1H3C*). Notably, these mutations are not exclusive to diffuse midline gliomas. Over the past few years, a number of tumors that are not diffuse midline gliomas have been reported with the same H3 K27M mutation, including ependymomas, pilocytic astrocytomas, pediatric diffuse astrocytomas, and gangliogliomas. Therefore these mutations cannot be used in and of themselves to define a diffuse midline glioma, H3 K27M-mutant.

It predominates in children but can also be seen in adults, with the most common locations being brain stem, thalamus, and spinal cord. Classic clinical symptoms include the triad of multiple cranial neuropathies, long tract signs, and ataxia, typically developing over a short period of time (1-2 months). The prognosis is poor, despite current therapies, with a 2-year survival rate of <10%. Correspondingly, H3 K27M-mutant diffuse midline glioma is WHO grade 4. The mere grading criterion of an entity based on a specific mutation means the histological features do not predict the outcome. Indeed, about 10% pontine examples lack mitotic figures, microvascular proliferation, and necrosis, and thus are histologically consistent with WHO grade 2. The remaining cases are histologically high grade, with 25% containing mitotic figures and the remainder containing mitotic figures as well as foci of necrosis and microvascular proliferation. The use of H3 K27M-mutant specific immunohistochemistry is useful to identify the mutation and specifically for diagnosis of diffuse midline glioma, H3 K27M-mutant. The K27M substitution results in a decrease in H3K27me3 (trimethylated), thought to be due to inhibition of PRC2 activity [26]. Antibody that has also been used to guide diagnosis of these

tumors is against H3 K27me3. H3 K27me3 immunohistochemistry, however, should only be used in conjunction with H3K27M immunohistochemistry, since loss of H3 K27me3 expression is by itself not specific.

## 7. Other astrocytic tumors

Pleomorphic xanthoastrocytoma is rare (constituting <1% of all astrocytic neoplasms) and most commonly affects children and young adults, with a median patient age at diagnosis of 22 years [27]. A superficial location, involving the leptomeninges and cerebrum is characteristic of this neoplasm. Approximately 98% of cases occur supratentorially, most commonly in the temporal lobe. Due to the superficial cerebral location of the lesion, many patients present with a fairly long history of seizures. On MRI, the solid portion of the tumor is hyperintense on T2 FLAIR images. Postcontrast enhancement is moderate or strong.

The adjective "pleomorphic" refers to the variable histological appearance of the tumor, in which spindled cells are intermingled with mononucleated or multinucleated giant astrocytes. The term "xanthoastrocytoma" refers to the presence of large, often multinucleated xanthomatous cells that have intracellular accumulation of lipids. Granular bodies are a nearly invariable finding. Focal collections of small lymphocytes are also frequent. The third histological hallmark of pleomorphic xanthoastrocytoma is the presence of reticulin fibers. Despite its alarming histological appearance, pleomorphic xanthoastrocytoma has relatively favorable prognosis compared with diffusely infiltrative astrocytoma, with 70.9% recurrence-free and 90.4% overall survival rates at 5 years, corresponding to WHO grade 2. Patients with anaplastic pleomorphic xanthoastrocytoma have significantly worse survival than those whose tumors show <5 mitoses per 10 HPFs. Necrosis may be present. *BRAF V600E* mutations occurs in approximately 50-78% of cases [28]. The frequency of *BRAF V600E* mutation is lower among anaplastic pleomorphic xanthoastrocytoma than among WHO grade 2 pleomorphic xanthoastrocytoma, but the prognostic significance of the mutation is unknown.

## 8. Ependymal tumors

Ependymomas are tumors that can arise anywhere along the ependymal-lined ventricular spaces of the neuraxis, including the brain and spinal cord. Like the other gliomas, this is a heterogeneous class of tumors that ranges from benign (subependymoma and myxopapillary ependymoma) to malignant (anaplastic ependymoma). Due to their location, even biologically benign examples can cause malignant clinical sequelae, including recurrent obstructive hydrocephalus and even death. The age of the patient seems to affect prognosis, with adults doing better than children, probably due in part to a predominant spinal cord involvement in adults. Histologically, these tumors are characterized by solid or pseudo-papillary proliferations of small to medium sized, hyperchromatic, oval to spindled cells with conspicuous pseudo-rosettes (cells palisading/lining up like a picket fence around a central capillary) and/or, less commonly, true ependymal rosettes (cells palisading around a hollow canal in an attempt to recapitulate the embryonic central canal). There are three histologic variants of WHO grade II ependymoma: papillary, clear cell (which tends to be biologically more aggressive), and tanycytic. However, the criteria for defining anaplastic ependymoma are not as well developed as those of astrocytomas as no association between grade and biological behavior or survival has been definitively established.

Advances in the understanding of the biological basis and molecular characteristics of ependymal tumors have prompted the cIMPACT-NOW group to recommend a new classification. Separation of ependymal tumors by anatomic site is an important principle of the new classification and was prompted by methylome profiling data to indicate that molecular groups of ependymal tumors in the posterior fossa and supratentorial and spinal compartments are distinct [8]. A supratentorial ependymoma characterized by a *C11orf95-RELA* fusion gene accounts for approximately 70% of all childhood supratentorial tumors and a lower proportion of such ependymomas in adult patients [29]. It forms in the context of chromothripsis, a shattering and reassembly of the genome that rearranges genes and produces oncogenic gene products. Rarely, *C11orf95* or *RELA* can be fused with other genes as a result of chromothripsis. *RELA* fusion-positive ependymomas show constitutive activation of the NF-kappaB pathway. Immunohistochemistry to assess the expression of L1CAM correlates well with the presence of a *RELA* fusion in these tumors. Importantly, *RELA* fusion-positive ependymomas have been reported to have the worst outcome among the supratentorial ependymomas [30].

## 9. Conclusions

Since 2016, ongoing discoveries in molecular pathology have advanced our understanding of many of the entities organized under the WHO 2016 classification. Most of these changes carry important implications for clinical practice and for the design and interpretation of clinical trials. It is almost certain that our understanding of the biology of CNS tumors will continue to expand at a rapid pace. Thus continuation of the efforts of optimal (evidence-based, balanced, rapid) and timely translation of novel insights into clinical diagnostics, is the ultimate goal to provide the best possible care to CNS tumor patients.

## Conflict of interest

The author declares no conflict of interest.

## Author details

Liam Chen
University of Minnesota Medical School, Minneapolis, USA

*Address all correspondence to: llchen@umn.edu

## References

[1] Louis, D.N., et al., *The 2016 World Health Organization Classification of Tumors of the Central Nervous System: a summary.* Acta Neuropathol, 2016. **131**(6): p. 803-820.

[2] Louis, D.N., et al., *cIMPACT-NOW update 1: Not Otherwise Specified (NOS) and Not Elsewhere Classified (NEC).* Acta Neuropathol, 2018. **135**(3): p. 481-484.

[3] Louis, D.N., et al., *cIMPACT-NOW update 2: diagnostic clarifications for diffuse midline glioma, H3 K27M-mutant and diffuse astrocytoma/anaplastic astrocytoma, IDH-mutant.* Acta Neuropathol, 2018. **135**(4): p. 639-642.

[4] Brat, D.J., et al., *cIMPACT-NOW update 3: recommended diagnostic criteria for "Diffuse astrocytic glioma, IDH-wildtype, with molecular features of glioblastoma, WHO grade IV".* Acta Neuropathol, 2018. **136**(5): p. 805-810.

[5] Ellison, D.W., et al., *cIMPACT-NOW update 4: diffuse gliomas characterized by MYB, MYBL1, or FGFR1 alterations or BRAF(V600E) mutation.* Acta Neuropathol, 2019. **137**(4): p. 683-687.

[6] Brat, D.J., et al., *cIMPACT-NOW update 5: recommended grading criteria and terminologies for IDH-mutant astrocytomas.* Acta Neuropathol, 2020. **139**(3): p. 603-608.

[7] Louis, D.N., et al., *cIMPACT-NOW update 6: new entity and diagnostic principle recommendations of the cIMPACT-Utrecht meeting on future CNS tumor classification and grading.* Brain Pathol, 2020. **30**(4): p. 844-856.

[8] Ellison, D.W., et al., *cIMPACT-NOW update 7: advancing the molecular classification of ependymal tumors.* Brain Pathol, 2020. **30**(5): p. 863-866.

[9] Braunstein, S., et al., *Pediatric high-grade glioma: current molecular landscape and therapeutic approaches.* J Neurooncol, 2017. **134**(3): p. 541-549.

[10] Jones, C., et al., *Pediatric high-grade glioma: biologically and clinically in need of new thinking.* Neuro Oncol, 2017. **19**(2): p. 153-161.

[11] Ohgaki, H. and P. Kleihues, *The definition of primary and secondary glioblastoma.* Clin Cancer Res, 2013. **19**(4): p. 764-772.

[12] Dang, L., et al., *Cancer-associated IDH1 mutations produce 2-hydroxyglutarate.* Nature, 2009. **462**(7274): p. 739-744.

[13] Eckel-Passow, J.E., et al., *Glioma Groups Based on 1p/19q, IDH, and TERT Promoter Mutations in Tumors.* N Engl J Med, 2015. **372**(26): p. 2499-2508.

[14] Ostrom, Q.T., et al., *Alex's Lemonade Stand Foundation Infant and Childhood Primary Brain and Central Nervous System Tumors Diagnosed in the United States in 2007-2011.* Neuro Oncol, 2015. **16 Suppl 10**: p. x1-x36.

[15] Acker, T. and K.H. Plate, *Hypoxia and hypoxia inducible factors (HIF) as important regulators of tumor physiology.* Cancer Treat Res, 2004. **117**: p. 219-248.

[16] Sorensen, A.G., et al., *Increased survival of glioblastoma patients who respond to antiangiogenic therapy with elevated blood perfusion.* Cancer Res, 2012. **72**(2): p. 402-407.

[17] Aoki, K., et al., *Prognostic relevance of genetic alterations in diffuse lower-grade gliomas.* Neuro Oncol, 2018. **20**(1): p. 66-77.

[18] Aibaidula, A., et al., *Adult IDH wild-type lower-grade gliomas should be further stratified.* Neuro Oncol, 2017. **19**(10): p. 1327-1337.

[19] Hegi, M.E., et al., *MGMT gene silencing and benefit from temozolomide in glioblastoma.* N Engl J Med, 2005. **352**(10): p. 997-1003.

[20] Ohgaki, H. and P. Kleihues, *Population-based studies on incidence, survival rates, and genetic alterations in astrocytic and oligodendroglial gliomas.* J Neuropathol Exp Neurol, 2005. **64**(6): p. 479-489.

[21] Yip, S., et al., *Concurrent CIC mutations, IDH mutations, and 1p/19q loss distinguish oligodendrogliomas from other cancers.* J Pathol, 2012. **226**(1): p. 7-16.

[22] Suzuki, H., et al., *Mutational landscape and clonal architecture in grade II and III gliomas.* Nat Genet, 2015. **47**(5): p. 458-468.

[23] Koelsche, C., et al., *Distribution of TERT promoter mutations in pediatric and adult tumors of the nervous system.* Acta Neuropathol, 2013. **126**(6): p. 907-915.

[24] Khalid, L., et al., *Imaging characteristics of oligodendrogliomas that predict grade.* AJNR Am J Neuroradiol, 2012. **33**(5): p. 852-857.

[25] Hartmann, C., et al., *Molecular markers in low-grade gliomas: predictive or prognostic?* Clin Cancer Res, 2011. **17**(13): p. 4588-4599.

[26] Lewis, P.W., et al., *Inhibition of PRC2 activity by a gain-of-function H3 mutation found in pediatric glioblastoma.* Science, 2013. **340**(6134): p. 857-861.

[27] Giannini, C., et al., *Pleomorphic xanthoastrocytoma: what do we really know about it?* Cancer, 1999. **85**(9): p. 2033-2045.

[28] Schindler, G., et al., *Analysis of BRAF V600E mutation in 1,320 nervous system tumors reveals high mutation frequencies in pleomorphic xanthoastrocytoma, ganglioglioma and extra-cerebellar pilocytic astrocytoma.* Acta Neuropathol, 2011. **121**(3): p. 397-405.

[29] Parker, M., et al., *C11orf95-RELA fusions drive oncogenic NF-kappaB signalling in ependymoma.* Nature, 2014. **506**(7489): p. 451-455.

[30] Pajtler, K.W., et al., *Molecular Classification of Ependymal Tumors across All CNS Compartments, Histopathological Grades, and Age Groups.* Cancer Cell, 2015. **27**(5): p. 728-743.

Chapter 8

# Molecular Classification of Diffuse Gliomas

*Kanwalpreet Kaur*

## Abstract

In 2016 WHO classification of CNS tumors genotypic and phenotypic parameters were integrated to define a new nomenclature of diffuse gliomas on the basis of presence or absence of isocitrate dehydrogenase mutations. This resulted in more homogenous and narrowly defined categories with better accuracy of prognostic information, thus, playing a crucial role in patient management. Broadly, astrocytomas are now histologically and genetically distinct with IDH-mutant, ATRX-mutant, 1p/19q-intact and oligodendroglial tumors has IDH-mutant, ATRX-wildtype and 1p/19q-codeleted profile. Glioblastoma are now classified into primary and secondary on the basis of IDH mutations independent of clinical history.

**Keywords:** Diffuse glioma, astrocytoma, oligodendroglioma, IDH, 1p/19q codeletion, ATRX, TERT, EGFR, PTEN, CDKN2A, MGMT, H3F3K27M

## 1. Introduction

In 2016 World Health Organization (WHO) classification of tumors of central nervous system, there was a paradigm deviation from earlier morphology based classification of gliomas to a new classification and nomenclature by integrating the molecular and histomorphological parameters. This approach provided finely defined diagnostic categories resulting in better correlation with prognostic and treatment parameters. Now diffuse gliomas whether astrocytoma or oligodendroglioma are grouped together on the basis of their shared *IDH1* or *IDH2* mutation status. Oligodendrogliomas also show 1p/19q codeletion. So, in 2016 diffuse glioma category comprise of WHO grade II and III astrocyctic tumors, grade II and III oligodendroglioma and grade IV glioblastoma, IDH mutant and wildtype. Continuing evolving knowledge on pathology of glioma led to a pediatric midline glioma with mutations in histone H3 genes to be also included with these adult diffuse gliomas. This excludes astrocytoma with circumscribed growth pattern and lacking IDH mutations i.e. pilocycytic astrocytoma, pleomorphic xanthoastrocytoma, subependymal giant cell astrocytoma. So, diffuse astrocytoma and oligodendrogliomas are now nosologically more similar than are diffuse astrocytoma and pilocytic astrocytoma and family tree of tumors is being redrawn [1].

This new classification was testament to rapid advancement in the field of molecular biology and reducing cost, easy availability for masses in the present times. Now there is possibility of detecting some of these mutations on immunohistochemistry. This journey from discovery of isocitrate dehydrogenase mutations peculiar to gliomas leading to their radical reclassification and new taxonomy based on the presence or absence of mutations happened over a period of just 8 years [2].



IntechOpen

## 2. Principle mutations

### 2.1 Isocitrate dehydrogenase mutations

Metabolism in cancer cells is rewired compared to normal cells since challenge is production more building blocks for proteins, nucleic acids rather than production of more ATP molecules as cell fuel. But very few tumors show mutations in genes directly involved in metabolic pathways. Isocitrate dehydrogenase (IDH) is an enzyme in the tricarboxylic acid (TCA) cycle of aerobic respiration and catalyzes the oxidative carboxylation converting isocitrate to α –ketoglutarate (α –KT). It exists in 3 isoforms i.e. IDH1, IDH2 and IDH3; isoenzymes are multiple forms of an enzyme catalyzing the same reaction but differ in amino acid sequence and kinetic properties (**Table 1**).

Only IDH 3 is a part of TCA cycle and dependent on nicotinamide adenine dinucleotide (NAD) as co factor [3–5].

Isocitrate + $NAD^+ \rightarrow$ α-ketoglutarate + $CO_2$ + NADH+ $H^+$.

IDH 1 is found in cytosol and peroxisomes while IDH 2 in mitochondria,both using nicotinamide adenine dinucleotide phosphate (NADP) as cofactor. They both catalyze reversible reaction and prevent oxidative damage by generating NADPH [2].

Isocitrate + $NADP^+ \rightleftarrows$ α -ketoglutarate + $CO_2$ + NADPH+ $H^+$.

In diffuse gliomas, heterozygous mutations seen in cytosolic IDH1 or mitochondrial IDH2 are considered as driver mutations [1–6]. Active site of both enzymes is formed by many arginine residues which is a polar amino acid. It forms hydrophilic bonds with isocitrate which is negatively charged. Most common mutation in diffuse gliomas is heterozygous point mutation at nucleotide position 395 of the *IDH1* replaces guanine by adenine G395A resulting in replacement of arginine by histidine (less polar amino acid) at amino acid residue 132 of the protein (R132H). However, new enzyme IDH1-R132H homodimer is not completely inactive despite losing a critical substrate-binding amino acid residue. It gets a neomorphic activity resulting in reducing α-KG to D-2-hydroxyglutarate (D-2-HG) and oxidizing NADPH to NADP+ [3–5].

This mutation was first discovered in 2008 when next generation sequencing was used to study 22,661 protein coding genes in 22 glioblastomas and 5 of them

| | IDH1 | IDH2 | IDH3 |
|---|---|---|---|
| LOCATION | Cytosol Peroxisomes | Mitochondria | Mitochondria |
| COFACTOR | NADP+ | NADP+ | NAD+ |
| STRUCTURE | Homodimer | Homodimer | Hetrooctamer (2 alpha, 1 beta, 1 gamma subunit) |
| REVERIBILITY OF REACTION | Reversible | reversible | irreversible |
| MAJOR ROLE | Prevent oxidative damage by generating NADPH | Prevent oxidative damage by generating NADPH | Catalytic role in TCA cycle (citric acid cycle) |
| GENES | IDH 1 gene: 2q33 | IDH 2 gene: 15q26.1 | IDH3A: 15q25.1–25.2<br>IDH3B: 20p13<br>IDH3G: Xq28 |

**Table 1.**
*Properties of three isoforms of IDH.*

showed expressed IDH mutations all at this same codon [2]. Subsequently, Yan and colleagues (26) analyzed IDH1 and IDH2 loci of nearly 1,000 central nervous system (CNS) tumors and found mutually exclusive mutations of IDH1 or IDH2 in more than 70% of WHO grade II and III astrocytomas and oligodendrogliomas and in secondary GBMs that developed from these lower-grade lesions [6]. Since then, numerous studies throughout the world substantiated the similar findings with heterozygous mutations in IDH 1 or less commonly in IDH2 been identified in nearly 74% diffuse astrocytoma WHO grade II, 59% anaplastic astrocytoma WHO grade III, all secondary glioblastoma, 76% oligodendroglioma WHO grade II and 67% anaplastic oligodendroglioma WHO grade III. Most common hot spot mutations identified are R132C, R132S, R132G, R132L in IDH1 and R172K, R172M, R172W and R172G in IDH2 [1, 5].

Mechanism of oncogenesis of IDH is still under research. These IDH mutations result in metabolic dysregulation in tumor glial cells affecting glucose sensing, glutamine metabolism, lipogenesis, and regulation of cellular redox status. In normal cells, IDH 1and 2 wild type (wt) are an important source of NADPH. They are responsible for nearly 65% of total NADPH production in the cytoplasm of IDH wildtype (IDHwt) glioblastoma [3–5]. Glioma cells overexpressing IDH1-R132H or other mutations in IDH 1 or 2 had decreased NADPH levels so consequently, levels of reactive oxygen species (ROS) increased and GSH decreased. Apart from role of ROS, increased production of D-2-HG also has its implications on the tumor cell. D-2-HG and α-KG are structurally similar; only differ for the C2-linked oxygen atom in α-KG, which is replaced by a hydroxyl group in D-2-HG. So D-2-HG causes competitive inhibition of α-KG–dependent dioxygenases thus exerting its direct oncogenic effects. Approximately 60 dioxygenases regulate diverse and important cellular processes by hydroxylating target acceptor proteins by using α-KG as the donor substrate. Important among these are prolyl hydroxylases that regulate hypoxia-inducible factor (HIF) 1α, chromatin-modifying enzymes like histone N-methyl-lysine demethylases and ten-eleven translocations (TET) 5-methylcytosine hydroxylases. The global histone demethylation by D-2-HG causes hypermethylation at a number of gene loci forming glioma-CpG island methylation phenotype and affect chromatin modification. D-2-HG also inhibits TET-mediated 5-methylcytosine hydroxylases levels which affect the expression of many regulatory proteins and possibly tumor suppressors that also contribute to tumorigenesis [5].

IDH mt gliomas can occur anywhere in the central nervous system but are preferentially located supratentorially in the frontal lobes [1, 7, 8]. Hence it is hypothesized IDH mt gliomas arise from a neural precursor population that is spatially and temporally restricted in the brain.

Since IDH mutations play a key role in tumourogenesis. Their diagnostic and prognostic role is well incorporated into routine neuropathology. IDH 1/2 mutations can be detected by Direct Sanger sequencing, pyrosequencing, allele-specific hybridization polymerase chain reaction (PCR), Real-time PCR, digital droplet PCR and high-throughput next-generation sequencing. IDH1 R132H accounts for nearly 90% of all IDH associated mutations in gliomas, so a monoclonal antibody has been developed against the mutant protein, allowing its use in paraffin-embedded specimens [1]. IHC IDH R132H mutation (clone H09) has shown sensitivity of 94% and a specificity of 100%. Positive staining is strong cytoplasmic and weak nuclear in tumor cells. Endothelial cells, perivascular lymphocytes, residual glial cells should be negative. Weak background staining and staining of macrophages is negative. Normal brain does not show staining for mIDH1 R132H IHC but granular staining in the neurons can be seen due to non specific binding to lipofuscin. One caveat to kept in mind while interpreting IHC is that macrophages can show strong cytoplasmic

granular staining even in IDH wt tumors. IHC is very useful for small samples where quantity of DNA extracted is too low for definite results by sequencing since it can highlight single infiltrating tumor cells [9]. IDH helps to separate gliosis (IDH negative) from low grade astrocytoma (IDH mt), if there is doubt in grade I and grade II glioma, IDH presence indicates we are dealing with grade II astrocytoma and also primary glioblastoma (IDH wt) from secondary glioblastoma (IDH mt). If IHC is negative, DNA sequencing is a must before calling a glioma IDH wt.

In all studies IDH mt gliomas have shown better improved progression free survival, longer time for treatment failure and extended overall survival in each of three treatment arms: radiotherapy, radiotherapy with PCV (procarbazine, lomustine and vincristine) or radiotherapy plus temozolomide [5]. So in addition to traditional good prognostic factors i.e. age < 40 years, lower tumor grade, tumor not crossing midline, absence of neurologic deficit before resection and tumor <6 cm, IDH mutation status has emerged as most important favorable prognostic factor in current times. Some studies have reported median survival of 10.9 years in IDH mt diffuse astrocytomas [1, 2, 6, 10].

Due to role of key role IDH mutations in glioma tumorogenesis, many isocitrate dehydrogenase inhibitors like hydroxypyridin-2-one, bis-imidazole phenol, tetrahydropyrazolopyridine are some of the drug under trails [5].

### 2.2 1p/19q codeletion

Nearly 60–80% of oligodendroglial neoplasms show co-deletion of 1p/19q: unbalanced translocation t(1;19)(q10;p10) after which only one copy of the short arm of chromosome 1 and one copy of the long arm of chromosome 19 remain and der (1;19) (q10;p10) is produced. It is hypothesized that translocation creates two derivative chromosomes, der(1;19)(p10;q10) and der(1;19)(q10;p10), and is followed by loss of the derivative chromosome containing 1p and 19q [11–16]. IDH wild type gliomas do not have 1p/19q codeletion.

Polysomy of 1p, 19q or both is also noted in a subset of oligodendrogliomas and has been associated with a poor prognosis, independent of deletion status [12, 13]. Oligodendrogliomas of grades II and III that have 1p/19q co-deletion also have a high frequency of TERT promoter mutations, CIC mutations on the remaining chromosome 1p allele and FUBP1 mutation on the remaining 19q allele (**Figure 1**) [14].

1p/19q codeletion are an essential part of molecular diagnostics of oligodendroglioma. Fluorescence in situ hybridisation (FISH), Cytogenomic microarray (CMA), Loss of heterozygosity and next generation sequencing are used to detect 1p/19q co-deletion. FISH is a reliable and validated most commonly used laboratory technique among these. Normal cells show a 2O2G signal (two test and two control probes, test: control ratio = 1.0). Loss of a test signal yields a 1O2G signal pattern (ratio = 0.5) and represents absolute deletion of a chromosome. Presence of aneuploidy, polyploidy and polysomy affects the interpretation since it become unclear what percentage of nuclei are displaying genuine co-deleted signals, so a ratio is calculated dividing total number of test signals by total number of control signals. Atleast 60 non-overlapping nuclei are counted and ratio < 0.8 should be both chromosomes for 1p/19co-deletion. Ratio of 0.75–0.90 is considered borderline [11].

PCR-LOH analysis can be used for borderline cases, it has better specificity than FISH because it tests for multiple loci in a single assay. But PCR is more labour intensive, requires more tissue, a higher proportion of neoplastic cells (at least about 70%) [11].

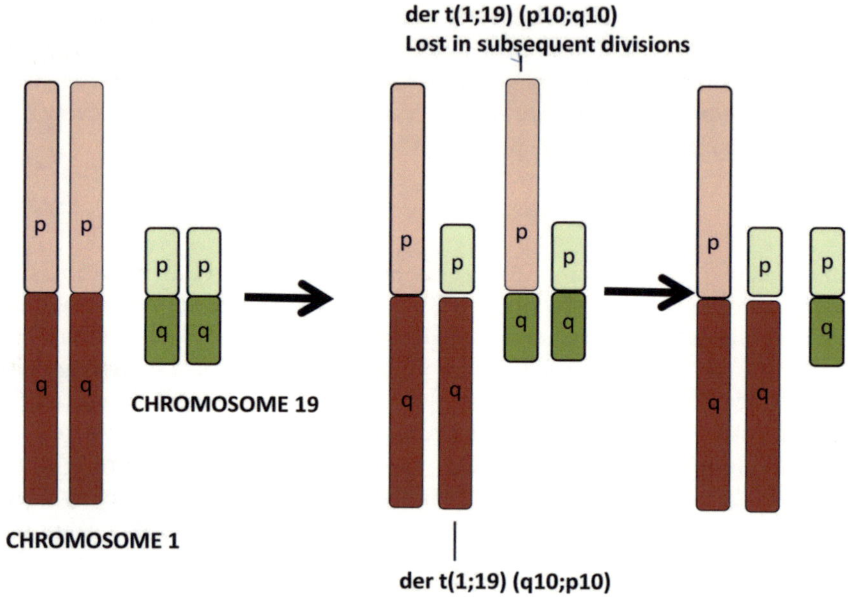


**Figure 1.**
*Unbalanced whole-arm translocation between chromosomes 1 and 19 [t(1,19)(q10;p10)] resulting in 1p/19q codeletion in glioma(11,15,16).*

The 1p/19q codeletion confers a favorable prognosis and is predictive of responses to alkylating chemotherapy and combination of radiotherapy and chemotherapy [1, 11–16].

### 2.3 Alpha Thalassemia/Mental Retardation Syndrome X-linked (ATRX)

Another critical marker that defined molecular classification of gliomas is ATRX gene present on Xq21.1. It is named so since it was first discovered through a study of assessing patients with the X-linked mental retardation syndrome presenting with α-thalassemia, severe psychomotor impairments, urogenital abnormalities, and patterns of characteristic facial dysmorphism. This gene encodes a protein which belongs to a chromatin-remodeling pathway (ATRX-DAXX) and is required for genomic stability by the incorporation of H3.3 at telomeres [17]. ATRX inactivation within gliomas can be due to mutations, deletions, gene fusions, or any combination of these. These mutations induce abnormal telomeres that are characteristic of a telomerase-independent telomere maintenance mechanism termed ALT (alternative lengthening of telomeres) [18].

Numerous studies have shown that ATRX mutations have a strong association with IDH mutations but never with 1p/19q codeletion. This property is exploited as diagnostic marker since ATRX inactivation indicates astrocytic lineage and rules out oligodendroglioma. ATRX mutations can be detected by direct Sanger sequencing, pyrosequencing, allele-specific hybridization polymerase chain reaction (PCR), Real-time PCR and high-throughput next-generation sequencing. ATRX IHC: clone CL0537 when show loss of nuclear expression >90% tumor nuclei is indicative of mutated ATRX. Nuclei of non-neoplastic cells such as endothelia, microglia, lymphocytes and reactive astrocytes are strongly positive and serve as positive internal control. When tumor cells show retained nuclear expression of ATRX IHC it indicates wild type ATRX [1, 17–20].

Low-grade glioma patients with ATRX retention and IDH mutations have lower progression-free survival and overall survival (OS) than tumors with 1p/19q codeletion and IDH mutations and longer time to treatment failure than those patients with IDH mutation and wild-type ATRX (55.6 vs. 31.8 months, respectively). Thus ATRX mutation infer a favorable prognosis to tumor [1, 19, 20].

### 2.4 TP53

Mutations of *TP53* are found in over 60–80% of infiltrative astrocytomas, anaplastic astrocytomas and secondary GBMs, yet are rare in oligodendrogliomas. There is a strong association between IDH1 mutation and *TP53* mutation in diffuse astrocytomas, and this combination of mutations is helpful in distinguishing astrocytomas from oligodendroglimas [1].

*TP53* mutations can be analyzed by direct Sanger sequencing, pyrosequencing, PCR, allele-specific hybridization, real-time PCR and high-throughput next-generation sequencing. P53 IHC is also easily available and widely used. Immunostain reacts with both the normal and mutant forms of p53. Wild type P53 is rapidly degraded and has short half-life, hence is not detected by p53 IHC. Mutant p53 degrade more slowly, accumulate within nucleus of tumor cells creating a stable target for IHC. IHC detection of overexpressed protein is thus used as a surrogate method for mutation analysis, But it is not sensitive or specific. Over the last 25 years, studies have shown concordance rates between p53 IHC and TP53 mutation status ranging from 55 to 89% in grade I–IV gliomas [1, 21, 22].

TP53 alterations are usually missense producing stable full-length protein. Nonsense, frameshift, or deletion mutations results in incomplete translation of p53 gene producing a truncated protein product or loss of protein expression. This anomalous p53 structure may not be recognized during p53 IHC analysis resulting in false negativity. Some studies considered >10% tumor nuclei staining as positive for TP53 mutation status while others consider >50% as positive [21, 22].

### 2.5 *TERT* promotor mutations

One of the hallmarks of cancer is its ability to proliferate indefinitely. In normal somatic cells, the number of cell division is limited by the telomere length of chromosomes as it decreases with each replicative cycle. Cancer cells often overcome this limit by activating their telomerase. Telomerase consists of an RNA subunit and a reverse transcriptase catalytic subunit (TERT), which adds telomeric repeats to chromosome ends, therefore, maintaining telomere length. *TERT* gene on 5p15.33 encodes catalytic active site of telomerase and one of the mechanisms of telomerase activation in gliomas is somatic mutations in the promoter region of *TERT*. Most common mutations are C228T and C250T. The frequency of mutation was nearly 72% of IDH wt glioblastomas and in 95% of IDH mt oligodendrogiomas while relatively low in diffuse astrocytomas and anaplastic astrocytomas (19 and 25%, respectively) [23]. ATRX mutations are mutually exclusive of TERT gene mutations [1].

TERT mutations are detected by sequencing. IDH mutation, with 1p/19q codeletion and TERT mutation is characteristic of oligodendroglioma. TERT mutation in absence of IDH mutation indicates astrocytoma. In IDH wt gliomas, one with TERT mutation is associated with reduced overall survival compared to those lacking it. TERT mutation in IDH mt gliomas carries good prognosis [24].

### 2.6 EGFR

Epidermal growth factor receptor (EGFR) is a transmembrane receptor tyrosine kinase, whose ligands include EGF and TGF-α. Most frequently amplified oncogene in astrocytic tumors. EGFR amplification is seen in nearly 40% of primary/ IDH wt glioblastoma and rarely in secondary/ IDH mt glioblastoma [1]. There are also specific EGFR mutations (the vIII mutant), which produce a truncated transmembrane receptor with constitutive activity. Both EGFR amplification and the EGFRvIII mutant are mutually exclusive with IDH mutations [25].

### 2.7 PTEN

Loss of large regions at 10p, 10q23 and 10q25–26 loci, or loss of an entire copy of chromosome 10 is the most frequent genetic alterations in primary glioblastoma. It is specific for astrocytic differentiation and are rare in oligodendrogliomas [25].

### 2.8 *CDKN2A:*

Cyclin-dependent kinase inhibitor 2A (CDKN2A) is a gene located at chromosome 9, band p21.3. CDKN2A homozygous deletion is associated with poor prognosis among IDH-mutant gliomas [26, 27].

### 2.9 MGMT methylation

MGMT (O6-methylguanine-DNA methyltransferase) is a DNA repair enzyme and reverses the damage caused by alkylating agent temozolomide(TMZ) which adds methyl group at O6 position of guanine and this alkylation forms cross-links between adjacent strands of DNA. The MGMT protein rapidly reverses alkylation at the O6 position of guanine thereby averting the formation of lethal cross-links resulting in TMZ resistance. Promotor methylation of MGMT inactivates the gene so patients with MGMT promotor methylation are more benefitted with TMZ than patients without it [28].

MGMT promotor methylation is an essential part of molecular workup of all grade III and IV gliomas. Promoter methylation of O6-methylguanine–DNA methyltransferase (MGMT) is detected by methylation specific PCR, pyrosequencing or array based studies. MGMT determination by immunohistochemistry lacks standardization, reproducibility and, most importantly, correlation with clinical outcome so it is no longer recommended.

MGMT promotor methylation is commonly associated with IDH mutations and genome wide epigenetic changes (G-CIMP).

## 3. Diffuse gliomas

**Difuse astrocytoma, IDH mutant, and WHO grade II:** Diffuse astrocytoma composed of well differentiated fibrillary astrocytes in loose microcystic matrix. They show nuclear atypia in the form of variation in nuclear shape or size with accompanying hyperchromasia. All show mutation in *IDH 1* or *IDH2* supported by presence of *ATRX* characterized by gemistocytes forming nearly 20% of the tumor cells is a variant of IDH mt diffuse astrocytoma [1, 29, 30].

**Difuse astrocytoma, IDH wild type, and WHO grade II:** diffusely infiltrating astrocytoma without mutations in the IDH genes. It is extremely rare.

**Anaplastic astrocytoma, IDH mutant**: Diffusely infiltrating astrocytoma with focal or dispersed anaplasia, significant mitotic activity and mutation in *IDH 1* or *IDH.* TP53 or ATRX mutations are found in majority of tumors.

**Glioblastoma, IDH wild type/ primary glioblastoma:** They are high grade astrocytoma with nuclear atypia, cellular pleomorphism, mitosis, microvascular proliferation and necrosis. They lack IDH mutations but show TERT promotor mutations (80% cases), homozygyous deletion of CDKN2A/CDKN2B (60% cases), loss of chromosome 10p (50% cases), 10q (70%), EGFR alterations (55% cases) and PTEN (40% cases) [14, 15]. They account for nearly 90% of all glioblastoma [1].

**Glioblastoma, IDH mutant/ secondary glioblastoma:** IDH mutations in glioblastomas are considered as a marker for glioblastoma that arise by transformation from lower-grade gliomas, regardless of clinical history. IDH mt/secondary glioblastomas differ from IDH wt/primary glioblastoma in preferential frontal location and lesser extent of necrosis. Radiologically IDHmt glioblastoma exhibited more frequent non-enhancing tumor component, larger size at diagnosis, lesser extent of edema, and increased prevalence of cystic and diffuse components [31, 32]. Median age of IDHmt glioblastoma at diagnosis is 43 years while that of primary IDH wt glioblastoma is nearly 60 years [1].

Hence in routine histopathology practice, for older patients >55 years old, glioblastoma not in midline location and no prior history of lower grade glioma, IDH wt type designation can be given solely on the basis of negative IDH R132H immunohistochemistry. Sequencing is not required as the probability of an alternate IDH mutation is <1% [1, 31, 32].

IDH mt glioblastoma manifest longer overall survival and showed more frequent promoter methylation of MGMT [6].

**Oligodendroglioma:** Diffusely infiltrating slow growing glioma composed of monomorphic cells with uniform round nuclei and variable perinuclear haloes with IDH1 or IDH2 mutation and codeletion of chromosomes arms 1p and 19q.

IDH mutant gliomas which do not show ATRX loss on IHC should be considered for 1p/19qcodeletion studies even in absence of clear cut oligodendroglial histology [33].

Rarely tumors with oligodendroglial morphology but lacking IDH mutations or 1p/19q codeletion are noted. This group belongs to pediatric type oligodendroglioma. It is important to rule out histological mimics like dysembryoplastic neuroectodermal tumor, extraventricular neurocytoma, clear cell ependymoma and pilocyctic astrocytoma before rendering diagnosis of pediatric type oligodendroglioma [34, 35]. They show FGFR1 duplications or rearrangements of MYB related MYBL1 translocation [33].

Tumors with 1p/19 q codeletion without IDH mutations are usually IDH wt high grade astrocytomas and must be evaluated for possibility of incomplete deletion of on 1p and 19q [1].

**Diffuse midline glioma:** They are Infiltrative midline high grade glioma with astrocytic differentiation and mutations in histone proteins. Pons, thalamus, spinal cord are the common locations. Median age is 5–11 years. They are always IDH wild type and are considered grade IV tumors. In humans, there are main three histone H3 proteins: H3.1 encoded by HIST1H3B and HIST1H3C, H3.2 encoded by HIST2H3C and H3.3 encoded by H3F3A and H3F3B. Most common histone mutation is H3K27M (lysine to methionine substitution in H3F3A gene) which inhibits trimethylation of H3.3 histone resulting in decrease in H3K27me3. Other less frequent mutations occur in *HIST1H3B* or *HIST1H3C*. This can be detected by Sequencing for H3F3A and HIST1H3B. However, monoclonal H3F3A K27M

antibody is also available and intense nuclear staining in more than 80% of cells is taken as positive. Concordance between immunohistochemistry and sequencing is nearly 95%. H3 K27M mutated tumors show loss of H3K27me3 staining which can also be detected by IHC but it is not specific [1, 36].

**Not otherwise specified (NOS) designation:** It is used in tumors when either molecular testing is not available (e.g., in low-resource settings), or was performed but did not yield adequate results (assay failure), or was deliberately not done (e.g., not testing IDH status in an elderly patient with glioblastoma because of lack of implications for therapeutic management. But when molecular tests have been performed but results do not lead to a precise categorization of the tumor within the framework of the WHO 2016 classification, then term not elsewhere classified (NEC) is used [1, 26].

Final histopathological report:

- Layer 1: Integrated diagnosis
- Layer 2: Histological classification (i.e. cellularity, mitosis, necrosis, vascular endothelial proliferations, variants)
- Layer 3: Histologic (WHO) grade (based on morphology)
- Layer 4: Biomarker studies (IDH, ATRX, p53, 1p/19q codel, EGFR)

Example:

- **Integrated diagnosis**: Diffuse Astrocytoma IDH mt, WHO grade II
- **Histological diagnosis**: Diffuse astrocytoma, WHO (histological) grade II
- **Molecular information**:
- **IDH**: positive (R132H immunohistochemistry; consistent with mutant type)
- **ATRX**: nuclear expression loss (immunohistochemistry; consistent with mutant type)
- **p53**: positive, >60% (immunohistochemistry; consistent with mutant type)

**Key points**

- Astrocytoma= *IDH+/ATRX* loss / mutated *TP53*
- Oligodendroglioma = *IDH* mutant/*ATRX* retained/1p/19q co-deleted
- Primary GBM: no IDH mutation/ EGFR/ TERT/PTEN/ TP53
- Secondary GBM: *IDH+/ATRX* loss / mutated *TP53*
- ATRX mutations are strongly associated with IDH mutations and are mutually exclusive with 1p/19q codeletion.

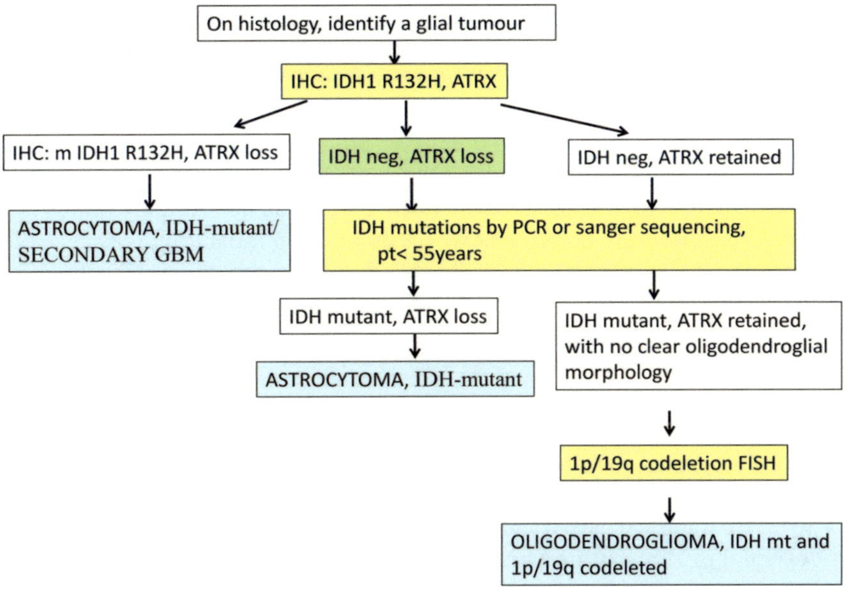


## Author details

Kanwalpreet Kaur
Department of Oncopathology, Gujarat Cancer and Research Institute, Ahmedabad, India

*Address all correspondence to: kanwalpreet.15@gmail.com

## References

[1] Louis D.N.,von Deimling A. Cavenee W.K. Diffuse astrocytic and oligodendroglial tumours. In: Louis D, Ohgaki H, Weistler O, Cavenee W, (eds). WHO Classification of Tumours of the Central Nervous System, 4th edn. Lyon: IARC, 2016; 57

[2] Parsons DW, Jones S, Zhang X, Lin JC, Leary RJ, et al. 2008. An integrated genomic analysis of human glioblastoma multiforme. Science 321:1807-1812

[3] Lenting K, Khurshed M, Peeters TH, Corina N. A. M. van den Heuvel , van Lith SAM et al. Isocitrate dehydrogenase 1–mutated human gliomas depend on lactate and glutamate to alleviate metabolic stress. The FASEB Journal 33(1): fj.201800907RR

[4] Bleeker, F.E.,Atai,N. A., Lamba, S., Jonker,A., Rijkeboer, D.,Bosch, K. S., Tigchelaar, W., Troost, D., Vandertop, W. P., Bardelli, A., and Van Noorden, C. J (2010) The prognostic IDH1( R132 ) mutation is associated with reduced NADP+-dependent IDH activity in glioblastoma. Acta Neuropathol. 119, 487-494

[5] Dang L and Michael Su S. Isocitrate dehydrogenase mutation and (R)-2-Hydroxyglutarate: From basic discovery to therapeutics development. Annu. Rev. Biochem. 2017. 86:18.1-18.27

[6] Yan H, Parsons DW, Jin G, McLendon R, Rasheed BA, et al. 2009. IDH1 and IDH2 mutations in gliomas. N. Engl. J. Med. 360:765-773

[7] Stockhammer F, Misch M, Helms HJ, Lengler U, Prall F, von Deimling A, et al. (2012). IDH1/2 mutations in WHO grade II astrocytomas associated with localization and seizure as the initial symptom. Seizure. 21(3):194-197. PMID:22217666.

[8] Lai A, Kharbanda S, Pope WB, Tran A, Solis OE, Peale F, et al. (2011). Evidence for sequenced molecular evolution of IDH1 mutant glioblastoma from a distinct cell of origin. J ClinOncol. 29(34):4482-90. PMID:22025148

[9] Capper D, Weissert S, Balss J, Habel A, Meyer J, Jäger D, Ackermann U, Tessmer C, Korshunov A, Zentgraf H, Hartmann C, von Deimling A. Characterization of R132H mutation-specific IDH1 antibody binding in brain tumors. Brain Pathol. 2010 Jan;20(1):245-254. doi: 10.1111/j.1750-3639.2009.00352.x. Epub 2009 Oct 27. PMID: 19903171.

[10] Reuss DE, Mamatjan Y, Schrimpf D, Capper D, Hovestadt V, Kratz A, et al. (2015). IDH mutant diffuse and anaplastic astrocytomas have similar age at presentation and little difference in survival: A grading problem for WHO. Acta Neuropathol. 129(6):867-873. PMID:25962792

[11] Pinkham MB, et al., FISHing tips: What every clinician should know about 1p19q analysis in gliomas using fluorescence in situ hybridisation, Clinical Oncology (2015), http://dx.doi.org/10.1016/j.clon.2015.04.008

[12] Wiens AL, Cheng L, Bertsch EC, Johnson KA, Zhang S, Hattab EM. Polysomy of chromosomes 1 and/or 19 is common and associated with less favorable clinical outcome in oligodendrogliomas: Fluorescent in situ hybridization analysis of 84 consecutive cases. J Neuropathol Exp Neurol. 2012;71(7):618-624.

[13] Snuderl M, Eichler AF, Ligon KL, et al. Polysomy for chromosomes 1 and 19 predicts earlier recurrence in anaplastic oligodendrogliomas with concurrent 1p/19q loss. Clin Cancer Res. 2009;15 (20):6430-6437.

[14] Yip S, Butterfield YS, Morozova O, et al. Concurrent CIC mutations, IDH mutations, and 1p/19q loss distinguish oligodendrogliomas from other cancers. J Pathol. 2012;226(1):7-16

[15] Marko NF, Weil RJ. A case for reclassifying infiltrating gliomas in adults. J Neurooncol 2012;109(3): 587e591.

[16] Jenkins RB, Blair H, Ballman KV, et al. A t(1;19)(q10;p10) mediates the combined deletions of 1p and 19q and predicts a better prognosis of patients with oligodendroglioma. CancerRes 2006;66(20):9852e9861.

[17] Nandakumar P, Mansouri A and Das S. The role of ATRX in glioma biology. Front. Oncol. 2013.7:236.

[18] Heaphy CM, de Wilde RF, Jiao Y, Klein AP, Edil BH, Shi C, et al. (2011). Altered telomeres in tumors with ATRX and DAXX mutations. Science. 333(6041 ):425. PMID:21719641

[19] Leeper HE, Caron AA, Decker PA, Jenkins RB, Lachance D, Giannini C. IDH mutation, 1p19q codeletion and ATRX loss in WHO grade II gliomas. Oncotarget (2015) 6(30):30295-30305. doi:10.18632/oncotarget.4497.

[20] Wiestler B, Capper D, Holland-Letz T, Korshunov A, Von Deimling A, Pfister SM, et al. ATRX loss refines the classification of anaplastic gliomas and identifies a subgroup of IDH mutant astrocytic tumors with better prognosis. Acta Neuropathol (2013) 126(3):443-451. doi:10.1007/s00401-013-1156-z

[21] Roshandel AK, Busch CM, Mullekom JV, Cuoco JA, Rogers CM, Apfel LS, Marvin EA, Sontheimer HW, Umans RA. The predictive capability of immunohistochemistry and DNA sequencing for determining TP53 functional mutation status: a comparative study of 41 glioblastoma patients. Oncotarget. 2019 Oct 22;10(58):6204-6218. doi: 10.18632/oncotarget.27252. PMID: 31692772; PMCID: PMC6817445.

[22] Murnyák B, Hortobágyi T. Immunohistochemical correlates of TP53 somatic mutations in cancer. Oncotarget. 2016 Oct 4;7(40):64910-64920. doi: 10.18632/oncotarget.11912. PMID: 27626311; PMCID: PMC5323125.

[23] Arita H, Narita Y, Fukushima S, Tateishi K, Matsushita Y, Yoshida A, Miyakita Y, Ohno M, Collins VP, Kawahara N, Shibui S, Ichimura K. Upregulating mutations in the TERT promoter commonly occur in adult malignant gliomas and are strongly associated with total 1p19q loss. Acta Neuropathol. 2013 Aug;126(2):267-276. doi: 10.1007/s00401-013-1141-6. Epub 2013 Jun 14. PMID: 23764841.

[24] Eckel-Passow JE, Lachance DH, Molinaro AM, Walsh KM, Decker PA, Sicotte H, Pekmezci M, Rice T, Kosel ML, Smirnov IV, Sarkar G, Caron AA, Kollmeyer TM, Praska CE, Chada AR, Halder C, Hansen HM, McCoy LS, Bracci PM, Marshall R, Zheng S, Reis GF, Pico AR, O'Neill BP, Buckner JC, Giannini C, Huse JT, Perry A, Tihan T, Berger MS, Chang SM, Prados MD, Wiemels J, Wiencke JK, Wrensch MR, Jenkins RB. Glioma Groups Based on 1p/19q, IDH, and TERT Promoter Mutations in Tumors. N Engl J Med. 2015 Jun 25;372(26):2499-508. doi: 10.1056/NEJMoa1407279. Epub 2015 Jun 10. PMID: 26061753; PMCID: PMC4489704.

[25] Smith JS, Tachibana I, Passe SM, et al. PTEN mutation, EGFR amplification, and outcome in patients with anaplastic astrocytoma and glioblastoma multiforme. J Natl Cancer Inst. 2001;93(16):1246-1256.

[26] Gonzalez Castro LN, Wesseling P. The cIMPACT-NOW updates and their significance to current neuro-oncology

practice. Neurooncol Pract. 2020 Aug 29;8(1):4-10. doi: 10.1093/nop/npaa055. PMID: 33664964; PMCID: PMC7906262.

[27] Shirahata M, Ono T, Stichel D, et al. Novel, improved grading system(s) for IDH-mutant astrocytic gliomas. Acta Neuropathol. 2018;136(1):1-14. doi:10.1007/s00401-018-1849-4

[28] Esteller M, Garcia-Foncillas J, Andion E, Goodman SN, Hidalgo OF, Vanaclocha V, Baylin SB, Herman JG. Inactivation of the DNA-repair gene MGMT and the clinical response of gliomas to alkylating agents. N Engl J Med. 2000 Nov 9;343(19):1350-4. doi: 10.1056/NEJM200011093431901. Erratum in: N Engl J Med 2000 Dec 7;343(23):1740. PMID: 11070098.

[29] Brat DJ, Verhaak RG, Aldape KD, Yung WK, Salama SR, Cooper LA, et al.; Cancer Genome Atlas Research Network (2015). Comprehensive, Integrative Genomic Analysis of Diffuse Lower-Grade Gliomas. N Engl J Med.372(26):2481-98. PMID:26061751

[30] Chen L, Voronovich Z, Clark K, Hands I, Mannas J, Walsh M, et al. (2014). Predicting the likelihood of an isocitrate dehydrogenase 1 or 2 mutation in diagnoses of infiltrative glioma. Neuro Oncol. 16(11):1478-1483. PMID:24860178

[31] Brennan CW, Verhaak RG, McKenna A, Campos B, Noushmehr H, Salama SR, et al.; TCGA Research Network (2013). The somatic genomic landscape of glioblastoma. Cell. 155(2):462-77. PMID:24120142

[32] Ohgaki H, Kleihues P (2013). The definition of primary and secondary glioblastoma. ClinCancerRes. 19(4): 764-772. PMID:23209033

[33] Labussiere M, Idbaih A, Wang XW et al. All the 1p19q codeleted gliomas are mutated on IDH1 or IDH2. Neurology 2010, 74(23):1886-1890

[34] Keser H, Barnes M, Moes G, Lee HS, Tihan T (2014). Well-differentiated pediatric glial neoplasms with features of oligodendroglioma, angiocentric glioma and dysembryoplastic neuroepithelial tumors: A morphological diagnostic challenge. Turk Patoloji Derg. 30(1 ):23-29. PMID:24448703

[35] Zhang J, Wu G, Miller CP, Tatevossian RG, Dalton JD, Tang B, et al.; St. Jude Children's Research Hospital-Washington University Pediatric Cancer Genome Project (2013). Whole-genome sequencing identifies genetic alterations in pediatric low-grade gliomas. Nat Genet. 45(6):602-12.PMID23583981

[36] Rao S, Kanuri NN, Nimbalkar V, Arivazhagan A, Santosh V. High frequency of H3K27M immunopositivity in adult thalamic glioblastoma. Neuropathology. 2019 Apr;39(2):78-84. doi: 10.1111/neup.12537. PMID: 30937985.

Section 5

# Genetics of CNS Tumors

Chapter 9

# Annexin A1-Binding Carbohydrate Mimetic Peptide Targets Drugs to Brain Tumors

*Michiko N. Fukuda, Misa Suzuki-Anekoji and Motohiro Nonaka*

## Abstract

Annexin A1 (Anxa1) is expressed specifically on the surface of the tumor vasculature. Previously, we demonstrated that a carbohydrate-mimetic peptide, designated IF7, bound to the Anxa1 N-terminal domain. Moreover, intravenously injected IF7 targeted the tumor vasculature in mouse and crossed tumor endothelia cells to stroma via transcytosis. Thus, we hypothesized that IF7 could overcome the blood–brain barrier to reach brain tumors. Our studies in brain tumor model mice showed that IF7 conjugated with the anti-cancer drug SN38 suppressed brain tumor growth with high efficiency. Furthermore IF7-SN38-treated mice mounted an immune response to brain tumors established by injected tumor cells and shrank those tumors in part by recruiting cytotoxic T-cells to the injection site. These results suggest that Anxa1-binding peptide IF7 represents a drug delivery vehicle useful to treat malignant brain tumors. This chapter describes the unique development of IF7-SN38 as a potential breakthrough cancer chemotherapeutic.

**Keywords:** carbohydrate mimetic peptides, phage display, annexin 1(Anxa1), blood–brain barrier (BBB), glioblastoma, chemotherapy, SN-38, CPT-11, geldanamycin (GA), cytotoxic T cell, CD8

## 1. Introduction

Brain malignancies are difficult to treat due to the blood–brain barrier (BBB), a layer of endothelial cells that separates the circulation from the brain and protects the central nervous system from pathogens and toxic materials [1, 2]. Although brain tumor cells cultured *in vitro* respond to several anti-cancer drugs, brain tumors *in vivo* do not due to the BBB. Chemotherapeutic drugs capable of passing the BBB are small lipopholic molecules of less than 500 Da [3], as exemplified by temozolomide [4–6]. Numerous investigators have attempted to overcome this hurdle using brain vasculature surface receptor-mediated proteins [7, 8], tumor-penetrating peptides [4, 9, 10], or nanoparticles [11, 12]. However, these attempts have not yet achieved clinically satisfactory results. On the other hand, tumor vasculature surrounding a brain tumor is chaotic, allowing large molecules and nanoparticles to overcome the BBB by passing through gaps between endothelial cells [13]. However, as this approach relies on passive diffusion, drugs must be administered at the maximum tolerable dose, causing adverse side effects.


IntechOpen

Thus, efficient treatment of brain tumors requires both tumor vasculature targeting and penetration by a therapeutic to overcome the BBB. In this chapter, we describe the carbohydrate mimetic 7-mer peptide IF7, which serves as a highly specific tumor vasculature-targeting vehicle. When conjugated to the anti-cancer drug SN-38 and injected into mouse brain tumor models, IF7-SN38 has a potent anti-tumor effect. IF7-SN38 represents a potential breakthrough chemotherapeutic in brain malignancies.

## 2. IF7 peptide: how was it identified?

IF7 is a linear 7-mer peptide with the sequence IFLLWQR [14]. This peptide is considered a carbohydrate mimetic, as it was identified in studies of cancer cell surface carbohydrates [15, 16]. Epithelial cancer cells express complex carbohydrate antigens, and some serve as ligands for carbohydrate binding proteins known as selectins. We hypothesized that interaction between selectin and selectin ligand functions in carbohydrate-dependent tumor cells colonization to the lung [17], in a manner similar to that seen in selectin-dependent hematogenous liver metastasis [18, 19].

Our goal, however, was challenging, as chemical synthesis of oligosaccharides as elaborate as the selectin ligand involved tedious, time-consuming and therefore expensive steps. To overcome this problem, we used phage display technology to identify carbohydrate mimetic peptides that might function as an E-selectin ligand. However, initially when we used E-selectin as the target, we did not obtain a phage clone. We then took a different approach and screened peptides for ability to bind

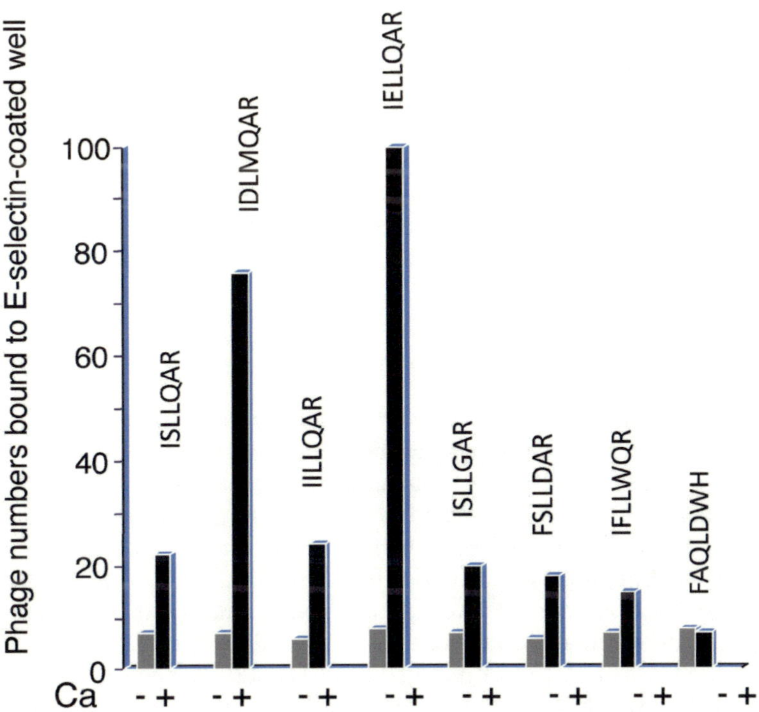


**Figure 1.**
*E-selectin binding of linear 7-mer peptide sequences. Phage clones were selected by mouse monoclonal anti-Lewis A antibody (clone 7LE). Each cloned phage was added to microtiter plate wells coated with E-selectin-IgG chimeric protein. Phage binding to E-selectin was tested in the presence or absence of 1 mM $CaCl_2$. The best binder, IELLQAR, was designated I-peptide.*

anti-carbohydrate antibodies that recognize E-selectin ligands or related carbohydrates. Using this approach, we succeeded in identifying a linear 7-mer peptide from a phage display library. Since carbohydrate antigen specificity is determined by 3–4 carbohydrate residues of 600–800 Da, we assumed that a 7-mer peptide of 770 Da would mimic a carbohydrate antigen. The phage library screening yielded a series of peptides with the consensus sequence IXLLXXR [15] (**Figure 1**).

Among those peptides, the strongest binder to E-selectin was IELLQAR, which we designated I-peptide. Chemically synthesized I-peptide inhibited hematogenous colonization of the tumor cells to the lung in mouse [15]. However, in E/P-selectin doubly-deficient mice, tumor cells expressing selectin ligand carbohydrate colonized the lung, and that colonization was inhibited by I-peptide [20]. These results indicated that I-peptide receptor is not an E- or P-selectin and raised the question of what receptor I-peptide bound to in lung vasculature?

To identify the I-peptide receptor, we injected mice intravenously with a biotinylation reagent plus I-peptide-displaying phage or controls. We then isolated lung tissue and immunoprecipitated lysates with rabbit anti-phage antibody or control IgG. When we resolved immunoprecipitates on SDS-PAGE, we detected two *in vivo* biotinylated proteins as 40 kDa and 20 kDa bands on a peroxidase avidin blot (**Figure 2**). We isolated respective candidate receptor proteins from lung membrane fractions using I-peptide affinity chromatography and proteomic analysis and

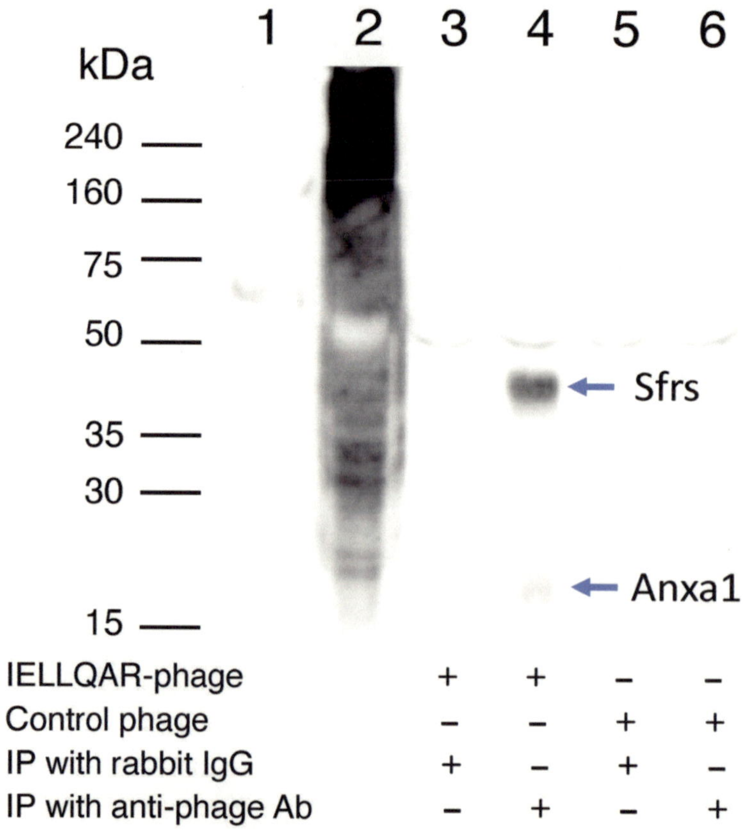


**Figure 2.**
*Detection of I-peptide receptor(s) on the surface of lung endothelial cells by* in vivo *biotinylation. Mice were injected intravenously with either PBS (lane 1) or a biotinylation reagent (lanes 2–6), followed by intravenous injection of I-peptide-displaying (lanes 3 and 4) or control (lanes 5 and 6) phage. After perfusion of mice with PBS, lungs were isolated and phage was immunoprecipitated with rabbit anti-phage antibody (lanes 4 and 6) or rabbit IgG (lane 3 and 5). Immunoprecipitates were resolved on SDS-PAGE and biotinylated proteins detected using a peroxidase avidin blot.*

found them to be the pre-mRNA splicing factor (Sfrs) and annexin A1 (Anxa1) [21]. Recombinant Sfrs proteins showed binding to I-peptide and a series of carbohydrates, whose structures overlapped with selectin ligand [21].

Full-length Anxa1 is 37 kDa; therefore, we considered the 20 kDa band seen in **Figure 2** to be a fragment of the full-length protein. By the time we identified Anxa1 fragments, Oh *et al.* had undertaken rigorous subtractive proteomics analysis and identified Anxa1 as a specific vasculature surface marker of malignant tumors [22]. Thus, we hypothesized that I-peptide or related peptides could serve as tumor vasculature-specific drug delivery vehicles via binding to Anxa1. We then rescreened a series of phage clones for tumor-targeting activity and identified an Anxa1-binding, but not Sfrs-binding, phage clone displaying IFLLWQR peptide (**Figure 3**). Moreover, tumor targeting was inhibited in the presence of an anti-Anxa1 antibody specific to the N-terminal region (**Figure 4**) [21].

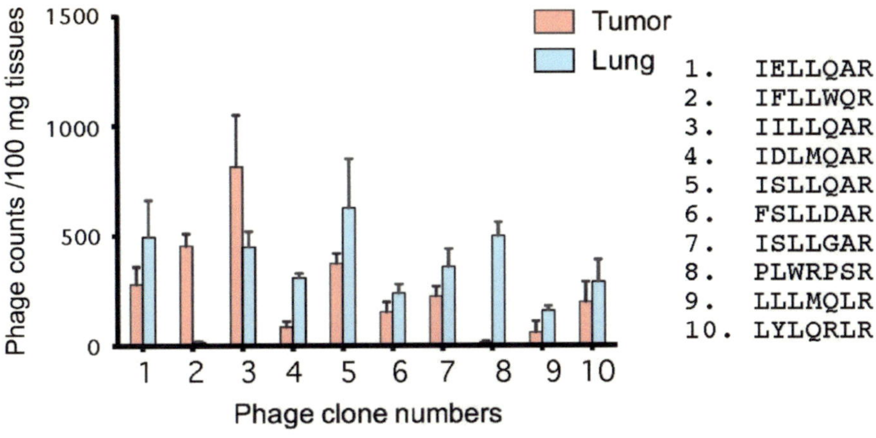


**Figure 3.**
In vivo *phage targeting specificity to tumor and normal lung. Subcutaneous B16 tumor-bearing mice were intravenously injected with each phage clone, and phage number in the tumor and lung was determined by a colony-forming assay. Note that IFLLWQR- or IF7 peptide-displaying phage exclusively targeted the tumor but not lung tissue.*

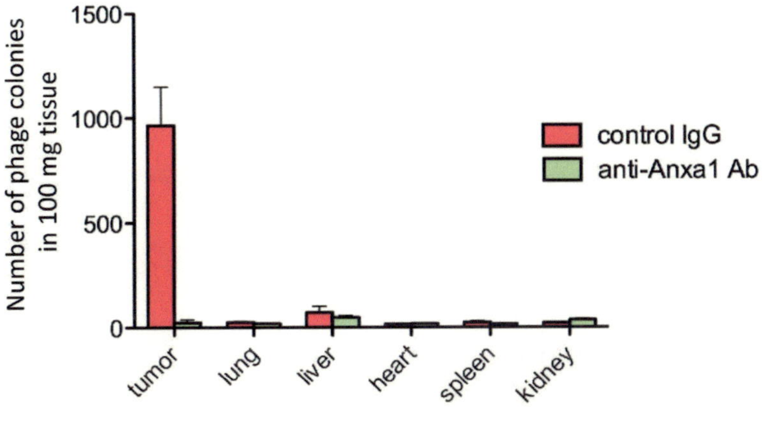


**Figure 4.**
In vivo *tumor and organ targeting by IF7-peptide-displaying phage. IF7-displaying phage were injected intravenously into subcutaneous B16 tumor-bearing mice. Note that IF7-displaying phage targeted the tumor but not normal organs. Tumor targeting by IF7 phage was inhibited by pre-injection of mice with rabbit polyclonal anti-Anxa1 (N-19) antibody directed to the Anxa1 N-terminal domain but not by injection with control rabbit IgG.*

## 3. Targeting the tumor vasculature by IF7 peptide

Next, to visualize tumor targeting by chemically synthesized IF7 peptide, we used intravital microscopy, in which tumor was implanted in a dorsal skinfold chamber [23] visualized tumor vasculature targeting of IF7 under fluorescence microscopy. Green fluorescent Alexa 488-labeled IF7 was injected intravenously and green fluorescent signals were recorded over time by video [14]. Fluorescence appeared in the tumor within 30 sec of injection and increased over time (**Figure 5**). Analysis of tumor tissue sections taken 15 minutes after A488-IF7 injection indicated fluorescent signals as a punctate staining pattern over endothelial cells (**Figure 6**, upper). By 40 min, green fluorescence had moved to the stroma (**Figure 6**, lower), suggesting that IF7 passed through endothelial cells and penetrated the tumor stroma where cancer cells reside. The punctate appearance of Alexa 488 staining suggests that IF7-bound to Anxa1 is internalized by endothelial cells, possibly in vesicles. Anxa1 on the tumor vasculature surface reportedly localizes in caveolae and, when bound by anti-Anxa1 antibody, the complex is internalized into vesicles transported to the basal surface via transcytosis [24]. Accordingly, we concluded that IF7 bound to Anxa1 on the tumor vasculature was transported from the luminal surface to the basal membrane via transcytosis through endothelial cells and likely released to the tumor stroma. Therefore, we asked whether IF7-conjugated chemotherapeutics could cross the BBB to deliver a cytotoxic drug to brain stroma.

To test this possibility we injected A488-IF7 through the tail vein into brain tumor-bearing mice and then prepared sections of mouse brain tissue 20 minutes later. Fluorescence microscopy analysis revealed bright fluorescence in tumor tissue [25]. At higher magnification A488-IF7 fluorescent signals were evident in cytoplasm and/or nuclei of cancer cells. Micrographs of representative organs from the same mouse showed no significant fluorescent signals in normal organs. Brain tumors and representative organs from an animal injected with A488-C(RR) peptide control showed background fluorescence. These results strongly suggest that intravenously-injected IF7 crosses the BBB to target and penetrate brain tumor vasculature and reach cancer cells [25].

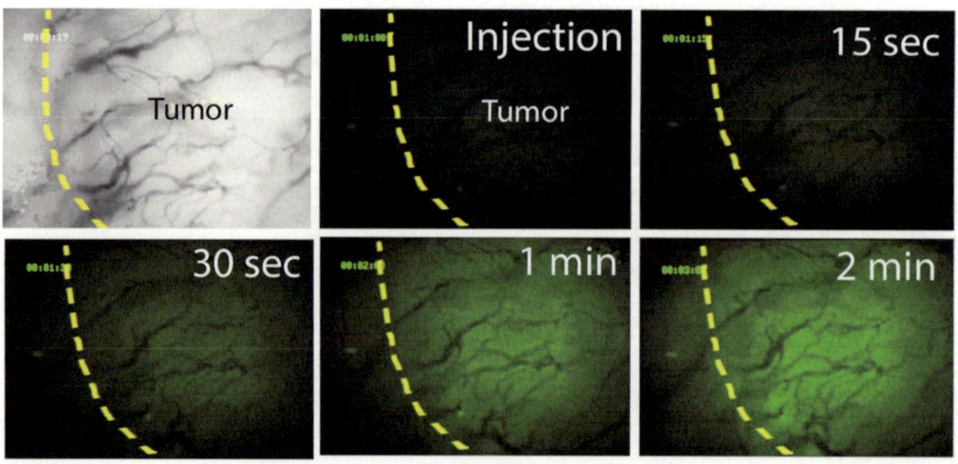


**Figure 5.**
*Intravital microscopy of Alexa 488-conjugated IF7 peptide. Mouse lung carcinoma LL/2 tumors were inoculated in the skin of nude mice of a dorsal skin-fold chamber [23]. A488-IF7 was injected intravenously and green fluorescent signals were video-recorded and detected at the indicated times.*

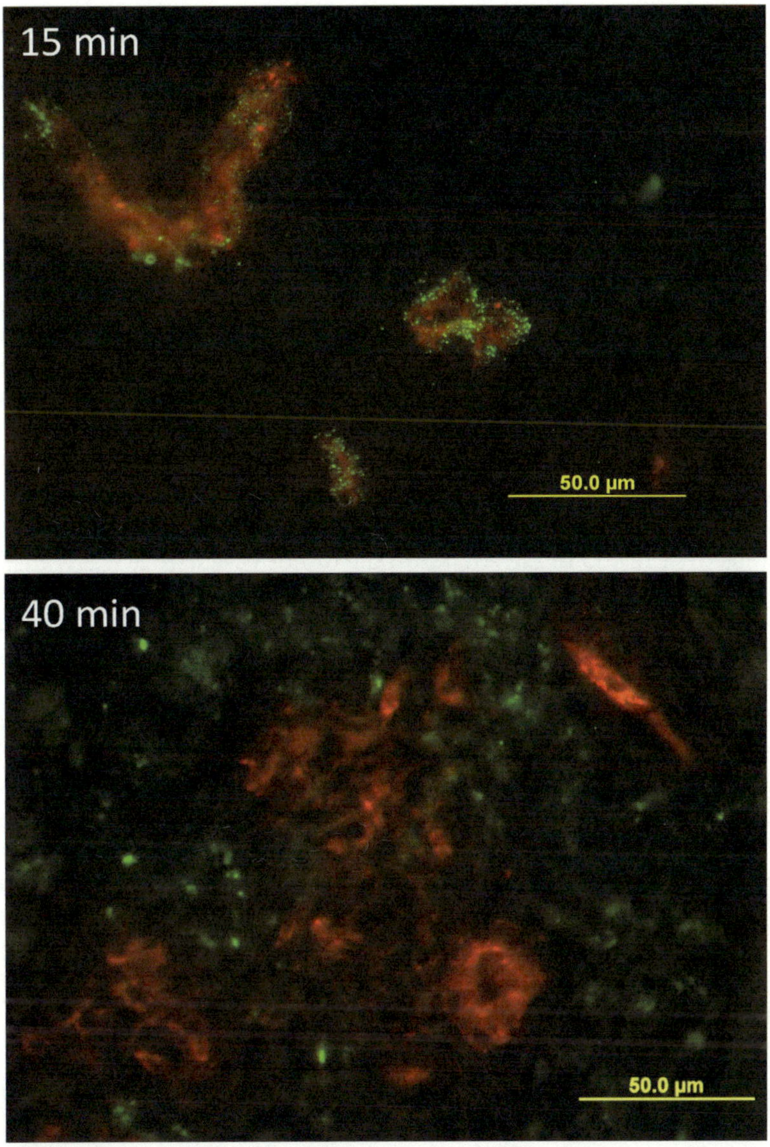


**Figure 6.**
*Fluorescence micrograms of subcutaneous B16 tumor sections from mice intravenously-injected with A488-IF7. Tissue sections taken at 15 (upper) and 40 (lower) min after A488-IF7 injection were stained by anti-CD34 antibody plus red fluorescence-conjugated secondary antibody to mark endothelial cells. Note that at 15 min, green IF7 signals are seen as punctate signals over endothelial cells, whereas at 40 min IF7 signals are in the stroma and seen as diffuse green fluorescence.*

## 4. The ANXA1 N-terminal domain is present on the tumor vasculature surface

Several lines of evidence suggest that IF7 binds to human and mouse Anxa1 at the N-terminal domain. First, an IF7 peptide-displaying phage clone failed to bind full-length recombinant ANXA protein when the N-terminus was blocked by a His6-tag, whereas IF7 bound to full-length ANXA1 that was C-terminally tagged with His6 [14]. Second, IF7 bound to full-length ANXA1 but not to an N-terminal deletion delta 27 mutant [14]. Third, when IF7 peptide-displaying phage was injected intravenously into a tumor-bearing mouse, phage targeted the tumor

vasculature, but that binding was blocked in comparable mice injected with an antibody raised against the ANXA1 N-terminal domain (**Figure 4**) [14]. Finally, *in vitro* binding assays showed that synthetic IF7 bound to a synthetic peptide representing the ANXA1 N-terminal domain (designated MC16), which includes 15 amino acids from $Met^{1}$ to $Glu^{15}$, plus a C-terminal Cys [25]. IF7 bound to both mouse and human MC16 peptides.

The molecular weight of full-length Anxa1 is 37 kDa, but Western blotting of endothelial plasma membranes and caveolae isolated from tumors detected a 34 kDa band [24]. Proteomics analysis of this 34 kDa protein suggested that it may lack the N-terminal domain. To determine whether the Anxa1 N-terminal domain is on the tumor vasculature surface, we generated a mouse monoclonal antibody specific to the human ANXA1 N-terminal domain (or MC16 peptide). Immunohistochemical analysis of various clinical specimens with anti-MC16 antibody revealed positive signals located at endothelial cells lining malignant tumor tissues in specimens from prostate, breast, lung, liver, ovarian and brain cancers [25], indicating that the ANXA1 N-terminus is present on endothelial cells in many human malignancies. Immunostaining alone did not reveal whether the antigen was on the cell surface or in the cytoplasm.

We confirmed that the MC16 domain was present on the luminal side of the plasma membrane by *in vivo* biotinylation of mouse brain tumors followed by immunoprecipitation by anti-MC16 antibody and proteomics analysis [25]. Plate binding assays of precipitates indicated high levels of biotinylated materials bound by the anti-MC16 antibody in tumor lysates, whereas biotinylated materials in tumor lysates treated with control antibody or those from normal liver tissue lysates showed significantly lower levels of biotinylated material. However, when immunoprecipitates from these tumors were analyzed on a protein gel followed by an avidin blot, we did not detect biotinylated proteins, whereas proteomics analysis had revealed predominantly Anxa1 peptide fragments [25]. We conclude that the Anxa1 N-terminal domain is cleaved from the rest of the protein and displayed on the tumor vasculature surface as a peptide fragment too small to be detected on a Western blot.

## 5. Therapeutic activity of IF7 conjugated to the anti-cancer drug SN-38 against brain tumors

Both we and others have reported that IF7-conjugated drugs show efficient anti-tumor activity in mouse models of tumors other than brain tumors. Examples include IF7-conjugated geldanamycin (GA) against prostate, lung, and breast cancers as well as melanoma [21], IF7-SN38 against colon cancer [21], IF7-taxol against breast cancer [26] and IF7-conjugated10B with boron neutron capture therapy against bladder carcinoma [27]. Below we focus on our studies of the effect of IF7-SN38 on mouse brain tumor models.

To target brain tumors, we chose to conjugate IF7 to SN-38, the active component of irinotecan (CPT-11), which is used clinically to treat brain cancer [28, 29]. To compare IF7-SN38 dosages we employed a dual-tumor model, in which a single mouse receives luciferase gene-transfected cancer cells in brain and under the skin (**Figure 7**). Growth of tumors in both regions was quantitatively monitored using an IVIS imager to detect photon numbers produced by luciferase. Once tumors were formed in the brain and under the skin, the dual tumor model mice were injected intravenously with IF7-SN38 and tumor growth in both locations was assessed *in vivo* by photon number. IF7-SN38 treatment significantly suppressed tumor growth relative to buffer controls in both brain and under the skin at a dosage of

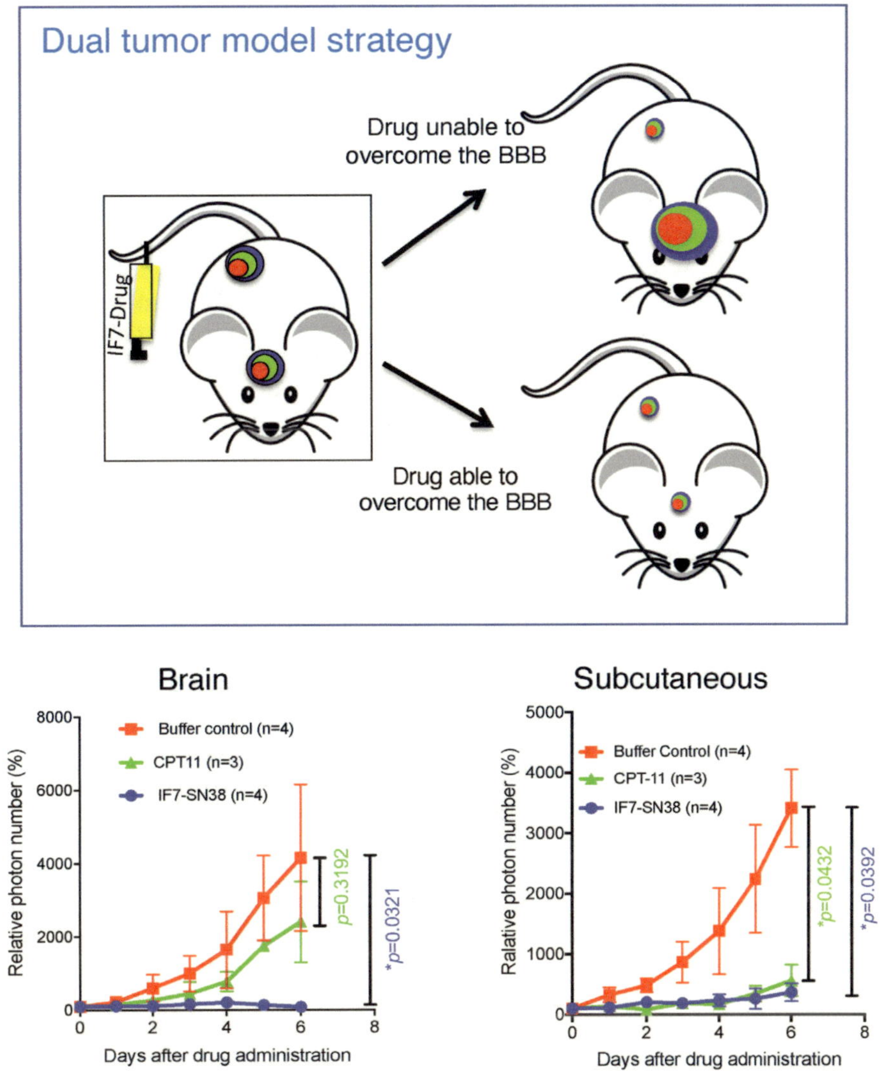


**Figure 7.**
*Analysis of whether IF7-SN38 overcomes the blood–brain barrier using a dual tumor mouse model. (upper) schematic showing that single mice established to harbor both brain and subcutaneous tumors are injected with IF7-conjugated drug through the tail vein. If the drug cannot overcome the BBB, only subcutaneous tumors are eradicated; if drug overcomes the BBB, growth of both is suppressed. (lower) graphs show that daily injection of IF7-SN38 (7.0 μmoles/kg) suppressed both brain (left) and subcutaneous (right) tumor growth. Moreover, CPT-11, the SN-38 pro-drug, suppressed growth of subcutaneous tumors at high dosage (50 μmoles/kg) [25].*

3.15 μmoles/kg. Moreover we found using either C6-Luc cells in SCID mice or B16-Luc cells in C57BL/6 mice, intravenously-injected IF7-SN38 significantly antagonized growth of brain and subcutaneous tumors relative to controls at a dosage of 7.0 μmoles/kg. When we performed similar experiments using the SN38 prodrug irinotecan alone at doses as high as 50 μmoles/kg, irinotecan suppressed subcutaneous tumor growth but only minimally suppressed brain tumor growth. Overall, these results indicate that in the mouse dual tumor models tested here, IF7-SN38 suppresses brain tumor growth as effectively as subcutaneous tumor growth.

For the dual tumor model experiments (**Figure** 7), we had dissolved IF7-SN38 in Cremophore EL, a non-ionic detergent used clinically to administer taxol, prior to injection. However, there are concerns about potential inflammatory effects of this detergent [30, 31]. Thus, we conducted experiments in which we dissolved

IF7-SN38 in 10% Solutol HS15, a non-ionic surfactant with low toxicity. The therapeutic effect of IF7-SN38 in 10% Solutol HS15 improved significantly relative to administration with Cremophore EL (**Figure 8A**): B16 brain tumors began shrinking during the first week of daily injections at dosages as low as 2.5 μmoles/kg, continued shrinking during the second week without drug injection, and then completely disappeared. Mice survived for more than 3 months after cessation of drug treatment without showing signs of B16-Luc cell growth in brain or other parts of their body, suggesting complete remission and potential involvement of host immune systems.

Relevant to potential immunogenicity, when we injected cells of either one of two isogenic lines, B16-Luc or LL/2-Luc, subcutaneously into naïve C57BL/6 mice, both lines produced tumors at injected site. By contrast, when either of these lines were injected into mice that had recovered from brain B16-Luc tumors, LL/2-Luc tumors grew but B16-Luc tumors did not (**Figure 8B**). The presence of tumor-infiltrating lymphocytes, especially $CD8^+$ cytotoxic T cells, is correlates with better

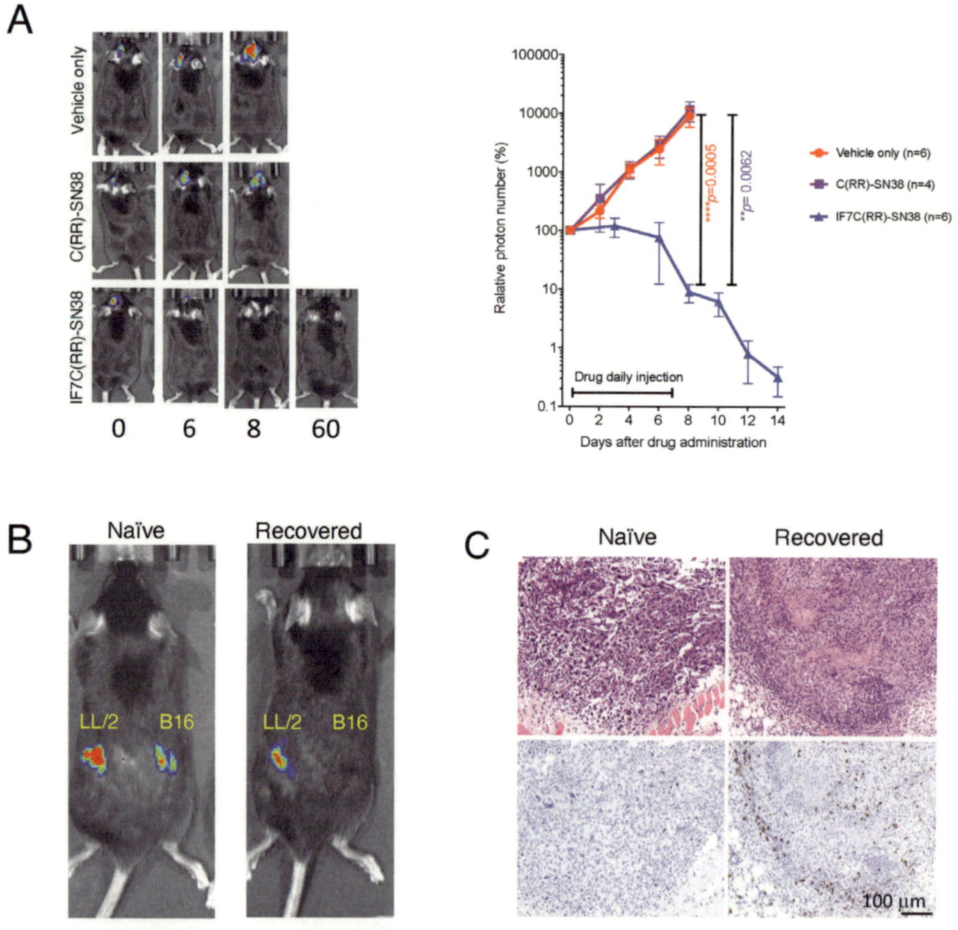


**Figure 8.**
*IF7-SN38 treatment promotes complete remission of B16 brain tumors and a host immune response against tumor cells. (A) Effect of IF7-SN38 on B16-Luc brain tumors in isogeneic C57BL/6 mice. Drug dosage was 2.5 μmoles/kg each for IF7-SN38 and control C(RR)-SN38 diluted with 10% Solutol HS15 in water and administered daily for 7 days. Note that brain tumors continued shrinking after cessation of IF7-SN38 administration in C56BL/6 mice. (B) Growth of two syngeneic cancer lines in naïve and brain-tumor-recovered mice 4 days after subcutaneous injection of LL/2-Luc and B16-Luc cells. (C) Immunohistochemistry with anti-CD8 antibody of B16-Luc cells at subcutaneous injection sites, 20 hours after B16-Luc cell injection.*

prognosis of various cancers [32, 33]. Immunohistochemistry of subcutaneous B16-Luc injection site using an anti-CD8 antibody 20 hours after injection of naïve C57BL/6 mice with B16-Luc cells revealed a minimal number of $CD8^{+}$ T cells at challenged sites. By contrast, we observed significant $CD8^{+}$ cell infiltration at injection sites of B16-Luc cells in C57BL/6 mice that had recovered from B16-Luc brain tumors following IF7-SN38 treatment (**Figure 8C**). Thus it is likely that IF7-SN38 therapy leads to complete remission in part by promoting immunological rejection of tumor cells by the host, preventing tumor recurrence elsewhere in the body.

## 6. Clinical application of IF7-SN38

As described, in mouse the Anxa1 N-terminal domain is present on the surface of tumor vasculature as peptide fragments. Nonetheless, such fragments should serve an IF7 receptor, as either the first 15 amino acid residues of ANXA1 or synthetic MC16 peptide is sufficient for IF7 binding [25]. IF7 binds both human and mouse MC16 peptides equally, suggesting that our results with IF7 in mouse tumor models are relevant to humans.

Although IF7-conjugated drugs are effective in various cancer types [14, 26, 27], their effectiveness against brain malignancies may be particularly high as gene expression data indicates *ANXA1* overexpression in brain tumors [34, 35], a finding supported by immunohistochemistry with anti-MC16 antibody [25]. Moreover, as IF7 targets tumor vasculature and overcomes the BBB, IF7-conjugated drug would accumulate in brain tumor cells, a critical advantage over low molecular weight drugs like temozolomide, which does not target brain tumors and must be administered at high doses (**Figure 9**).

We found the effective dosage of IF7-SN38 in the mouse brain tumor models to be 2.5 μmoles (5.35 mg)/kg (**Figure 8**), which translates into a human equivalent [36] of 0.43 mg/kg or SN-38 0.079 mg. This dosage is considerably lower than that currently recommended for CPT-11 (the SN-38 pro-drug) administered to cancer patients, namely, 120 ~ 200 mg/$m^2$ or 2.91 ~ 4.85 mg/kg [37, 38]. Anticipated doses of IF7-SN38 in humans are also unlikely to be toxic at pharmacologically active dosage.

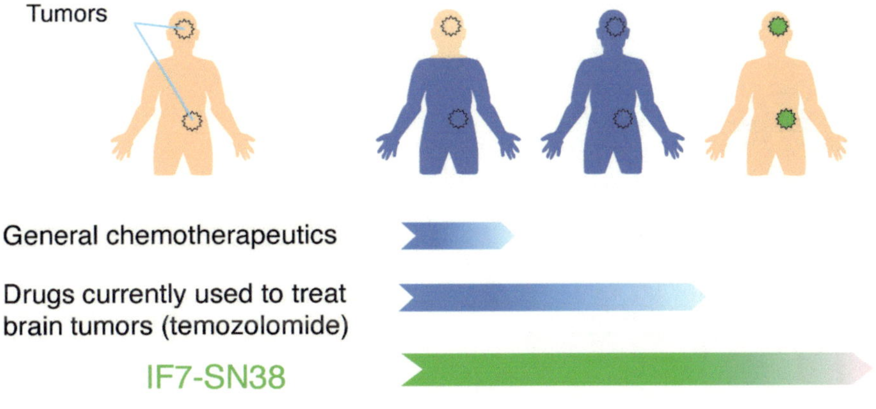


**Figure 9.**
*Mode of action of chemotherapeutics directed against brain tumors. General chemotherapeutics do not penetrate brain tumors due to the BBB and thus are administered to patients at high dosage. Some low molecular weight chemotherapeutics such as temozolomide penetrates the brain but requires high dosage, because temozolomide does not target brain tumors. IF7-SN38 targets brain tumors and overcomes the BBB. At low dosage, IF7-SN38 becomes concentrated in tumors, including brain tumors, and exhibits therapeutic activity.*

## 7. Conclusions and future perspectives

Historically, reagents like IF7 emerged with the advent of carbohydrate mimetic peptides [15, 16]. The surprising finding that Anxa1 is an I-peptide receptor led us to identify IF7 [14, 21]. When IF7 was injected intravenously into brain tumor-bearing mice, it targeted tumor vasculature by binding the Anxa1 N-terminal domain and then crossed the vasculature via transcytosis, to overcome the BBB. Due to its highly specific tumor vasculature targeting activity, IF7-SN38 eradicated brain tumors at low dosage, initiating an immune reaction against cancer cells, followed by complete remission of brain tumors [25]. A similar host immune reaction was also found in IF7-conjugated boron neutron capture therapy in a mouse bladder carcinoma model [27].

IF7-SN38 is, however, susceptible to esterases and proteases. To circumvent stability issues, we have developed an ANXA1-binding D-peptide, designated dTIT7 [39]. We have found that GA-dTIT7, in which geldanamycin is conjugated to dTIT7 through an esterase-resistant linker, is orally administrable and suppresses brain tumor growth in the mouse.

Cancer treatments are increasingly expensive due to development of sophisticated diagnostics and therapies. IF7-SN38 can be chemically synthesized cost-effectively and is stable as a dry powder. Furthermore, orally-administrable peptide-conjugated drugs would be advantageous in societies that lack infrastructure required for costly treatment. Further development of peptide-conjugated drugs could reveal additional candidates with clinical applications against intractable cancers.

## Acknowledgements

We thank Dr. Elise Lamar for her editing of the manuscript.

## Conflict of interest

The authors declare no conflict of interest.

## Author details

Michiko N. Fukuda*, Misa Suzuki-Anekoji and Motohiro Nonaka
Sanford-Burnham-Prebys Medical Discovery Institute, California, USA

*Address all correspondence to: michiko@sbpdiscovery.org

## References

[1] Abbott NJ, Patabendige AA, Dolman DE, Yusof SR, Begley DJ. Structure and function of the blood-brain barrier. Neurobiol Dis. 2010;37(1):13-25. doi: 10.1016/j.nbd.2009.07.030. PubMed PMID: 19664713.

[2] Pardridge WM. The blood-brain barrier: bottleneck in brain drug development. NeuroRx. 2005;2(1):3-14. doi: 10.1602/neurorx.2.1.3. PubMed PMID: 15717053; PubMed Central PMCID: PMC539316.

[3] Pardridge WM. CNS drug design based on principles of blood-brain barrier transport. J Neurochem. 1998;70(5):1781-1792. Epub 1998/05/08. doi: 10.1046/j.1471-4159.1998.70051781.x. PubMed PMID: 9572261.

[4] Przystal JM, Waramit S, Pranjol MZI, Yan W, Chu G, Chongchai A, et al. Efficacy of systemic temozolomide-activated phage-targeted gene therapy in human glioblastoma. EMBO Mol Med. 2019;11(4). Epub 2019/02/28. doi: 10.15252/emmm.201708492. PubMed PMID: 30808679; PubMed Central PMCID: PMCPMC6460351.

[5] Pesce GA, Klingbiel D, Ribi K, Zouhair A, von Moos R, Schlaeppi M, et al. Outcome, quality of life and cognitive function of patients with brain metastases from non-small cell lung cancer treated with whole brain radiotherapy combined with gefitinib or temozolomide. A randomised phase II trial of the Swiss Group for Clinical Cancer Research (SAKK 70/03). Eur J Cancer. 2012;48(3):377-384. Epub 2011/11/19. doi: 10.1016/j.ejca.2011.10.016. PubMed PMID: 22093943.

[6] Zhu W, Zhou L, Qian JQ, Qiu TZ, Shu YQ, Liu P. Temozolomide for treatment of brain metastases: A review of 21 clinical trials. World J Clin Oncol. 2014;5(1):19-27. Epub 2014/02/15. doi: 10.5306/wjco.v5.i1.19. PubMed PMID: 24527399; PubMed Central PMCID: PMCPMC3920177.

[7] Spencer BJ, Verma IM. Targeted delivery of proteins across the blood-brain barrier. Proc Natl Acad Sci U S A. 2007;104(18):7594-7599. doi: 10.1073/pnas.0702170104. PubMed PMID: 17463083; PubMed Central PMCID: PMC1857226.

[8] Hui EK, Boado RJ, Pardridge WM. Tumor necrosis factor receptor-IgG fusion protein for targeted drug delivery across the human blood-brain barrier. Mol Pharm. 2009;6(5):1536-1543. Epub 2009/07/25. doi: 10.1021/mp900103n. PubMed PMID: 19624167.

[9] Sugahara KN, Teesalu T, Karmali PP, Kotamraju VR, Agemy L, Greenwald DR, et al. Coadministration of a tumor-penetrating peptide enhances the efficacy of cancer drugs. Science. 2010;328(5981):1031-1035. Epub 2010/04/10. doi: science.1183057 [pii] 10.1126/science.1183057. PubMed PMID: 20378772.

[10] Agemy L, Friedmann-Morvinski D, Kotamraju VR, Roth L, Sugahara KN, Girard OM, et al. Targeted nanoparticle enhanced proapoptotic peptide as potential therapy for glioblastoma. Proc Natl Acad Sci U S A. 2011. Epub 2011/10/05. doi: 1114518108 [pii] 10.1073/pnas.1114518108. PubMed PMID: 21969599.

[11] Bhaskar S, Tian F, Stoeger T, Kreyling W, de la Fuente JM, Grazu V, et al. Multifunctional Nanocarriers for diagnostics, drug delivery and targeted treatment across blood-brain barrier: perspectives on tracking and neuroimaging. Part Fibre Toxicol. 2010;7:3. doi: 10.1186/1743-8977-7-3. PubMed PMID: 20199661; PubMed Central PMCID: PMC2847536.

[12] Zhou Y, Peng Z, Seven ES, Leblanc RM. Crossing the blood-brain barrier with nanoparticles. J Control Release. 2018;270:290-303. Epub 2017/12/23. doi: 10.1016/j.jconrel.2017.12.015. PubMed PMID: 29269142.

[13] Dhermain FG, Hau P, Lanfermann H, Jacobs AH, van den Bent MJ. Advanced MRI and PET imaging for assessment of treatment response in patients with gliomas. Lancet Neurol. 2010;9(9):906-920. Epub 2010/08/14. doi: 10.1016/S1474-4422(10)70181-2. PubMed PMID: 20705518.

[14] Hatakeyama S, Sugihara K, Shibata TK, Nakayama J, Akama TO, Tamura N, et al. Targeted drug delivery to tumor vasculature by a carbohydrate mimetic peptide. Proc Natl Acad Sci U S A. 2011;108(49):19587-19592. Epub 2011/11/25. doi: 1105057108 [pii] 10.1073/pnas.1105057108. PubMed PMID: 22114188; PubMed Central PMCID: PMC3241764.

[15] Fukuda MN, Ohyama C, Lowitz K, Matsuo O, Pasqualini R, Ruoslahti E, et al. A peptide mimic of E-selectin ligand inhibits sialyl Lewis X-dependent lung colonization of tumor cells. Cancer Res. 2000;60(2):450-456. PubMed PMID: 10667600.

[16] Fukuda MN. Peptide-displaying phage technology in glycobiology. Glycobiology. 2012;22(3):318-325. Epub 2011/09/21. doi: cwr140 [pii] 10.1093/glycob/cwr140. PubMed PMID: 21930649; PubMed Central PMCID: PMC3267529.

[17] Ohyama C, Tsuboi S, Fukuda M. Dual roles of sialyl Lewis X oligosaccharides in tumor metastasis and rejection by natural killer cells. Embo J. 1999;18(6):1516-1525. PubMed PMID: 10075923.

[18] Kannagi R. Carbohydrate-mediated cell adhesion involved in hematogenous metastasis of cancer. Glycoconj J. 1997;14(5):577-584. PubMed PMID: 9298690.

[19] Kannagi R, Izawa M, Koike T, Miyazaki K, Kimura N. Carbohydrate-mediated cell adhesion in cancer metastasis and angiogenesis. Cancer Sci. 2004;95(5):377-384. PubMed PMID: 15132763.

[20] Zhang J, Nakayama J, Ohyama C, Suzuki M, Suzuki A, Fukuda M, et al. Sialyl Lewis X-dependent lung colonization of B16 melanoma cells through a selectin-like endothelial receptor distinct from E- or P-selectin. Cancer Res. 2002;62(15):4194-4198. PubMed PMID: 12154017.

[21] Hatakeyama S, Sugihara K, Nakayama J, Akama TO, Wong SM, Kawashima H, et al. Identification of mRNA splicing factors as the endothelial receptor for carbohydrate-dependent lung colonization of cancer cells. Proc Natl Acad Sci U S A. 2009;106(9):3095-3100. PubMed PMID: 19218444; PubMed Central PMCID: PMC264266.

[22] Oh P, Li Y, Yu J, Durr E, Krasinska KM, Carver LA, et al. Subtractive proteomic mapping of the endothelial surface in lung and solid tumours for tissue-specific therapy. Nature. 2004;429(6992):629-635. PubMed PMID: 15190345.

[23] Lehr HA, Leunig M, Menger MD, Nolte D, Messmer K. Dorsal skinfold chamber technique for intravital microscopy in nude mice. Am J Pathol. 1993;143(4):1055-1062. PubMed PMID: 7692730.

[24] Oh P, Testa JE, Borgstrom P, Witkiewicz H, Li Y, Schnitzer JE. In vivo proteomic imaging analysis of caveolae reveals pumping system to penetrate solid tumors. Nat Med. 2014;20(9):1062-1068. doi: 10.1038/nm.3623. PubMed PMID: 25129480.

[25] Nonaka M, Suzuki-Anekoji M, Nakayama J, Mabashi-Asazuma H, Jarvis DL, Yeh JC, et al. Overcoming the blood-brain barrier by Annexin A1-binding peptide to target brain tumours. Br J Cancer. 2020;123(11):1633-1643. Epub 2020/09/15. doi: 10.1038/s41416-020-01066-2. PubMed PMID: 32921792.

[26] Yu DH, Liu YR, Luan X, Liu HJ, Gao YG, Wu H, et al. IF7-Conjugated Nanoparticles Target Annexin 1 of Tumor Vasculature against P-gp Mediated Multidrug Resistance. Bioconjug Chem. 2015;26(8):1702-1712. Epub 2015/06/16. doi: 10.1021/acs.bioconjchem.5b00283. PubMed PMID: 26076081.

[27] Yoneyama T, Hatakeyama S, Sutoh-Yoneyama M, Yoshiya T, Uemura T, Ishizu T, et al. Tumor vasculature-targeted (10)B delivery by an Annexin A1-binding peptide boosts effects of boron neutron capture therapy. BMC Cancer. 2021;21(1):72. Epub 2021/01/16. doi: 10.1186/s12885-020-07760-x. PubMed PMID: 33446132; PubMed Central PMCID: PMCPMC7809749.

[28] Prados MD, Lamborn K, Yung WK, Jaeckle K, Robins HI, Mehta M, et al. A phase 2 trial of irinotecan (CPT-11) in patients with recurrent malignant glioma: a North American Brain Tumor Consortium study. Neuro Oncol. 2006;8(2):189-193. doi: 10.1215/15228517-2005-010. PubMed PMID: 16533878; PubMed Central PMCID: PMC1871932.

[29] Kuroda J, Kuratsu J, Yasunaga M, Koga Y, Saito Y, Matsumura Y. Potent antitumor effect of SN-38-incorporating polymeric micelle, NK012, against malignant glioma. Int J Cancer. 2009;124(11):2505-11. Epub 2009/02/04. doi: 10.1002/ijc.24171. PubMed PMID: 19189401.

[30] Weiss RB, Donehower RC, Wiernik PH, Ohnuma T, Gralla RJ, Trump DL, et al. Hypersensitivity reactions from taxol. J Clin Oncol. 1990;8(7):1263-1268. Epub 1990/07/11. doi: 10.1200/JCO.1990.8.7.1263. PubMed PMID: 1972736.

[31] Gelderblom H, Verweij J, Nooter K, Sparreboom A. Cremophor EL: the drawbacks and advantages of vehicle selection for drug formulation. Eur J Cancer. 2001;37(13):1590-1598. Epub 2001/08/31. PubMed PMID: 11527683.

[32] Salgado R, Loi S. Tumour infiltrating lymphocytes in breast cancer: increasing clinical relevance. Lancet Oncol. 2018;19(1):3-5. Epub 2017/12/14. doi: 10.1016/S1470-2045(17)30905-1. PubMed PMID: 29233560.

[33] Savas P, Salgado R, Denkert C, Sotiriou C, Darcy PK, Smyth MJ, et al. Clinical relevance of host immunity in breast cancer: from TILs to the clinic. Nat Rev Clin Oncol. 2016;13(4):228-241. Epub 2015/12/17. doi: 10.1038/nrclinonc.2015.215. PubMed PMID: 26667975.

[34] Sun L, Hui AM, Su Q, Vortmeyer A, Kotliarov Y, Pastorino S, et al. Neuronal and glioma-derived stem cell factor induces angiogenesis within the brain. Cancer Cell. 2006;9(4):287-300. doi: 10.1016/j.ccr.2006.03.003. PubMed PMID: 16616334.

[35] Bredel M, Bredel C, Juric D, Harsh GR, Vogel H, Recht LD, et al. Functional network analysis reveals extended gliomagenesis pathway maps and three novel MYC-interacting genes in human gliomas. Cancer Res. 2005;65(19):8679-8689. doi: 10.1158/0008-5472.CAN-05-1204. PubMed PMID: 16204036.

[36] Nair AB, Jacob S. A simple practice guide for dose conversion between animals and human. J Basic Clin Pharm. 2016;7(2):27-31. Epub 2016/04/09. doi: 10.4103/0976-0105.177703. PubMed

PMID: 27057123; PubMed Central PMCID: PMCPMC4804402.

[37] Stupp R, Hegi ME, Gilbert MR, Chakravarti A. Chemoradiotherapy in malignant glioma: standard of care and future directions. J Clin Oncol. 2007;25(26):4127-4136. Epub 2007/09/11. doi: 10.1200/JCO.2007.11.8554. PubMed PMID: 17827463.

[38] Lu CY, Huang CW, Wu IC, Tsai HL, Ma CJ, Yeh YS, et al. Clinical Implication of UGT1A1 Promoter Polymorphism for Irinotecan Dose Escalation in Metastatic Colorectal Cancer Patients Treated with Bevacizumab Combined with FOLFIRI in the First-line Setting. Transl Oncol. 2015;8(6):474-9. Epub 2015/12/23. doi: 10.1016/j.tranon.2015.11.002. PubMed PMID: 26692528; PubMed Central PMCID: PMCPMC4700286.

[39] Nonaka M, Mabashi-Asazuma H, Jarvis DL, Yamasaki K, Akama TO, Nagaoka M, et al. Development of an orally-administrable tumor vasculature-targeting therapeutic using annexin A1-binding D-peptides. PLoS One. 2021;16(1):e0241157. Epub 2021/01/07. doi: 10.1371/journal.pone.0241157. PubMed PMID: 33406123; PubMed Central PMCID: PMCPMC7787448.

Chapter 10

# DNA Damage Repair Genes and Noncoding RNA in High-Grade Gliomas and Its Clinical Relevance

*Tanvi R. Parashar, Febina Ravindran and Bibha Choudhary*

## Abstract

Gliomas are the most common malignant tumors originating from the glial cells in the central nervous system. Grades III and IV, considered high-grade gliomas occur at a lower incidence (1.5%) but have higher mortality. Several genomic alterations like IDH mutation, MGMT mutation, 1p19q Codeletion, and p53 mutations have been attributed to its pathogenicity. Recently, several noncoding RNAs have also been identified to alter the expression of crucial genes. Current chemotherapeutic drugs include temozolomide targeting hypermethylated MGMT, a DNA repair protein; or bevacizumab, which targets VEGF. This book chapter delves deeper into the DNA damage repair pathway including its correlation with survival and the regulation of these genes by noncoding RNAs. Novel therapeutic drugs being developed are also highlighted.

**Keywords:** DDR in glioblastoma, noncoding RNA in gliomas, targeted therapy

## 1. Introduction and epidemiology

Gliomas are the brain's solid tumors that arise from the glial cells, which are the non-neuronal cells of the central nervous system (CNS). Neurons function in synaptic interactions, whereas glial cells provide protective and structural support to the neurons. According to the 2020 GLOBOCAN, cancer of the brain and central nervous system rank at 19th and 12th, respectively [1]. The age-standardized incidence of these tumors is 3.9 per 100,000 in males and 3.0 in females globally. In comparison, the mortality is 3.5 per 100,000 in males vs. 2.8 in females worldwide. These cancers are prevalent in countries with a high human development index [1]. In 2020 alone, 308102 worldwide brain and central nervous system cases were reported. More than half were reported from Asia (54.2%) [1]. The number of deaths reported in the same year was 251329 worldwide, pushing the mortality rate to 81.57% [1]. The survival rate of gliomas vary based on their grade; the median survival time for high-grade glioma is 14 to 16 months. It ranges from 3–15 years for low-grade gliomas [2].

One of the only risk factors identified for the development of high-grade gliomas is exposure to high-dose of ionizing radiation [3]. However, environmental factors, toxins, infections, cell phone usage, or head trauma have not been correlated to the development of gliomas. Only 5% of cases of brain tumors have been linked to

hereditary genetic syndromes [4]. Some of which are Li-Fraumeni cancer syndrome (associated with a germline mutation in the TP53 gene), neurofibromatosis, Turcot syndrome, and Lynch syndrome (constitutional mismatch repair deficiency), tuberous sclerosis, melanoma-neural system tumor syndrome, Ollier disease and Rubinstein-Taybi syndrome [4–7].

Gliomas are diagnosed when the patients become symptomatic, exhibiting recurrent headaches, the onset of seizures, personality changes, weakness in limbs, or language disturbances [8]. Elevated intracranial pressure is also a common feature in gliomas [9]. Infantile spasms and seizures have also been noted in infants [9]. Gliomas are generally diagnosed by computed tomography (CT), and Magnetic Resonance Imaging (MRI) scans [10]. The current treatment regimen is based on the tumor grade and includes either or combinations of surgical resection, radiation, and chemotherapy [11]. The chemotherapeutic drugs used for glioma treatment fall under the category of alkylating agents that induce double-stranded breaks in the DNA, thereby inhibiting tumor proliferation [12]. The standard chemotherapeutic drug used for high-grade glioma is temozolomide (TMZ), and for low-grade gliomas are carmustine, procarbazine, and lomustine [13]. Metastasis of malignant gliomas is rare, primarily due to the low survival of the patients and also due to the blood–brain barriers [14]. However, in certain rare cases of high-grade gliomas, metastasis to the lung, pleura, lymph nodes, bone, and liver have been reported [15]. Recurrence post-treatment is reported in most gliomas and can be attributed mainly to surgical brain injury (SBI) and TMZ chemoresistance [16].

The following sections describe the glioma subtypes, their molecular characterization, and their deregulated signaling pathways. This chapter's primary focus is on the DNA damage response (DDR) pathway, and noncoding RNAs in high-grade glioma called glioblastoma multiforme (GBM). The role of noncoding RNAs affecting chemosensitivity and other novel therapeutic drugs being developed for gliomas are also highlighted.

## 2. Glioma classification

The Glial cells are classified as astrocytes, oligodendrocytes, and ependymal cells [17]. The astrocytes function in providing mechanical support to the neurons; oligodendrocytes are involved in myelin production, a component of the myelin sheath and ependymal cells play essential roles in the transport of CSF and brain homeostasis [18]. Based on the cellular origins, gliomas are classified as astrocytoma (derived from astrocytes), oligodendrogliomas (derived from oligodendrocytes), and ependymoma [2].

Until 2016, the World Health Organization (WHO) had categorized gliomas entirely based on histological features and graded them according to their malignancy profile [19]. **Table 1** represents this WHO grading of gliomas where grades I and II are considered low-grade gliomas (LGGs) that are slow-growing with a better prognosis. The Grade I tumors are mainly diagnosed in children and curable with just surgical resection. On the contrary, the most aggressive tumors are referred to as high-grade gliomas (grade III and IV). Grade III tumors are termed 'anaplastic' as they have lost their characteristic cellular features to become malignant. The grade IV in this category, which accounts for 90% of gliomas, is GBM, the most aggressive and deadly tumor of all gliomas, with an abysmal survival rate. About 90% of GBM cases are de novo and develop in older patients [20]. On the contrary, secondary GBM, which arises from LGG, manifests mostly in younger patients and has a better prognosis [20].

| WHO grade | | Astrocytoma | Oligodendroglioma | Oligoastrocytoma | Prognosis | Incidence |
|---|---|---|---|---|---|---|
| Low grade | I | Pilocytic astrocytoma, subependymal giant cell astrocytoma | | | Good | Predominant in children <1 year |
| | II | Low-grade astrocytoma | Low-grade oligoastrocytoma | Low-grade oligodendroglioma | Favorable | Median age of 35 |
| High grade | III | Anaplastic astrocytoma | Anaplastic oligoastrocytoma | Anaplastic oligodendroglioma | Poor | Predominant in adults |
| | IV | Glioblastoma | | | Very poor | Predominant in adults |

**Table 1.**
*Glioma classification based on histology and malignancy scale.*

## 2.1 Molecular classification of gliomas

A more recent WHO classification in 2016 includes genetic screening to histopathological analysis, which integrates the tumor's morphological and genetic considerations [21]. The status of the following molecular alterations has been incorporated in this classification and are critical to diagnosis and further treatment.

IDH mutation: The most prevalent genetic mutation is the Isocitrate dehydrogenase (IDH) mutation accounting for a single point mutation in around 80% of glioma cases [22]. It is identified to be one of the earliest mutations for gliomagenesis and has been implemented primarily to classify gliomas as either IDH mutant or IDH wildtype. IDH mutation is considered to be a favorable prognostic marker with increased survival [23]. It is a metabolic enzyme that catalyzes the oxidative decarboxylation of isocitrate to α-ketoglutarate (α-KG) and produces NADPH from NADP without the Kreb cycle's involvement. This mutated IDH produces high levels of 2-hydroxyglutarate (2-HG) instead of the α-KG which is implicated in glioma invasion as well in epigenetic alterations leading to a glioma CpG island methylator (G-CIMP) phenotype (G-CIMP) [24].

Codeletion 1p19q: Post IDH mutation status, the gliomas are further classified based on this chromosomal co-deletion of 1p19q where the short arm chromosome 1 (1p) and the long arm of chromosome 19 (19q) are lost. It is observed in more than 70% oligodendrogliomas and 50% mixed oligoastrocytomas [25]. Clinically, IDH mutants with co-deletion 1p19q are linked to better prognosis and chemotherapy response [26].

TERT promoter mutations: Telomerase reverse transcriptase (TERT) promoter mutations are reported in several cancers leading to enhanced activity of TERT resulting in tumor cell survival and its progression [27]. It is present in 55% GBM and its prevalence is inversely correlated with IDH mutation [27, 28]. This TERT mutation serves as a prognostic biomarker and is associated with poor survival [29].

MGMT promoter methylation: MGMT (O[6]-methylguanine-DNA methyltransferase) is a DNA damage repair protein that removes alkyl groups added to nucleotides preventing mutation. Chemotherapeutic drugs like TMZ blocks cell growth by alkylating DNA. Hypermethylation of MGMT promoter regions renders this enzyme inactive and is reported in 40% GBM cases [30]. IDH mutant-MGMT promoter methylation cases are associated with increased PFS (Progression-free

survival) whereas MGMT promoter methylation with TP53 mutation has favorable outcome irrespective of IDH status [31].

ATRX mutation: The alpha thalassemia/mental retardation syndrome X-linked (ATRX) is a chromatin remodeling enzyme involved in incorporating histone H3.3 at telomeres and pericentromeric heterochromatin. Loss of function mutations of ATRX is reported in gliomas which correspond to alternative lengthening of telomeres (ALT) phenotype [32]. ATRX and TERT mutations occur in 90% diffuse IDH mutant gliomas with both being mutually exclusive which confer better progression-free and overall survival [33].

H3K27M mutations: H3K27M (methionine substitution of lysine at residue 27 of histone H3) are mutations that occur in Histone 3 of H3F3A or HIST1H3B/C gene. These mutations are predominantly present in pediatric cases with IDH-wildtype and lack 1p/19q co-deletion and are associated with poor prognosis [34]. The H3K27M mutant protein has a dominant-negative effect on EZH2 protein, a histone methyltransferase impacting the epigenetic landscape of tumor genes [35].

Besides the above, other somatic and germline mutations are also reported in gliomas. More than 25 gene loci are linked to an increased risk of development of gliomas. Somatic mutations of cyclin-dependent kinase inhibitor 2A and B (CDKN2A, CDKN2B), epidermal growth factor receptor (EGFR), pleckstrin homology-like domain family B member 1 (PHLDB1), and regulator of telomere elongation helicase 1 (RTEL1) are reported in gliomas [36]. In case of GBM, the frequent genetic alterations in the decreasing order are LOH 10q (69%), EGFR amplification (34%), TP53 mutations (31%), p16INK4a deletions (31%) and PTEN mutations (24%) [37].

## 3. Deregulated pathways in glioblastomas

GBMs are the most fatal of all glial cancers. Secondary GBMs arising from LGG constitute 10% whereas the remaining 90% GBMs arise de novo. The genomic alterations of oncogenes and tumor suppressors are the fundamental cause of cancer development. These alterations further lead to deregulation of several signaling pathways aiding in tumor progression manifesting in metastasis and chemoresistant cancers. GBMs were one of the first tumors to be studied by the TCGA [38] and some of the key signaling pathways reported to be deregulated are as follows:

RTK/RAS/PI3K pathway: This pathway is majorly involved in growth and proliferation and is dysregulated in 88% of GBM cases. This dysregulation occurs by amplification and mutational activation of receptor tyrosine kinase (RTK) genes – EGFR, ERBB2, PDGFRA, MET. A variant of the protein – EGFRvIII that occurs due to intragenic deletions is also a common feature. Activation of the phosphatidylinositol 3-kinase (PI3K) pathway are achieved by PTEN deletion, activating mutations in PIK3CA or PIK3R, AKT3 amplification, NF1 mutation, RAS mutation, FOXO mutation.

p53 pathway: Inactivation of the p53 pathway occurs in about 87% of the GBM cases. TP53, termed as "the guardian of the genome", is a tumor suppressor gene and is frequently mutated or deleted in most cancers [39, 40]. The pathway is involved in several processes like cell cycle arrest, DNA repair, apoptosis, autophagy, differentiation, senescence, and self-renewal [41]. Mutations in the TP53 gene lead to nonfunctional proteins. Several missense mutations, particularly in IDH-wildtype GBM (primary GBM), have been reported, resulting in accumulating the protein in the nucleus [42]. Additionally, deletions in ARF (ADP-ribosylation factor) at 55%, amplification of MDM2 (Mouse double minute 2 homolog)at 11%, and amplification of MDM4 (Double minute 4 protein) at 4% contribute to the inactivation of the P53 pathway [38]. TP53 is the most frequent and the earliest detectable alteration in the transition from low grade to high-grade [43].

Rb pathway: This retinoblastoma (Rb) pathway is dysregulated in 78% of GBM cases and is a vital regulator of the cell cycle and controls progression through the G1 to S phase of the cell cycle at the G1 checkpoint [44]. The Rb gene promoter is methylated frequently in secondary than primary GBMs and is associated with its low gene expression. There are two significant genetic alterations seen in the pathway– deletion of the CDKN2A/CDKN2B locus on chromosome 9p21 and the amplification of the CDK4 locus [38]. Such a loss of CDKN2A, RB or CDK4 amplification disrupts the p16INK4A-CDK4-RB tumor suppressor pathway. It has been shown to correlate with decreased expression and survival.

## 4. Significance of DDR pathway in glioblastoma

Recent studies have implicated the DNA damage response (DDR) pathway in modulating GBM chemoresistance. GBMs being the most aggressive gliomas with the least survival rate with treatment options being only radiation and chemotherapy using TMZ. These tumors ultimately gain resistance, leading to cancer relapse. This chemoresistant phenotype is attributed to enhanced DDR with alterations in DNA-repair and cell-cycle genes [12]. DNA repair mechanisms have evolved to counteract this damage based on the type of damage the DNA experiences (**Figure 1**). Some of the commonly observed damage and repair mechanisms are:

1. Methylated O6 or N7 Guanine is repaired directly by MGMT (O-6-Methylguanine-DNA Methyltransferase)
2. Oxidized/Deaminated bases by Base excision repair
3. Bulky DNA lesions or DNA-protein adducts by Nucleotide excision repair
4. Mismatched bases by Mismatch repair
5. Double-strand breaks by Homologous recombination or Nonhomologous end-joining or Alternate End Joining or Single-strand annealing
6. Inter-strand crosslinks by Fanconi Anemia pathway

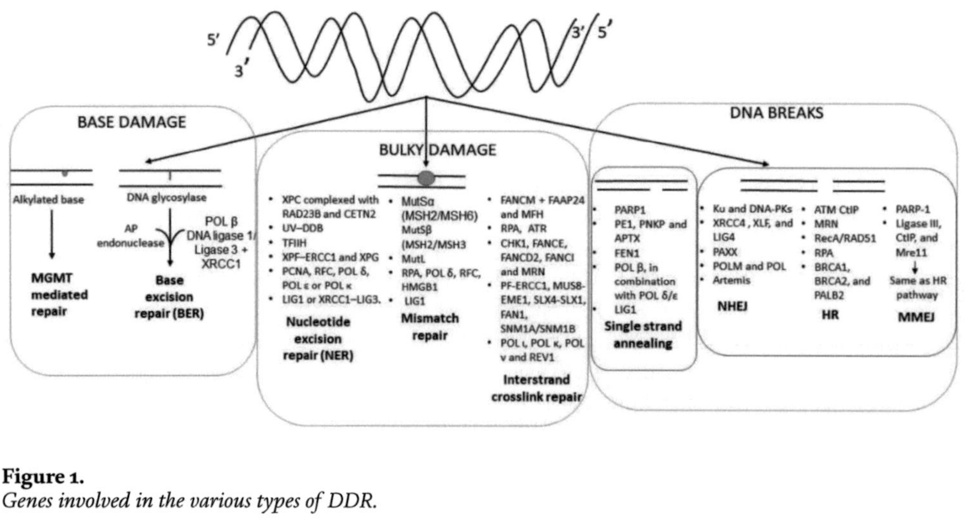


**Figure 1.**
*Genes involved in the various types of DDR.*

### 4.1 Frequently mutated genes of DDR pathway in glioblastoma

Besides mutations in IDH, TP53, and TERT promoter in GBMs, the mutation in genes that function in various DDR pathways have been reported:

MGMT-mediated DNA repair: As previously explained, MGMT is a DNA repair enzyme involved in DNA damage repair induced by alkylating drugs like TMZ. It is involved in the repair of DNA lesions. MGMT enzyme reverses O-alkylated DNA lesions of the alkylated bases [45]. MGMT is mostly hypermethylated in GBM; ~1.6% of the patient's mutation is observed (The results are in whole or part based upon data generated by the TCGA Research Network: https://www.cancer.gov/tcga).

Base excision repair: BER corrects base damage that does not cause significant distortions to the DNA helix. The enzymes involved in repair are DNA glycosylase, AP endonuclease, POL β, DNA ligase 1, or a complex of DNA ligase 3 and XRCC1 [46]. Unlike direct repair by MGMT, there are very few BER machinery components that showed a mutation in GBM.

Nucleotide excision repair: NER is the pathway chosen to remove bulky lesions. The damage is sensed by XPC complexed with RAD23B and CETN2. The other pathway proteins are the UV–DDB complex consisting of DDB1, DDB2, and TFIIH complex. Endonuclease XPF–ERCC1 and XPG, the replicative proteins PCNA, RFC, POL δ, POL ε or POL κ, and LIG1, XRCC1–LIG3 [47]. Of these genes, 5.6% of the cases had a mutation in POLE [48].

Mismatch repair (MMR): The mismatches incorporated during replication are recognized by MutSα heterodimer (MSH2/MSH6) or MutSβ heterodimer (MSH2/MSH3). The other proteins involved are POL δ, RFC, HMGB1, and LIG1 [49]. Of these, 3.8% of patients had a mutation in MSH6 and 1.6% in the MSH2 gene [48].

Double-strand breaks repair: The Double-Stranded Breaks (DSBs) are majorly repaired by nonhomologous end-joining (NHEJ) [50] and homologous recombination (HR) [51]. The alternate less-characterized pathway is microhomology-mediated end joining (MMEJ) or alternative end-joining (AEJ) [52]. While HR is restricted to the cell-cycle S and G2 phases, NHEJ and MMEJ are free to get employed in any cell cycle phase [53]. In response to DSBs, three proteins of the phosphoinositide 3-kinase-related kinase (PIKK) family are activated – ATM, ATR, and DNA-PK, downstream they phosphorylate other substrates, activating them [12]. The additional factors that are subsequently recruited include XRCC4, XLF, DNA ligase IV (LIG4), ARTEMIS, and PAXX which plays a key role in stabilizing the complex chromatin [54]. Other proteins that facilitate the pathway are DNA polymerases like POLM and POLL. Multiple proteins in this pathway are mutated in GBM. The ATR gene is mutated in 4.5% patients followed by 2.9% in PRKDC (DNA-PK), 2.5% in ATM, 1.9% ARTEMIS, 1.94% in XRCC5 (Ku80) and POLL [48].

The HR preferentially repairs the DSBs, which occur at the replication fork [55]. The pre-requisite for the homologous recombination repair pathway is the end-processing of DSBs by helicases and nucleases to produce single-stranded DNA. ATM, CtIP, MRN complex(MRE11-RAD50-NBS1) is involved in generating ssDNA [56]. This ssDNA binds with the RecA/RAD51 complex, stimulated by RPA, promotes DNA pairing and strand exchange in an ATP-dependent fashion [57]. Additionally, the tumor suppressor proteins – BRCA1, BRCA2, and PALB2 are involved in HR [58]. In GBM patients, 3.55% BRCA1, 1.86% MRE11A and RAD50, 1.4% NBN, and ~ 1% RPA1 mutations have been reported [48].

The MMEJ pathway is promoted by PARP-1, Ligase III, CtIP, and Mre11. It uses the same machinery as the HR pathway to form a 3′ single-stranded overhang at the

region of DSB [52, 59]. Mutations in Ligase III (3.49%) PARP1 (3.33%) and CtIP (2.5%) have been reported in GBM patients [48].

Single strand annealing (SSBR): The single-strand breaks are detected by PARP1, followed by end-processing by PE1, PNKP, and APTX. FEN1 acts as an endonuclease to create a gap. POL β, in combination with POL δ/ε, fills the gap and is ligated by LIG1 [60]. Mutations, although at a much lower frequency, have been reported in all the components of SSBR, APTX (1.17%), FEN1 and PNKP (0.78%), and POLB (0.39%) [48].

Inter-strand crosslink repair (ICL): ICLs are resolved by complex FANCM and FAAP24. MFH stimulates the remodeling of the replication fork. The RPA protein binds to ssDNA and activates ATR, CHK1, FANCE, FANCD2, FANCI, and MRN consecutively. Further, excision is carried out by PF-ERCC1, MUS8-EME1, SLX4-SLX1, FAN1, SNM1A/SNM1B. The polymerase which acts to repair includes POL ι, POL κ, POL ν, and REV1 [61]. 4.42% mutations in FANCD2, 2.26% in FANCI, 1.61% in FANCE, 2.7% and 1.91% in SNM1A and SNM1B, respectively have been reported in GBM patients [48].

Depending on the type of damage a cell encounters, any of these pathways can be activated to restore the damage sites. One of the most deleterious repairs found in cancer cells is MMEJ which results in large deletions and translocations, destabilizing the genome. In GBM, HR and c-NHEJ have higher mutation rates than in MMEJ, making MMEJ the preferred pathway for DNA repair. **Figure 2** represents the frequently mutated genes of the various DDR pathways along with their impact

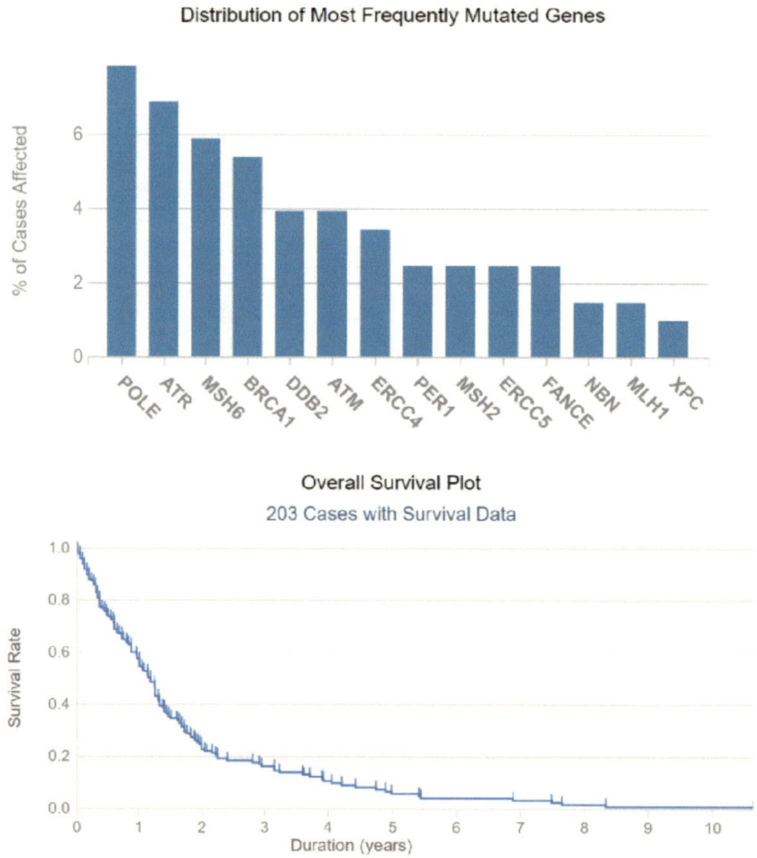


**Figure 2.**
*Frequently mutated genes of DDR pathway in glioblastomas obtained from GEPIA database.*

on overall survival obtained from NCI - GDC Database [62]. As can be observed, the mutations in these genes reduce patients' survival in GBM (14–16 months).

## 4.2 Altered gene expressions of DDR pathway genes in glioblastoma

The various genomic mutations like the overexpression of oncogenes and under expression of tumor suppressor genes lead to altered genomic and epigenomic changes favoring cancer growth. In GBM several genes that encode proteins in the DNA repair pathway have altered expression. **Figure 3** represents some of the altered gene expressions in the different DDR pathways in GBMs. This data is obtained from GEPIA database which compares normal patient samples with GBM tumor samples [63].

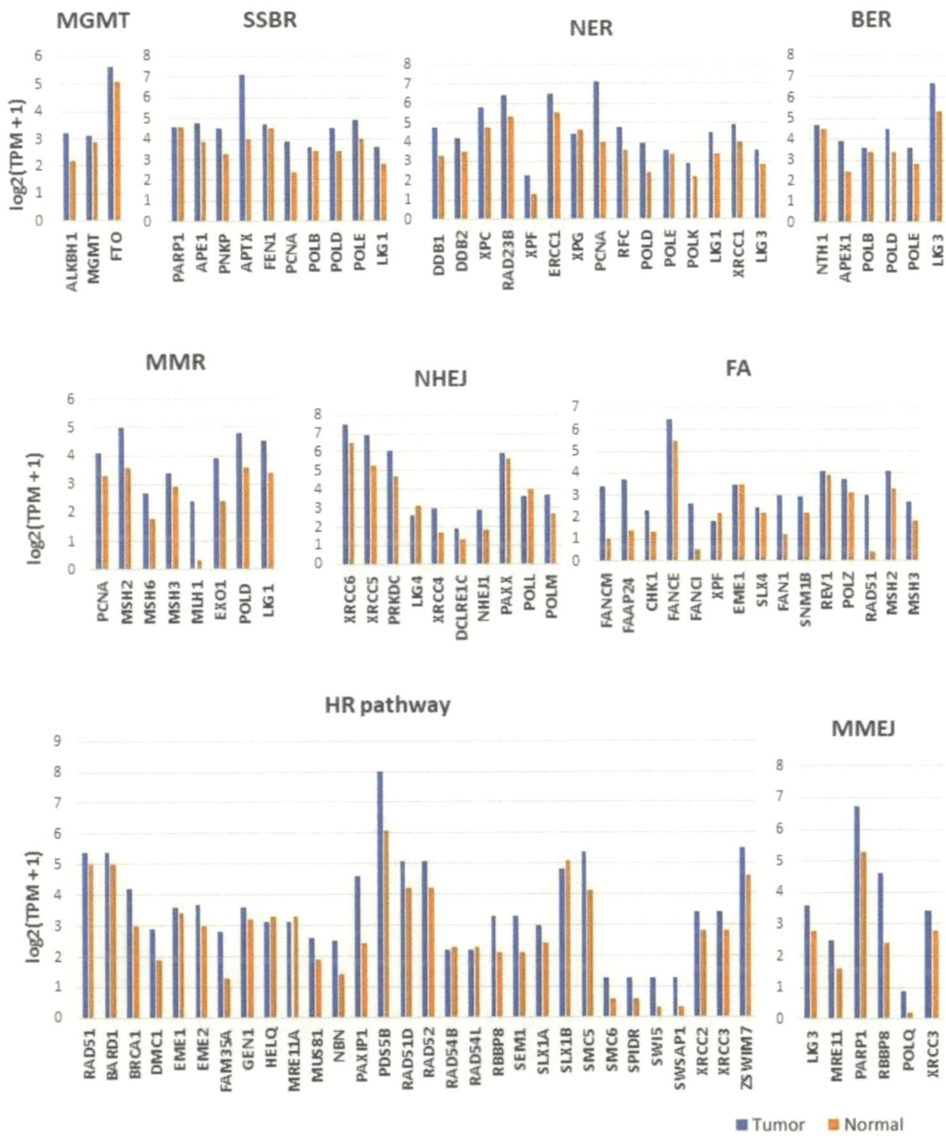


**Figure 3.**
*Altered gene expressions in the various DDR pathway in glioblastoma.*

The DDR genes are significantly upregulated and include HR factors - RAD51 recombinase, the chromatin remodelers RAD54B and RAD54L, enzymes in the HOLLIDAY JUNCTION resolution (EME1/MUS81 complex), NER (ERCC3 (XPB), ERCC4 (XPF). Also, expression of genes encoding DNA glycosylase NEIL3, Fanconi Anemia factors (FANCD2, UBE2T), the ubiquitin-protein ligase UBE3B, and two specialized DNA polymerases POLM and POLQ in the NHEJ pathway are increased significantly [64]. Coincident with the least mutation, MMEJ transcripts show relatively higher expression than other pathways. Closer observation shows elevated MMR transcripts, but a higher mutation rate has been observed of some of the genes like MSH2 and MSH6 in GBM. Among HR gene expression, PDS5B is highly expressed, which is required for proper segregation.

Additionally, these signatures also suggest the sensitivity of the tumor to therapeutic drugs. Upregulation of the TOP2A gene, which encodes topoisomerase II, might be more sensitive to topoisomerase II inhibitors like etoposide. Similarly, the decreased expression of NER genes like ERCC3/XPB and ERCC4/XPF can be more sensitive to cisplatin. Cisplatin acts by causing inter-strand crosslinking, and its repair requires NER [64]. Targeting RAD51 is also a potential therapeutic option that can either target the HR pathway or sensitize the cancer cells to irradiation and chemotherapeutic agents that cause DSBs [65].

### 4.3 Drugs targeting DDR kinases

In tumors treated with DNA damaging agents, efficient DNA repair systems become the primary cause for treatment failure. GBM's ability to resist DNA insults is directly attributable to its upregulation of DNA repair pathways. Hence, along with the standard care regimen, DDR kinase inhibitors are being investigated to overcome chemo- and radio-resistance. **Table 2** represents inhibitors that are being developed to target kinases in the DNA damage response pathway.

| Kinase | Inhibitor | Phase | Reference |
|---|---|---|---|
| ATM | KU60019 | Preclinical | [54] |
| | CP466722 | Pre-clinical +temozolomide | [66] |
| | AZ32 | Preclinical + IR | [67] |
| | AZD1390 | Phase-I + IR | [68] |
| ATR | VE-821 | Preclinical +cisplatin | [55] |
| | AZ20 | Preclinical | [56, 57] |
| DNA-PK | CC-115 | Phase-I + neratinib +temozolomide | [58] |
| Chk2 | PV1019 | Pre-clinical - + IR + topotecan | [59] |
| | CCT241533 | Pre-clinical - bleomycin +olaparib +IR | [61] |
| Wee1 | MK-1775 | Phase-I monotherapy +IR + temozolomide | [60] |
| PARP | Niraparib | Phase II monotherapy +temozolomide +bevacizumab +carboplatin | [69] |
| | Veliparib | Phase III + IR + temozolomide | [70] |
| | Olaparib | Phase II monotherapy +bevacizumab +IR + temozolomide | [71] |

**Table 2.**
*List of drugs developed targeting DDR kinases in gliomas.*

## 4.4 miRNAs involved in DDR

MicroRNAs are a group of noncoding RNAs ~18–22 nucleotides in length. miRNA regulates gene expression at both transcriptional and post-transcriptional levels. It modulates transcription by binding to the 5' UTR of the gene. The binding of miRNA at 3' UTR regions (untranslated regions) reduces mRNA stability or inhibits translation [72, 73]. Dysregulated miRNA expression is one of the hallmarks of cancer. They have been shown to affect several crucial processes like proliferation, invasion, and metastasis [74]. Hence, they are potential biomarkers and targets for therapeutic intervention. The aberrant expression of miRNAs in GBM is well documented. 256 upregulated miRNAs and 95 downregulated miRNAs are reported in GBM compared to normal brain tissue [72]. Here, we focus on the deregulated miRNAs involved in DDR pathways leading to chemoresistant or chemosensitive phenotype (**Table 3**).

| miRNA | Target | Activity | Reference |
|---|---|---|---|
| MiR-338-5p | Ndfip1, Rheb, ppp2R5a | Radio sensitivity | [75] |
| MiR-10b | p-AKT | Decreases sensitivity to radiation | [76] |
| miR-26a, miR-100 | ATM | Radio sensitivity | [77] |
| miR-30b-3p | HIF1α, STAT3 | Chemo resistance | [78] |
| miR-1193 | FEN1 | Chemo sensitivity | [79] |
| miR-96 | PDCD4 | Radio resistance | [80] |
| miR-17 | ATG7 | Chemo and radio sensitivity | [81] |
| miR-21 | PDCD4, TPM1, PTEN | Chemoresistance | [82] |
| miR-143 | N-RAS | Chemo sensitivity | [83] |
| miR200a, miR-603, miR-181d, miRNA-370-3p, miR-198, miR-142-3p | MGMT | Chemo sensitivity | [84] |
| miR195 | SIAH1,WEE1 RANBP3 | Chemoresistance | [85] |
| miR-455-3p | LTBR, EI24, SMAD2 | Chemoresistance | |
| miR-10a | EPHX1 and BRD7 | Chemoresistance | |
| miR-222 | GAS5, MGMT | Increase the DNA damage effect induced by TMZ | [86] |
| miR-29c | Sp1, MGMT | Chemo sensitivity | [87] |
| miR-99 | SNF2H/SMARCA5 | Radio sensitivity | [88] |
| miR210-3p | HIF1α/HIF2α | Chemo resistance | [89] |
| miR-136 | AEG-1 | Chemo sensitivity | [90] |
| miR-155 | p38 | Chemo sensitivity | [91] |
| miR-181b | MEK1 | Chemo sensitivity | [92] |
| miR-29b | STAT3 | Chemo sensitivity | [93] |
| miR-101 | DNA-PKcs, ATM | Radio sensitivity | [94] |
| miR-137 | CAR, MDR1 | Chemo sensitivity | [95] |
| miR-204 | FAP-α | Reverses chemo resistance | [96] |
| MiR-181a | Bcl-2 | Radio sensitivity | [97] |
| miR-132 | TUSC3 | Chemo resistance | [98] |

| miRNA | Target | Activity | Reference |
|---|---|---|---|
| miR-138 | BIM | Chemo resistance | [99] |
| miR-221, miR-222 | DNA-PKcs | Radio resistance | [100] |
| miR-1238 | CAV1 | Chemo resistance | [101] |
| miR-26a | Bax, Bad, HIF-1α | Chemo resistance | [102] |
| miR-9 | PTCH1 | Chemo resistance | [103] |
| miR-124, miR-128, miR-137 | EZH2, BMI1, LSD1 | Chemo resistance | [104] |
| miR-151a | XRCC4 | Chemo sensitivity | [105] |

**Table 3.**
*Deregulated miRNAs involved in DNA damage response in GBM.*

### 4.5 lncRNAs in gliomas

The noncoding RNAs are a diverse group of transcribed RNAs, with long-non coding RNA or lncRNA being the largest sub-type in this category [106]. Long noncoding RNA can regulate gene expression by binding to the gene's promoter and recruiting activators or repressors, or chromatin modifiers and activating or repressing transcription, respectively [106, 107]. Alternatively, they can work as antisense and bind to the transcripts, thereby inhibiting translation or destabilizing the transcript. They can also act as miRNA sponges, altering gene expression post-transcriptionally [108]. LncRNA deregulation is involved in cancer development, progression, and metastasis. It is a potential target for therapeutic interventions. Their expression pattern in response to chemotherapeutic treatment has prognostic value and serves as predictive biomarkers [106, 107].

lncRNAs are abundantly expressed in the brain as compared to other parts of the body [109]. Glioma subclassification has also been done based on the lncRNA profile into three groups: (i) astrocytic tumor with high EGFR amplification (ii) neuronal-type tumor (iii) oligodendrocytic tumor enriched with an IDH-1 mutation and 1p19q co-deletion. Such a classification has been shown to correspond to patient survival where lncRNAs like PART1, MGC21881, MIAT, GAS5, and PAR5 were correlated with prolonged survival. At the same time, KIAA0495 was associated with poor survival [109]. **Table 4** represents the lncRNAs studied in gliomas that are involved in chemoresistance or chemosensitivity.

### 4.6 Circular RNAs in gliomas

Circular RNA is yet another group of noncoding RNA produced from pre-mRNA back-splicing [137]. They inhibit miRNA and upregulate the expression of genes at the transcriptional and post-transcriptional levels [138, 139]. CircRNAs have also been shown to bind to different proteins to form circRNA-protein complexes (circRNPs) that regulate the action of associated proteins, the subcellular localization of proteins, and the transcription of parental or related genes [140]. circRNAs play significant roles in tumor growth, metastasis, EMT transformation, and therapy resistance [141]. circRNAs are the most abundant in the brain and play a crucial role in the brain's functioning [142]. In glioma, they are expressed aberrantly and play a key role in tumor initiation and progression [143]. In GBM, several studies have identified the upregulated and the down-regulated circRNAs. Identifying these circRNAs is valuable for further understanding the molecular mechanism of glioma and developing novel targeted treatments [144]. **Table 5** represents the circRNAs studied in gliomas with their targets.

| lncRNA | Target | Activity | Reference |
|---|---|---|---|
| ADAMTS9-AS2 | FUS | Chemo-resistance | [110] |
| AHIF | HIF1a, p53 | Radio-resistance | [111] |
| CASC-2 | miR 181a, PTEN | Chemo-resistance | [112] |
| CCAT2 | miR-424, CHK1 | Chemo-resistance | [113] |
| H19 | MDR, MRP, and ABCG2 | Chemo-resistance, Stemness in GSCs | [114] |
| HMMR-AS1 | HMMR mRNA stabilization, ATM, RAD51, BMI1 | Radio-resistance | [115] |
| HOTAIR | miR-519a-3p, RRM1 | Chemo resistance | [116] |
| LINC00174 | miR-138-5, SOX9 | Chemo resistance | [117] |
| LINC01057 | IKKα | Radio resistance | [118] |
| MALAT1 | miR-203, miR-101, Thymidylate synthase (TS) | Reduction of cell proliferation | [119, 120] |
| MIR155HG | PTBP1 | Chemo-resistance | [121] |
| NCK1-AS1 | miR-137, TRIM24 | Chemo-resistance | [122] |
| PCAT1 | miR-129-5p, HMGB1 | Radio-resistance | [123] |
| PSMB8-AS1 | MiRNA-22-3p, DDIT4 | Radio resistance | [124] |
| RA1 | H2B | Radio resistance | [125] |
| SBF2-AS1 | miR-151a-3p, XRCC4 | Chemo-resistance | [126] |
| SNHG18 | Sema5A | Radio resistance | [127] |
| SOX2OT | ALKBH5, SOX2, Wnt5a/β-catenin | Chemo-resistance | [128] |
| TALC | miR-20b-3p, Stat3/p300 complex, MGMT | Chemo-resistance | [129] |
| TALNEC2 | G1/S transition, mesenchymal transformation | Radio-resistance | [130] |
| TP53TG1 | miR-524-5p, RAB5A | Radio-resistance | [131] |
| TP73-AS1 | Metabolism related genes, ALDH1A1 | Chemo-resistance | [132] |
| TPTEP1 | miR-106a-5p, MAPK14 | Radio-resistance | [133] |
| TUSC7 | miR-10a MDR1 | Chemo resistance | [134] |
| UCA1 | Wnt/β-catenin | Chemo-resistance | [135] |
| Xist | miR-29c, SP1, MGMT | Chemo-resistance | [136] |

**Table 4.**
*lncRNAs in glioma involved in chemoresistance or chemosensitivity.*

| circRNA | Target | Activity | Reference |
|---|---|---|---|
| NFIX | miR-132 | Chemo resistance | [145] |
| circ_0005198 | miR-198 TRIM14 | Chemo resistance | [146] |
| CEP128 | miR-145-5p | Chemo resistance | [147] |
| VCAN | miR-1183 | Radio resistance | [148] |
| circPITX1 | MiR-329-3p NEK2 | Radio resistance | [149] |
| CircATP8B4 | miR-766-5p | Radio resistance | [150] |
| CDR1as | miR-7, p53 | Protects from DNA damage | [151] |

**Table 5.**
*circRNAs involved in chemoresistance/chemosensitivity in gliomas.*

## 5. Novel therapeutic drugs being developed for gliomas

The standard chemotherapeutic drugs used for gliomas are alkylating agents (TMZ, procarbazine, vincristine, carmustine). More recently, GLIADEL wafer containing carmustine is approved for GBM as an adjunct to surgery and radiation [152]. Humanized monoclonal IgG1 antibody Bevacizumab targeting VEGF is used for recurrent GBM [153]. Surpassing the blood–brain barrier makes treating gliomas difficult [154]. Several inhibitors targeting enzymes like topoisomerase II, [155], immunotherapeutic agents like α-type-1 dendritic cell vaccine [156], autologous cytokine-induced killer cell immunotherapy [157], autologous dendritic cell vaccine [158], and immunomodulatory drugs [159] are in clinical trials phases I and II. Additionally, many of these drugs in combination with the standard chemotherapeutic drug are also in trials, including Giladel wafers with dendritic cell vaccine [160], Lomustine-temozolomide [160, 161], Bevacizumab + radiation therapy + temozolomide [162], Irinotecan + bevacizumab + temozolomide [163]. The **Table 6** lists some of the drugs which are in phase 3 trial for glioma treatment.

| Drug | Status | Activity | Reference |
|---|---|---|---|
| Cilengitide | Did not improve outcomes | αvβ3 and αvβ5 integrin inhibitor | [164] |
| Rindopepimut | Did not improve outcomes | Targets EGFRvIII | [165] |
| DCVax®-L | Feasible and safe, May extend survival | Autologous tumor lysate-pulsed dendritic cell vaccine | [166] |
| Nivolumab | Did not improve overall survival | PD-1 inhibitor | [167] |
| Lomustine (CCNU) -temozolomide | Might improve survival | Nitrosourea Alkylating agent | [161] |
| Tumor treating fields | Significantly improved OS and PFS (with TMZ) | Alternating electric fields targeting microtubules and septin fibers | [168] |
| Sitimagene ceradenovec | Can increase time to death or re-intervention but did not improve overall survival | Adenovirus-mediated gene therapy | [169] |
| CIK cell immunotherapy | Along with TMZ improves PFS, but not OS | Autologous cytokine-induced killer cell immunotherapy | [157] |

**Table 6.**
*Novel drugs in clinical trials for glioma treatment.*

## 6. Conclusion

Gliomas are the most common malignant brain cancers constituting 80% of all brain & central nervous system cancers. Even though gliomas represent a small percentage of all cancers, they account for disproportionally high morbidity and mortality. Despite the emphasis on new therapeutic interventions, the standard care regimen has not changed drastically. However, there has been more emphasis on understanding molecular pathogenesis and its clinical relevance. Emerging preclinical and clinical data points to a shift towards more personalized therapies, and targeting the DDR pathway and its related noncoding genes is on the horizon. **Figure 4** summarizes the interplay of noncoding in DDR and drug resistance in gliomas.

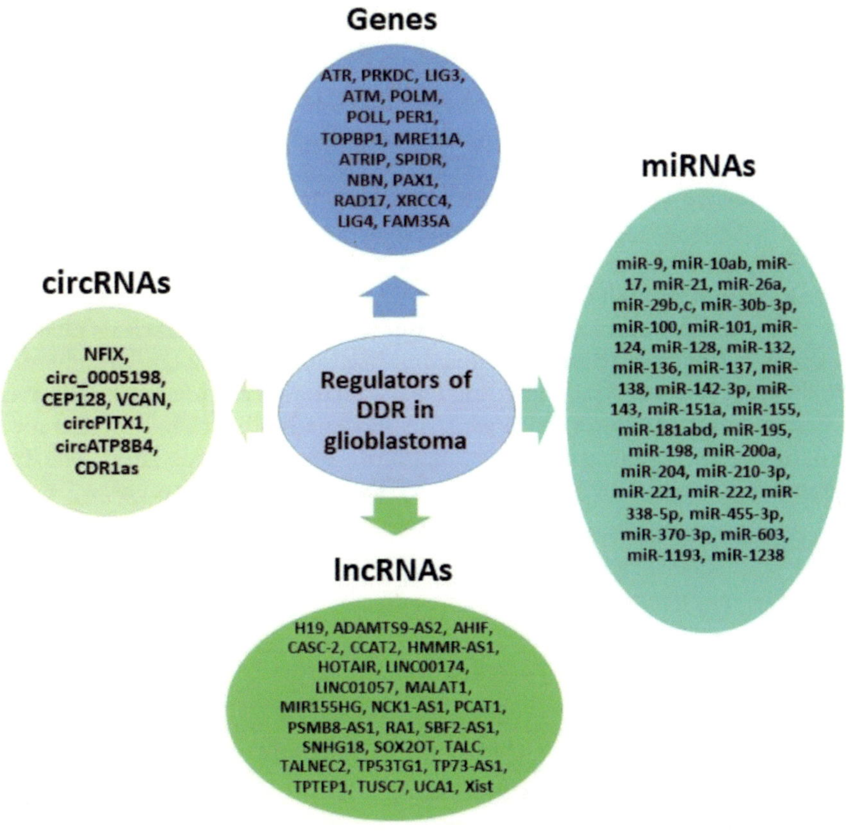


**Figure 4.**
*Representative genes and non-coding RNAs in glioblastomas.*

## Acknowledgements

We acknowledge the support from the Department of Science and Technology Fund for Improvement of S&T Infrastructure in Higher Educational Institutions (Grant no. SR/FST/LSI-5361/2012), the Department of Biotechnology, India, Glue grant (BTIPR23078/MED/29/1253/2017), and the Departments Information Technology, Biotechnology and Science and Technology, Government of Karnataka, India.

## Author details

Tanvi R. Parashar, Febina Ravindran and Bibha Choudhary*
Institute of Bioinformatics and Applied Biotechnology, Bangalore, India

*Address all correspondence to: vibha@ibab.ac.in

## References

[1] Cancer today [Internet]. [cited 2021 Feb 16]. Available from: http://gco.iarc.fr/today/home

[2] de Groot JF. High-grade gliomas. Continuum. 2015 Apr;21(2 Neuro-oncology):332-44.

[3] Wrensch M, Fisher JL, Schwartzbaum JA, Bondy M, Berger M, Aldape KD. The molecular epidemiology of gliomas in adults [Internet]. Vol. 19, Neurosurgical Focus. 2005. p. 1-11. Available from: http://dx.doi.org/10.3171/foc.2005.19.5.6

[4] Nayak L, Reardon DA. High-grade Gliomas [Internet]. Vol. 23, CONTINUUM: Lifelong Learning in Neurology. 2017. p. 1548-63. Available from: http://dx.doi.org/10.1212/con.0000000000000554

[5] Michaeli O, Tabori U. Pediatric High Grade Gliomas in the Context of Cancer Predisposition Syndromes. J Korean Neurosurg Soc. 2018 May;61(3):319-332.

[6] Vijapura C, Saad Aldin E, Capizzano AA, Policeni B, Sato Y, Moritani T. Genetic Syndromes Associated with Central Nervous System Tumors. Radiographics. 2017 Jan;37(1):258-280.

[7] Rice T, Lachance DH, Molinaro AM, Eckel-Passow JE, Walsh KM, Barnholtz-Sloan J, et al. Understanding inherited genetic risk of adult glioma – a review. Neurooncol Pract. 2015 Aug 25;3(1):10-16.

[8] Holland EC. Gliomagenesis: genetic alterations and mouse models. Nat Rev Genet [Internet]. 2001 Feb [cited 2021 Feb 16];2(2). Available from: https://pubmed.ncbi.nlm.nih.gov/11253051/

[9] Rajesh Y, Pal I, Banik P, Chakraborty S, Borkar SA, Dey G, et al. Insights into molecular therapy of glioma: current challenges and next generation blueprint [Internet]. Vol. 38, Acta Pharmacologica Sinica. 2017. p. 591-613. Available from: http://dx.doi.org/10.1038/aps.2016.167

[10] Wang R-J, Shen G-Q, Shiroishi MS, Gao B. Current concepts of imaging genomics in glioma. Glioma. 2018 Jan 1;1(1):9.

[11] Turek G, Pasterski T, Bankiewicz K, Dzierzęcki S, Ząbek M. Current strategies for the treatment of malignant gliomas – experience of the Department of Neurosurgery, Brodno Masovian Hospital in Warsaw [Internet]. Vol. 92, Polish Journal of Surgery. 2020. p. 1-5. Available from: http://dx.doi.org/10.5604/01.3001.0014.2473

[12] Ferri A, Stagni V, Barilà D. Targeting the DNA Damage Response to Overcome Cancer Drug Resistance in Glioblastoma [Internet]. Vol. 21, International Journal of Molecular Sciences. 2020. p. 4910. Available from: http://dx.doi.org/10.3390/ijms21144910

[13] McDuff SGR, Dietrich J, Atkins KM, Oh KS, Loeffler JS, Shih HA. Radiation and chemotherapy for high-risk lower grade gliomas: Choosing between temozolomide and PCV [Internet]. Vol. 9, Cancer Medicine. 2020. p. 3-11. Available from: http://dx.doi.org/10.1002/cam4.2686

[14] Wirsching H-G, Galanis E, Weller M. Glioblastoma [Internet]. Handbook of Clinical Neurology. 2016. p. 381-97. Available from: http://dx.doi.org/10.1016/b978-0-12-802997-8.00023-2

[15] Schweitzer T, Vince GH, Herbold C, Roosen K, Tonn JC. Extraneural metastases of primary brain tumors. J Neurooncol [Internet]. 2001 Jun [cited 2021 Feb 16];53(2). Available

from: https://pubmed.ncbi.nlm.nih.gov/11716064/

[16] Hamard L, Ratel D, Selek L, Berger F, van der Sanden B, Wion D. The brain tissue response to surgical injury and its possible contribution to glioma recurrence. J Neurooncol. 2016 May;128(1):1-8.

[17] Jessen KR. Glial cells [Internet]. Vol. 36, The International Journal of Biochemistry & Cell Biology. 2004. p. 1861-7. Available from: http://dx.doi.org/10.1016/j.biocel.2004.02.023

[18] Yao Y, Mack SC, Taylor MD. Molecular genetics of ependymoma [Internet]. Vol. 30, Chinese Journal of Cancer. 2011. p. 669-81. Available from: http://dx.doi.org/10.5732/cjc.011.10129

[19] Louis DN, Ohgaki H, Wiestler OD, Cavenee WK, Burger PC, Jouvet A, et al. The 2007 WHO Classification of Tumours of the Central Nervous System. Acta Neuropathol. 2007 Aug;114(2):97.

[20] Wen PY, Kesari S. Malignant gliomas in adults. N Engl J Med [Internet]. 2008 Jul 31 [cited 2021 Feb 16];359(5). Available from: https://pubmed.ncbi.nlm.nih.gov/18669428/

[21] International Agency for Research on Cancer, Wiestler OD. WHO Classification of Tumours of the Central Nervous System. International Agency for Research on Cancer; 2016. 408 p.

[22] Han S, Liu Y, Cai SJ, Qian M, Ding J, Larion M, et al. IDH mutation in glioma: molecular mechanisms and potential therapeutic targets. Br J Cancer. 2020 Apr 15;122(11):1580-1589.

[23] Cohen A, Holmen S, Colman H. IDH1 and IDH2 Mutations in Gliomas. Curr Neurol Neurosci Rep. 2013 May;13(5):345.

[24] Huang J, Yu J, Tu L, Huang N, Li H, Luo Y. Isocitrate Dehydrogenase Mutations in Glioma: From Basic Discovery to Therapeutics Development. Front Oncol [Internet]. 2019 [cited 2021 Feb 15];9. Available from: https://www.ncbi.nlm.nih.gov/pmc/articles/PMC6584818/

[25] Yao J, Hagiwara A, Raymond C, Shabani S, Pope WB, Salamon N, et al. Human IDH mutant 1p/19q co-deleted gliomas have low tumor acidity as evidenced by molecular MRI and PET: a retrospective study. Sci Rep. 2020 Jul 17;10(1):1-12.

[26] Felsberg J, Erkwoh A, Sabel MC, Kirsch L, Fimmers R, Blaschke B, et al. Oligodendroglial tumors: refinement of candidate regions on chromosome arm 1p and correlation of 1p/19q status with survival. Brain Pathol [Internet]. 2004 Apr [cited 2021 Feb 15];14(2). Available from: https://pubmed.ncbi.nlm.nih.gov/15193024/

[27] Bell RJA, Rube HT, Xavier-Magalhães A, Costa BM, Mancini A, Song JS, et al. Understanding TERT Promoter Mutations: A Common Path to Immortality. Mol Cancer Res. 2016 Apr;14(4):315-323.

[28] Nonoguchi N, Ohta T, Oh J-E, Kim Y-H, Kleihues P, Ohgaki H. TERT promoter mutations in primary and secondary glioblastomas. Acta Neuropathol. 2013 Dec;126(6):931-937.

[29] Clinical implications of TERT promoter mutation on IDH mutation and MGMT promoter methylation in diffuse gliomas. Pathology - Research and Practice. 2018 Jun 1;214(6):881-8.

[30] Wick W, Weller M, van den Bent M, Sanson M, Weiler M, von Deimling A, et al. MGMT testing--the challenges for biomarker-based glioma treatment. Nat Rev Neurol. 2014 Jul;10(7):372-385.

[31] Wang K, Wang Y-Y, Ma J, Wang J-F, Li S-W, Jiang T, et al. Prognostic value of

MGMT promoter methylation and TP53 mutation in glioblastomas depends on IDH1 mutation. Asian Pac J Cancer Prev. 2014;15(24):10893-10898.

[32] Oppel F, Tao T, Shi H, Ross KN, Zimmerman MW, He S, et al. Loss of atrx cooperates with p53-deficiency to promote the development of sarcomas and other malignancies. PLoS Genet. 2019 Apr 10;15(4):e1008039.

[33] Haase S, Garcia-Fabiani MB, Carney S, Altshuler D, Núñez FJ, Méndez FM, et al. Mutant ATRX: uncovering a new therapeutic target for glioma. Expert Opin Ther Targets. 2018 Jul;22(7):599.

[34] Adult H3K27M-mutant diffuse midline glioma with gliomatosis cerebri growth pattern: Case report and review of the literature. Int J Surg Case Rep. 2020 Jan 1;68:124-128.

[35] Mohammad F, Weissmann S, Leblanc B, Pandey DP, Højfeldt JW, Comet I, et al. EZH2 is a potential therapeutic target for H3K27M-mutant pediatric gliomas. Nat Med. 2017 Feb 27;23(4):483-492.

[36] Ghasimi S, Wibom C, Dahlin AM, Brännström T, Golovleva I, Andersson U, et al. Genetic risk variants in the CDKN2A/B, RTEL1 and EGFR genes are associated with somatic biomarkers in glioma. J Neurooncol. 2016 Feb 2;127(3):483-492.

[37] Ohgaki H, Dessen P, Jourde B, Horstmann S, Nishikawa T, Di Patre PL, et al. Genetic pathways to glioblastoma: a population-based study. Cancer Res [Internet]. 2004 Oct 1 [cited 2021 Feb 16];64(19). Available from: https://pubmed.ncbi.nlm.nih.gov/15466178/

[38] Cancer Genome Atlas Research Network. Comprehensive genomic characterization defines human glioblastoma genes and core pathways. Nature. 2008 Oct 23;455(7216):1061-1068.

[39] Eléonore Toufektchan FT. The Guardian of the Genome Revisited: p53 Downregulates Genes Required for Telomere Maintenance, DNA Repair, and Centromere Structure. Cancers [Internet]. 2018 May [cited 2021 Feb 15];10(5). Available from: https://www.ncbi.nlm.nih.gov/pmc/articles/PMC5977108/

[40] Toshinori Ozaki AN. Role of p53 in Cell Death and Human Cancers. Cancers. 2011 Mar;3(1):994.

[41] Aubrey BJ, Strasser A, Kelly GL. Tumor-Suppressor Functions of the TP53 Pathway. Cold Spring Harb Perspect Med [Internet]. 2016 May 2;6(5). Available from: http://dx.doi.org/10.1101/cshperspect.a026062

[42] Takami H, Yoshida A, Fukushima S, Arita H, Matsushita Y, Nakamura T, et al. RevisitingTP53Mutations and Immunohistochemistry-A Comparative Study in 157 Diffuse Gliomas [Internet]. Vol. 25, Brain Pathology. 2015. p. 256-65. Available from: http://dx.doi.org/10.1111/bpa.12173

[43] Ohgaki H, Kleihues P. Genetic pathways to primary and secondary glioblastoma. Am J Pathol. 2007 May;170(5):1445-1453.

[44] Biasoli D, Kahn SA, Cornélio TA, Furtado M, Campanati L, Chneiweiss H, et al. Retinoblastoma protein regulates the crosstalk between autophagy and apoptosis, and favors glioblastoma resistance to etoposide. Cell Death Dis. 2013 Aug 15;4(8):e767–e767.

[45] Christmann M, Verbeek B, Roos WP, Kaina B. O(6)-Methylguanine-DNA methyltransferase (MGMT) in normal tissues and tumors: enzyme activity, promoter methylation and immunohistochemistry. Biochim Biophys Acta. 2011 Dec;1816(2):179-190.

[46] Krokan HE, Bjørås M. Base excision repair. Cold Spring Harb Perspect Biol. 2013 Apr 1;5(4):a012583.

[47] Schärer OD. Nucleotide excision repair in eukaryotes. Cold Spring Harb Perspect Biol. 2013 Oct 1;5(10):a012609.

[48] The Cancer Genome Atlas program [Internet]. 2018 [cited 2021 Mar 6]. Available from: https://www.cancer.gov/tcga

[49] Li G-M. Mechanisms and functions of DNA mismatch repair. Cell Res. 2007 Dec 24;18(1):85-98.

[50] Lieber MR. The mechanism of human nonhomologous DNA end joining. J Biol Chem. 2008 Jan 4;283(1):1-5.

[51] San Filippo J, Sung P, Klein H. Mechanism of eukaryotic homologous recombination. Annu Rev Biochem. 2008;77:229-257.

[52] McVey M, Lee SE. MMEJ repair of double-strand breaks (director's cut): deleted sequences and alternative endings. Trends Genet. 2008 Nov;24(11):529-538.

[53] Jackson SP, Bartek J. The DNA-damage response in human biology and disease. Nature. 2009 Oct 22;461(7267):1071-1078.

[54] Golding SE, Rosenberg E, Valerie N, Hussaini I, Frigerio M, Cockcroft XF, et al. Improved ATM kinase inhibitor KU-60019 radiosensitizes glioma cells, compromises insulin, AKT and ERK prosurvival signaling, and inhibits migration and invasion. Mol Cancer Ther. 2009 Oct;8(10):2894-2902.

[55] Charrier J-D, Durrant SJ, Golec JMC, Kay DP, Knegtel RMA, MacCormick S, et al. Discovery of potent and selective inhibitors of ataxia telangiectasia mutated and Rad3 related (ATR) protein kinase as potential anticancer agents. J Med Chem. 2011 Apr 14;54(7):2320-2330.

[56] Foote KM, Blades K, Cronin A, Fillery S, Guichard SS, Hassall L, et al. Discovery of 4-{4-[(3R)-3-Methylmorpholin-4-yl]-6-[1-(methylsulfonyl)cyclopropyl]pyrimidin-2-yl}-1H-indole (AZ20): a potent and selective inhibitor of ATR protein kinase with monotherapy in vivo antitumor activity. J Med Chem. 2013 Mar 14;56(5):2125-2138.

[57] Ning J, Wakimoto H, Martuza RL, Rabkin SD. Abstract 1122: ATR inhibitors synergize with PARP inhibitors in killing glioblastoma stem cells and treating glioblastoma. Cancer Res. 2017 Jul 1;77(13 Supplement):1122-1122.

[58] Munster P, Mita M, Mahipal A, Nemunaitis J, Massard C, Mikkelsen T, et al. First-In-Human Phase I Study Of A Dual mTOR Kinase And DNA-PK Inhibitor (CC-115) In Advanced Malignancy. Cancer Manag Res. 2019 Dec 13;11:10463-10476.

[59] Jobson AG, Lountos GT, Lorenzi PL, Llamas J, Connelly J, Cerna D, et al. Cellular inhibition of checkpoint kinase 2 (Chk2) and potentiation of camptothecins and radiation by the novel Chk2 inhibitor PV1019 [7-nitro-1H-indole-2-carboxylic acid {4-[1-(guanidinohydrazone)-ethyl]-phenyl}-amide]. J Pharmacol Exp Ther. 2009 Dec;331(3):816-826.

[60] Alexander B, Supko J, Agar N, Ahluwalia M, Desai A, Dietrich J, et al. ACTR-14. PHASE I STUDY OF AZD1775 WITH RADIATION THERAPY (RT) AND TEMOZOLOMIDE (TMZ) IN PATIENTS WITH NEWLY DIAGNOSED GLIOBLASTOMA (GBM) AND EVALUATION OF INTRATUMORAL DRUG DISTRIBUTION (IDD) IN PATIENTS

WITH RECURRENT GBM. Neuro Oncol. 2018 Nov;20(Suppl 6):vi13.

[61] Anderson VE, Walton MI, Eve PD, Boxall KJ, Antoni L, Caldwell JJ, et al. CCT241533 is a potent and selective inhibitor of CHK2 that potentiates the cytotoxicity of PARP inhibitors. Cancer Res. 2011 Jan 15;71(2):463-472.

[62] Grossman RL, Heath AP, Ferretti V, Varmus HE, Lowy DR, Kibbe WA, et al. Toward a Shared Vision for Cancer Genomic Data. N Engl J Med. 2016 Sep 22;375(12):1109-12.

[63] Tang Z, Li C, Kang B, Gao G, Li C, Zhang Z. GEPIA: a web server for cancer and normal gene expression profiling and interactive analyses. Nucleic Acids Res. 2017 Jul 3;45(W1):W98-102.

[64] Gobin M, Nazarov PV, Warta R, Timmer M, Reifenberger G, Felsberg J, et al. A DNA Repair and Cell-Cycle Gene Expression Signature in Primary and Recurrent Glioblastoma: Prognostic Value and Clinical Implications. Cancer Res. 2019 Mar 15;79(6):1226-1238.

[65] Brown JS, O'Carrigan B, Jackson SP, Yap TA. Targeting DNA Repair in Cancer: Beyond PARP Inhibitors. Cancer Discov. 2017 Jan;7(1):20-37.

[66] Rainey MD, Charlton ME, Stanton RV, Kastan MB. Transient inhibition of ATM kinase is sufficient to enhance cellular sensitivity to ionizing radiation. Cancer Res. 2008 Sep 15;68(18):7466-7474.

[67] Karlin J, Allen J, Ahmad SF, Hughes G, Sheridan V, Odedra R, et al. Orally Bioavailable and Blood-Brain Barrier-Penetrating ATM Inhibitor (AZ32) Radiosensitizes Intracranial Gliomas in Mice. Mol Cancer Ther. 2018 Aug;17(8):1637-1647.

[68] Durant ST, Zheng L, Wang Y, Chen K, Zhang L, Zhang T, et al. The brain-penetrant clinical ATM inhibitor AZD1390 radiosensitizes and improves survival of preclinical brain tumor models. Sci Adv. 2018 Jun;4(6):eaat1719.

[69] Sun K, Mikule K, Wang Z, Poon G, Vaidyanathan A, Smith G, et al. A comparative pharmacokinetic study of PARP inhibitors demonstrates favorable properties for niraparib efficacy in preclinical tumor models. Oncotarget. 2018 Dec 14;9(98):37080-37096.

[70] Gupta SK, Kizilbash SH, Carlson BL, Mladek AC, Boakye-Agyeman F, Bakken KK, et al. Delineation of MGMT Hypermethylation as a Biomarker for Veliparib-Mediated Temozolomide-Sensitizing Therapy of Glioblastoma. J Natl Cancer Inst [Internet]. 2016 May;108(5). Available from: http://dx.doi.org/10.1093/jnci/djv369

[71] Hanna C, Kurian KM, Williams K, Watts C, Jackson A, Carruthers R, et al. Pharmacokinetics, safety, and tolerability of olaparib and temozolomide for recurrent glioblastoma: results of the phase I OPARATIC trial. Neuro Oncol. 2020 Dec 18;22(12):1840-1850.

[72] Zhang Y, Cruickshanks N, Pahuski M, Yuan F, Dutta A, Schiff D, et al. Noncoding RNAs in Glioblastoma. Exon Publications. 2017 Sep 20;95-130.

[73] O'Brien J, Hayder H, Zayed Y, Peng C. Overview of MicroRNA Biogenesis, Mechanisms of Actions, and Circulation. Front Endocrinol [Internet]. 2018 [cited 2021 Feb 16];9. Available from: https://www.frontiersin.org/articles/10.3389/fendo.2018.00402/pdf

[74] Peng Y, Croce CM. The role of MicroRNAs in human cancer. Signal Transduction and Targeted Therapy. 2016 Jan 28;1(1):1-9.

[75] Besse A, Sana J, Lakomy R, Kren L, Fadrus P, Smrcka M, et al. MiR-338-5p

sensitizes glioblastoma cells to radiation through regulation of genes involved in DNA damage response. Tumour Biol. 2016 Jun;37(6):7719-7727.

[76] Zhen L, Li J, Zhang M, Yang K. MiR-10b decreases sensitivity of glioblastoma cells to radiation by targeting AKT. J Biol Res. 2016 Dec;23:14.

[77] Guo P, Lan J, Ge J, Nie Q, Guo L, Qiu Y, et al. MiR-26a enhances the radiosensitivity of glioblastoma multiforme cells through targeting of ataxia-telangiectasia mutated. Exp Cell Res. 2014 Jan 15;320(2):200-208.

[78] Yin J, Ge X, Shi Z, Yu C, Lu C, Wei Y, et al. Extracellular vesicles derived from hypoxic glioma stem-like cells confer temozolomide resistance on glioblastoma by delivering miR-30b-3p. Theranostics. 2021 Jan 1;11(4):1763-1779.

[79] Zhang J, Jing L, Tan S, Zeng E-M, Lin Y, He L, et al. Inhibition of miR-1193 leads to synthetic lethality in glioblastoma multiforme cells deficient of DNA-PKcs. Cell Death Dis. 2020 Jul 30;11(7):602.

[80] Guo P, Yu Y, Tian Z, Lin Y, Qiu Y, Yao W, et al. Upregulation of miR-96 promotes radioresistance in glioblastoma cells via targeting PDCD4. Int J Oncol. 2018 Oct;53(4):1591-1600.

[81] Comincini S, Allavena G, Palumbo S, Morini M, Durando F, Angeletti F, et al. microRNA-17 regulates the expression of ATG7 and modulates the autophagy process, improving the sensitivity to temozolomide and low-dose ionizing radiation treatments in human glioblastoma cells. Cancer Biol Ther. 2013 Jul;14(7):574-586.

[82] Wong STS, Zhang X-Q, Zhuang JT-F, Chan H-L, Li C-H, Leung GKK. MicroRNA-21 inhibition enhances in vitro chemosensitivity of temozolomide-resistant glioblastoma cells. Anticancer Res. 2012 Jul;32(7):2835-2841.

[83] Wang L, Shi Z-M, Jiang C-F, Liu X, Chen Q-D, Qian X, et al. MiR-143 acts as a tumor suppressor by targeting N-RAS and enhances temozolomide-induced apoptosis in glioma. Oncotarget. 2014 Jul 30;5(14):5416-5427.

[84] Berthois Y, Delfino C, Metellus P, Fina F, Nanni-Metellus I, Al Aswy H, et al. Differential expression of miR200a-3p and miR21 in grade II-III and grade IV gliomas: evidence that miR200a-3p is regulated by O6-methylguanine methyltransferase and promotes temozolomide responsiveness. Cancer Biol Ther. 2014 Jul;15(7):938-950.

[85] miR-195, miR-455-3p and miR-10a∗ are implicated in acquired temozolomide resistance in glioblastoma multiforme cells. Cancer Lett. 2010 Oct 28;296(2):241-8.

[86] Huang H, Jiang R, Lian Z, Zhang W, Hu Z, Hu D. miR-222/GAS5 is involved in DNA damage and cytotoxic effects induced by temozolomide in T98G cell line. J Appl Toxicol. 2019 May;39(5):726-734.

[87] Xiao S, Yang Z, Qiu X, Lv R, Liu J, Wu M, et al. miR-29c contribute to glioma cells temozolomide sensitivity by targeting O6-methylguanine-DNA methyltransferases indirectely. Oncotarget. 2016 Aug 2;7(31):50229-50238.

[88] Mueller AC, Sun D, Dutta A. The miR-99 family regulates the DNA damage response through its target SNF2H. Oncogene. 2013 Feb 28;32(9):1164-1172.

[89] Wang P, Yan Q, Liao B, Zhao L, Xiong S, Wang J, et al. The HIF1α/HIF2α-miR210-3p network regulates glioblastoma cell proliferation, dedifferentiation and chemoresistance

through EGF under hypoxic conditions. Cell Death Dis. 2020 Nov 18;11(11):992.

[90] Wu H, Liu Q, Cai T, Chen Y-D, Liao F, Wang Z-F. MiR-136 modulates glioma cell sensitivity to temozolomide by targeting astrocyte elevated gene-1. Diagn Pathol. 2014 Sep 30;9:173.

[91] Liu Q, Zou R, Zhou R, Gong C, Wang Z, Cai T, et al. miR-155 Regulates Glioma Cells Invasion and Chemosensitivity by p38 Isforms In Vitro. J Cell Biochem. 2015 Jul;116(7):1213-1221.

[92] Wang J, Sai K, Chen F-R, Chen Z-P. miR-181b modulates glioma cell sensitivity to temozolomide by targeting MEK1. Cancer Chemother Pharmacol. 2013 Jul;72(1):147-158.

[93] Xu J-X, Yang Y, Zhang X, Luan X-P. MicroRNA-29b promotes cell sensitivity to Temozolomide by targeting STAT3 in glioma. Eur Rev Med Pharmacol Sci. 2020 Feb;24(4):1922-1931.

[94] Yan D, Ng WL, Zhang X, Wang P, Zhang Z, Mo Y-Y, et al. Targeting DNA-PKcs and ATM with miR-101 sensitizes tumors to radiation. PLoS One. 2010 Jul 1;5(7):e11397.

[95] Wang Y, Chen R, Zhou X, Guo R, Yin J, Li Y, et al. miR-137: A Novel Therapeutic Target for Human Glioma. Mol Ther Nucleic Acids. 2020 Sep 4;21:614-622.

[96] Yang Y-N, Zhang X-H, Wang Y-M, Zhang X, Gu Z. miR-204 reverses temozolomide resistance and inhibits cancer initiating cells phenotypes by degrading FAP-α in glioblastoma. Oncol Lett. 2018 May;15(5):7563-7570.

[97] Chen G, Zhu W, Shi D, Lv L, Zhang C, Liu P, et al. MicroRNA-181a sensitizes human malignant glioma U87MG cells to radiation by targeting Bcl-2. Oncol Rep. 2010 Apr;23(4):997-1003.

[98] Cheng Z-X, Yin W-B, Wang Z-Y. MicroRNA-132 induces temozolomide resistance and promotes the formation of cancer stem cell phenotypes by targeting tumor suppressor candidate 3 in glioblastoma. Int J Mol Med. 2017 Nov;40(5):1307-1314.

[99] Stojcheva N, Schechtmann G, Sass S, Roth P, Florea A-M, Stefanski A, et al. MicroRNA-138 promotes acquired alkylator resistance in glioblastoma by targeting the Bcl-2-interacting mediator BIM. Oncotarget. 2016 Mar 15;7(11):12937-12950.

[100] Li W, Guo F, Wang P, Hong S, Zhang C. miR-221/222 confers radioresistance in glioblastoma cells through activating Akt independent of PTEN status. Curr Mol Med. 2014 Jan;14(1):185-195.

[101] Yin J, Zeng A, Zhang Z, Shi Z, Yan W, You Y. Exosomal transfer of miR-1238 contributes to temozolomide-resistance in glioblastoma. EBioMedicine. 2019 Apr;42:238-251.

[102] Ge X, Pan M-H, Wang L, Li W, Jiang C, He J, et al. Hypoxia-mediated mitochondria apoptosis inhibition induces temozolomide treatment resistance through miR-26a/Bad/Bax axis. Cell Death Dis. 2018 Nov 13;9(11):1128.

[103] Munoz JL, Rodriguez-Cruz V, Ramkissoon SH, Ligon KL, Greco SJ, Rameshwar P. Temozolomide resistance in glioblastoma occurs by miRNA-9-targeted PTCH1, independent of sonic hedgehog level. Oncotarget. 2015 Jan 20;6(2):1190-1201.

[104] Bhaskaran V, Nowicki MO, Idriss M, Jimenez MA, Lugli G, Hayes JL, et al. The functional synergism of microRNA clustering provides therapeutically relevant epigenetic interference in glioblastoma. Nat Commun. 2019 Jan 25;10(1):442.

[105] Zeng A, Wei Z, Yan W, Yin J, Huang X, Zhou X, et al. Exosomal transfer of miR-151a enhances chemosensitivity to temozolomide in drug-resistant glioblastoma. Cancer Lett. 2018 Nov 1;436:10-21.

[106] Rynkeviciene R, Simiene J, Strainiene E, Stankevicius V, Usinskiene J, Kaubriene EM, et al. Non-Coding RNAs in Glioma [Internet]. Vol. 11, Cancers. 2018. p. 17. Available from: http://dx.doi.org/10.3390/cancers11010017

[107] Stackhouse CT, Gillespie GY, Willey CD. Exploring the Roles of lncRNAs in GBM Pathophysiology and Their Therapeutic Potential. Cells [Internet]. 2020 Oct 28;9(11). Available from: http://dx.doi.org/10.3390/cells9112369

[108] Quinn JJ, Chang HY. Unique features of long non-coding RNA biogenesis and function. Nat Rev Genet. 2016 Jan;17(1):47-62.

[109] Kiang K, Zhang X-Q, Leung G. Long Non-Coding RNAs: The Key Players in Glioma Pathogenesis [Internet]. Vol. 7, Cancers. 2015. p. 1406-24. Available from: http://dx.doi.org/10.3390/cancers7030843

[110] Yan Y, Xu Z, Chen X, Wang X, Zeng S, Zhao Z, et al. Novel Function of lncRNA ADAMTS9-AS2 in Promoting Temozolomide Resistance in Glioblastoma via Upregulating the FUS/MDM2 Ubiquitination Axis. Front Cell Dev Biol. 2019 Oct 2;7:217.

[111] Dai X, Liao K, Zhuang Z, Chen B, Zhou Z, Zhou S, et al. AHIF promotes glioblastoma progression and radioresistance via exosomes. Int J Oncol. 2019 Jan;54(1):261-270.

[112] Liao Y, Shen L, Zhao H, Liu Q, Fu J, Guo Y, et al. LncRNA CASC2 Interacts With miR-181a to Modulate Glioma Growth and Resistance to TMZ Through PTEN Pathway. J Cell Biochem. 2017 Jul;118(7):1889-1899.

[113] Ding J, Zhang L, Chen S, Cao H, Xu C, Wang X. lncRNA CCAT2 Enhanced Resistance of Glioma Cells Against Chemodrugs by Disturbing the Normal Function of miR-424. Onco Targets Ther. 2020 Feb 17;13:1431-45.

[114] Jiang P, Wang P, Sun X, Yuan Z, Zhan R, Ma X, et al. Knockdown of long noncoding RNA H19 sensitizes human glioma cells to temozolomide therapy. Onco Targets Ther. 2016 Jun 13;9:3501-3509.

[115] Li J, Ji X, Wang H. Targeting Long Noncoding RNA HMMR-AS1 Suppresses and Radiosensitizes Glioblastoma. Neoplasia. 2018 May;20(5):456-466.

[116] Yuan Z, Yang Z, Li W, Wu A, Su Z, Jiang B. Exosome-Mediated Transfer of Long Noncoding RNA HOTAIR Regulates Temozolomide Resistance by miR-519a-3p/RRM1 Axis in Glioblastoma. Cancer Biother Radiopharm [Internet]. 2020 Jul 24; Available from: http://dx.doi.org/10.1089/cbr.2019.3499

[117] Li B, Zhao H, Song J, Wang F, Chen M. LINC00174 down-regulation decreases chemoresistance to temozolomide in human glioma cells by regulating miR-138-5p/SOX9 axis. Hum Cell. 2020 Jan;33(1):159-174.

[118] Tang G, Luo L, Zhang J, Zhai D, Huang D, Yin J, et al. lncRNA LINC01057 promotes mesenchymal differentiation by activating NF-κB signaling in glioblastoma. Cancer Lett. 2021 Feb 1;498:152-164.

[119] Chen W, Xu X-K, Li J-L, Kong K-K, Li H, Chen C, et al. MALAT1 is a prognostic factor in glioblastoma multiforme and induces chemoresistance to temozolomide through suppressing miR-203 and

promoting thymidylate synthase expression [Internet]. Vol. 8, Oncotarget. 2017. p. 22783-99. Available from: http://dx.doi.org/10.18632/oncotarget.15199

[120] Cai T, Liu Y, Xiao J. Long noncoding RNA MALAT1 knockdown reverses chemoresistance to temozolomide via promoting microRNA-101 in glioblastoma. Cancer Med. 2018 Apr;7(4):1404-1415.

[121] He X, Sheng J, Yu W, Wang K, Zhu S, Liu Q. LncRNA MIR155HG Promotes Temozolomide Resistance by Activating the Wnt/β-Catenin Pathway Via Binding to PTBP1 in Glioma. Cell Mol Neurobiol [Internet]. 2020 Jun 11; Available from: http://dx.doi.org/10.1007/s10571-020-00898-z

[122] Chen M, Cheng Y, Yuan Z, Wang F, Yang L, Zhao H. NCK1-AS1 Increases Drug Resistance of Glioma Cells to Temozolomide by Modulating miR-137/TRIM24 [Internet]. Vol. 35, Cancer Biotherapy and Radiopharmaceuticals. 2020. p. 101-8. Available from: http://dx.doi.org/10.1089/cbr.2019.3054

[123] Zhang P, Liu Y, Fu C, Wang C, Duan X, Zou W, et al. Knockdown of long non-coding RNA PCAT1 in glioma stem cells promotes radiation sensitivity. Med Mol Morphol. 2019 Jun;52(2):114-122.

[124] Hu T, Wang F, Han G. LncRNA PSMB8-AS1 acts as ceRNA of miR-22-3p to regulate DDIT4 expression in glioblastoma. Neurosci Lett. 2020 May 29;728:134896.

[125] Zheng J, Wang B, Zheng R, Zhang J, Huang C, Zheng R, et al. Linc-RA1 inhibits autophagy and promotes radioresistance by preventing H2Bub1/USP44 combination in glioma cells. Cell Death Dis. 2020 Sep 15;11(9):758.

[126] Zhang Z, Yin J, Lu C, Wei Y, Zeng A, You Y. Exosomal transfer of long non-coding RNA SBF2-AS1 enhances chemoresistance to temozolomide in glioblastoma. J Exp Clin Cancer Res. 2019 Apr 16;38(1):166.

[127] Zheng R, Yao Q, Ren C, Liu Y, Yang H, Xie G, et al. Upregulation of Long Noncoding RNA Small Nucleolar RNA Host Gene 18 Promotes Radioresistance of Glioma by Repressing Semaphorin 5A. Int J Radiat Oncol Biol Phys. 2016 Nov 15;96(4):877-887.

[128] Liu B, Zhou J, Wang C, Chi Y, Wei Q, Fu Z, et al. LncRNA SOX2OT promotes temozolomide resistance by elevating SOX2 expression via ALKBH5-mediated epigenetic regulation in glioblastoma. Cell Death Dis. 2020 May 21;11(5):384.

[129] Wu P, Cai J, Chen Q, Han B, Meng X, Li Y, et al. Lnc-TALC promotes O6-methylguanine-DNA methyltransferase expression via regulating the c-Met pathway by competitively binding with miR-20b-3p [Internet]. Vol. 10, Nature Communications. 2019. Available from: http://dx.doi.org/10.1038/s41467-019-10025-2

[130] Brodie S, Lee HK, Jiang W, Cazacu S, Xiang C, Poisson LM, et al. The novel long non-coding RNA TALNEC2, regulates tumor cell growth and the stemness and radiation response of glioma stem cells. Oncotarget. 2017 May 9;8(19):31785-31801.

[131] Gao W, Qiao M, Luo K. Long Noncoding RNA TP53TG1 Contributes to Radioresistance of Glioma Cells Via miR-524-5p/RAB5A Axis. Cancer Biother Radiopharm [Internet]. 2020 Aug 6; Available from: http://dx.doi.org/10.1089/cbr.2020.3567

[132] Mazor G, Levin L, Picard D, Ahmadov U, Carén H, Borkhardt A, et al. The lncRNA TP73-AS1 is linked to aggressiveness in glioblastoma and

promotes temozolomide resistance in glioblastoma cancer stem cells. Cell Death Dis. 2019 Mar 13;10(3):246.

[133] Tang T, Wang L-X, Yang M-L, Zhang R-M. lncRNA TPTEP1 inhibits stemness and radioresistance of glioma through miR-106a-5p-mediated P38 MAPK signaling. Mol Med Rep. 2020 Dec;22(6):4857-4867.

[134] Shang C, Tang W, Pan C, Hu X, Hong Y. Long non-coding RNA TUSC7 inhibits temozolomide resistance by targeting miR-10a in glioblastoma. Cancer Chemother Pharmacol. 2018 Apr;81(4):671-678.

[135] Zhang B, Fang S, Cheng Y, Zhou C, Deng F. The long non-coding RNA, urothelial carcinoma associated 1, promotes cell growth, invasion, migration, and chemo-resistance in glioma through Wnt/β-catenin signaling pathway [Internet]. Vol. 11, Aging. 2019. p. 8239-53. Available from: http://dx.doi.org/10.18632/aging.102317

[136] Du P, Zhao H, Peng R, Liu Q, Yuan J, Peng G, et al. LncRNA-XIST interacts with miR-29c to modulate the chemoresistance of glioma cell to TMZ through DNA mismatch repair pathway [Internet]. Vol. 37, Bioscience Reports. 2017. Available from: http://dx.doi.org/10.1042/bsr20170696

[137] Hao Z, Hu S, Liu Z, Song W, Zhao Y, Li M. Circular RNAs: Functions and Prospects in Glioma. J Mol Neurosci. 2019 Jan;67(1):72-81.

[138] Tay Y, Rinn J, Pandolfi PP. The multilayered complexity of ceRNA crosstalk and competition [Internet]. Vol. 505, Nature. 2014. p. 344-52. Available from: http://dx.doi.org/10.1038/nature12986

[139] Li Z, Huang C, Bao C, Chen L, Lin M, Wang X, et al. Exon-intron circular RNAs regulate transcription in the nucleus. Nat Struct Mol Biol. 2015 Mar;22(3):256-264.

[140] Schneider T, Hung L-H, Schreiner S, Starke S, Eckhof H, Rossbach O, et al. CircRNA-protein complexes: IMP3 protein component defines subfamily of circRNPs. Sci Rep. 2016 Aug 11;6:31313.

[141] Guarnerio J, Bezzi M, Jeong JC, Paffenholz SV, Berry K, Naldini MM, et al. Oncogenic Role of Fusion-circRNAs Derived from Cancer-Associated Chromosomal Translocations. Cell. 2016 Aug 11;166(4):1055-1056.

[142] Rybak-Wolf A, Stottmeister C, Glažar P, Jens M, Pino N, Giusti S, et al. Circular RNAs in the Mammalian Brain Are Highly Abundant, Conserved, and Dynamically Expressed. Mol Cell. 2015 Jun 4;58(5):870-885.

[143] Shang Q, Yang Z, Jia R, Ge S. The novel roles of circRNAs in human cancer [Internet]. Vol. 18, Molecular Cancer. 2019. Available from: http://dx.doi.org/10.1186/s12943-018-0934-6

[144] Sun J, Li B, Shu C, Ma Q, Wang J. Functions and clinical significance of circular RNAs in glioma. Mol Cancer. 2020 Feb 15;19(1):34.

[145] Ding C, Yi X, Wu X, Bu X, Wang D, Wu Z, et al. Exosome-mediated transfer of circRNA CircNFIX enhances temozolomide resistance in glioma. Cancer Lett. 2020 Jun 1;479:1-12.

[146] Deng Y, Zhu H, Xiao L, Liu C, Meng X. Circ_0005198 enhances temozolomide resistance of glioma cells through miR-198/TRIM14 axis. Aging. 2020 Dec 9;13(2):2198-2211.

[147] Hua L, Huang L, Zhang X, Feng H, Shen B. Knockdown of circular RNA CEP128 suppresses proliferation and improves cytotoxic efficacy of temozolomide in glioma cells by regulating miR-145-5p. Neuroreport. 2019 Dec 18;30(18):1231-1238.

[148] Zhu C, Mao X, Zhao H. The circ_VCAN with radioresistance contributes

to the carcinogenesis of glioma by regulating microRNA-1183. Medicine. 2020 Feb;99(8):e19171.

[149] Guan Y, Cao Z, Du J, Liu T, Wang T. Circular RNA circPITX1 knockdown inhibits glycolysis to enhance radiosensitivity of glioma cells by miR-329-3p/NEK2 axis. Cancer Cell Int. 2020 Mar 14;20:80.

[150] Zhao M, Xu J, Zhong S, Liu Y, Xiao H, Geng L, et al. Expression profiles and potential functions of circular RNAs in extracellular vesicles isolated from radioresistant glioma cells. Oncol Rep. 2019 Mar;41(3):1893-1900.

[151] Lou J, Hao Y, Lin K, Lyu Y, Chen M, Wang H, et al. Circular RNA CDR1as disrupts the p53/MDM2 complex to inhibit Gliomagenesis. Mol Cancer. 2020 Sep 7;19(1):138.

[152] Xing W-K, Shao C, Qi Z-Y, Yang C, Wang Z. The role of Gliadel wafers in the treatment of newly diagnosed GBM: a meta-analysis. Drug Des Devel Ther. 2015 Jun 29;9:3341-3348.

[153] Cohen MH, Shen YL, Keegan P, Pazdur R. FDA drug approval summary: bevacizumab (Avastin) as treatment of recurrent glioblastoma multiforme. Oncologist. 2009 Nov;14(11):1131-1138.

[154] Arvanitis CD, Ferraro GB, Jain RK. The blood-brain barrier and blood-tumour barrier in brain tumours and metastases. Nat Rev Cancer. 2020 Jan;20(1):26-41.

[155] Chastagner P, Devictor B, Geoerger B, Aerts I, Leblond P, Frappaz D, et al. Phase I study of non-pegylated liposomal doxorubicin in children with recurrent/refractory high-grade glioma. Cancer Chemother Pharmacol. 2015 Aug;76(2):425-432.

[156] Mitsuya K, Akiyama Y, Iizuka A, Miyata H, Deguchi S, Hayashi N, et al. Alpha-type-1 Polarized Dendritic Cell-based Vaccination in Newly Diagnosed High-grade Glioma: A Phase II Clinical Trial. Anticancer Res. 2020 Nov 1;40(11):6473-6484.

[157] Kong D-S, Nam D-H, Kang S-H, Lee JW, Chang J-H, Kim J-H, et al. Phase III randomized trial of autologous cytokine-induced killer cell immunotherapy for newly diagnosed glioblastoma in Korea. Oncotarget. 2017 Jan 24;8(4):7003-7013.

[158] Liau LM, Ashkan K, Tran DD, Campian JL, Trusheim JE, Cobbs CS, et al. First results on survival from a large Phase 3 clinical trial of an autologous dendritic cell vaccine in newly diagnosed glioblastoma. J Transl Med. 2018 May 29;16(1):142.

[159] Hipp SJ, Goldman S, Kaushal A, Krauze A, Citrin D, Glod J, et al. A phase I trial of lenalidomide and radiotherapy in children with diffuse intrinsic pontine gliomas or high-grade gliomas. J Neurooncol. 2020 Sep;149(3):437-445.

[160] Rudnick JD, Sarmiento JM, Uy B, Nuno M, Wheeler CJ, Mazer MJ, et al. A phase I trial of surgical resection with Gliadel Wafer placement followed by vaccination with dendritic cells pulsed with tumor lysate for patients with malignant glioma. J Clin Neurosci. 2020 Apr;74:187-193.

[161] Herrlinger U, Tzaridis T, Mack F, Steinbach JP, Schlegel U, Sabel M, et al. Lomustine-temozolomide combination therapy versus standard temozolomide therapy in patients with newly diagnosed glioblastoma with methylated MGMT promoter (CeTeG/NOA-09): a randomised, open-label, phase 3 trial. Lancet. 2019 Feb 16;393(10172):678-688.

[162] Grill J, Massimino M, Bouffet E, Azizi AA, McCowage G, Cañete A, et al. Phase II, Open-Label, Randomized, Multicenter Trial (HERBY) of Bevacizumab in Pediatric Patients With

Newly Diagnosed High-Grade Glioma. J Clin Oncol. 2018 Apr 1;36(10):951-958.

[163] Hummel TR, Salloum R, Drissi R, Kumar S, Sobo M, Goldman S, et al. A pilot study of bevacizumab-based therapy in patients with newly diagnosed high-grade gliomas and diffuse intrinsic pontine gliomas. J Neurooncol. 2016 Mar;127(1):53-61.

[164] Stupp R, Hegi ME, Gorlia T, Erridge SC, Perry J, Hong Y-K, et al. Cilengitide combined with standard treatment for patients with newly diagnosed glioblastoma with methylated MGMT promoter (CENTRIC EORTC 26071-22072 study): a multicentre, randomised, open-label, phase 3 trial. Lancet Oncol. 2014 Sep;15(10):1100-1108.

[165] Weller M, Butowski N, Tran DD, Recht LD, Lim M, Hirte H, et al. Rindopepimut with temozolomide for patients with newly diagnosed, EGFRvIII-expressing glioblastoma (ACT IV): a randomised, double-blind, international phase 3 trial. Lancet Oncol. 2017 Oct;18(10):1373-1385.

[166] Liau LM, Ashkan K, Tran DD, Campian JL, Trusheim JE, Cobbs CS, et al. Correction to: First results on survival from a large Phase 3 clinical trial of an autologous dendritic cell vaccine in newly diagnosed glioblastoma. J Transl Med. 2018 Jun 29;16(1):179.

[167] Reardon DA, Brandes AA, Omuro A, Mulholland P, Lim M, Wick A, et al. Effect of Nivolumab vs Bevacizumab in Patients With Recurrent Glioblastoma: The CheckMate 143 Phase 3 Randomized Clinical Trial. JAMA Oncol. 2020 Jul 1;6(7):1003-1010.

[168] Toms SA, Kim CY, Nicholas G, Ram Z. Increased compliance with tumor treating fields therapy is prognostic for improved survival in the treatment of glioblastoma: a subgroup analysis of the EF-14 phase III trial. J Neurooncol. 2019 Jan;141(2):467-473.

[169] Westphal M, Ylä-Herttuala S, Martin J, Warnke P, Menei P, Eckland D, et al. Adenovirus-mediated gene therapy with sitimagene ceradenovec followed by intravenous ganciclovir for patients with operable high-grade glioma (ASPECT): a randomised, open-label, phase 3 trial. Lancet Oncol. 2013 Aug;14(9):823-33. g;14(9):823-33.

Chapter 11

# The Dynamic m$^6$A Epitranscriptome in Glioma Stem Cell Plasticity and Function

*David Karambizi and Nikos Tapinos*


## Abstract

Glioblastoma multiforme is one of the most aggressive tumors of the central nervous system. The current standard-of-care includes maximal resection followed by chemotherapy, radiation and more recently, tumor treating fields (TTFs). Despite this multimodal approach, glioblastoma remains refractory to therapy. Glioblastoma resistance, recurrence and malignancy are believed to be driven by a subpopulation of glioma stem cells (GSCs) within the tumor bulk which are characterized by the retention of self-renewal potential as well as the capacity to recapitulate tumor heterogeneity. Within the dynamic intratumoral niche, GSCs demonstrate a high degree of cellular plasticity, reversibly interconverting between stem-like states and more differentiated states as a result of environmental cues/signaling fluctuations. Such plastic adaptive properties are mostly driven by multiple dynamic, reversible epigenetic modifications. We posit that reversible post-transcriptional methylation of RNA transcripts at the m$^6$A position may be one such regulatory mechanism employed by GSCs to efficiently maintain plasticity and adaptive phenotypic transitions. In this section, we discuss the concept of cellular plasticity, introduce dynamic m$^6$a epitranscriptomic mechanisms as potential key regulators of GSC plasticity and finally propose epigenetic based therapeutics as a mean of attenuating glioblastoma plasticity to improve patient outcome.


**Keywords:** glioma stem cell, plasticity, epigenetic landscape, epitranscriptome, cellular states, glioblastoma

## 1. Introduction

Glioblastoma is one of the most lethal malignant tumors of the central nervous system. Its treatment involves maximal resection followed by chemotherapy, radiation and tumor treating fields [1]. Despite this multimodal approach, GBM remains uniformly lethal, with a median survival of 15 to 16 months [1]. Histologically, GBM presents as a heterogenous mass with multifocal necrosis, hypervascularization, hemorrhage, pleiomorphic cells with notable mitotic activity and pseudo-palisading nuclei [2, 3]. Recent advances in whole genome sequencing allowed for better GBM characterization to compliment current medical knowledge.

The Cancer Genome Atlas (TCGA) initiative generated DNA, RNA and methylation sequencing data on multiple GBMs and lower grade gliomas [4], shedding light onto GBM specific structural, mutational and methylation alterations. It was

shown that NF1, IDH, PDGFRA and PARK2 were mutated and that AKT3 and EGFR were amplified in GBMs [5, 6]. Additionally, the vast majority of GBMs were shown to activate the RB, p53 and RTK/RAS/PI3K pathways [5]. Using tumor gene expression signatures, patients could be categorized into discrete subtypes, namely mesenchymal, proneural and classical [6]. However, subtyping did not directly relate to long term survival [7]. Tendencies towards survival were only observed when the data was restricted to patients with lowest simplicity score [7].

The TCGA derived data supplied useful information, but it simultaneously raised new questions. First, it was noted that 8% of the samples did not discretely fit within defined TCGA subtypes, but instead scored for multiple subtypes [6–8]. Second, tumors were shown to undergo subtype switching following recurrence [9]. Third, even with low mutational burden, GBM exhibited significant intra and inter tumoral heterogeneity. GBM's aggressiveness and recurrence is believed to be driven by a small subpopulation of stem like cells within the tumor niche [10–13]. These cells, generally referred to as glioma stem cells (GSCs), possess the ability to self-renew and can fully recapitulate the tumor bulk with fidelity to parental tissue properties following xenotransplantation [14]. Recent developments have helped to catapult GSCs at the nexus of GBM tumorigenesis. It has been shown that the adult human brain is not an entirely post-mitotic tissue and to possess specific regions with an enrichment for cells with stem like properties or neural stem cells (NSCs) [14, 15]. Interestingly, NSC markers such as CD133 and Nestin are frequently expressed in GSCs [16]. Such homology raised questions on GSCs relation to NSCs. Thus, "the cell of origin" theory emerged. The theory posited that GSCs, which are mutated NSCs are the cells of origin of GBM. Spatial studies demonstrated that GBMs exhibited a growth bias for the subventricular zone (SVZ), a region known to be enriched with NSCs [14]. Furthermore, multiple studies showed that *de novo* GBM tumorigenesis could be achieved by inducing tumor initiating mutations within the SVZ [8]. Together, these findings cemented GSCs as initiators and drivers of GBM, hence placing them center stage as key targets in GBM therapy. However, most therapies targeted at GSC continue to fail, likely due to GSCs' high adaptability potential and tendency to continuously fuel tumor niche dynamic heterogeneity by undergoing reversible multilineage differentiation.

The aforementioned complex cell dynamics likely rely on coordinated genetic and epigenetic processes. Here, we focus on epigenetic processes, more specifically post transcriptional chemical decorum on mRNA adenosine or mRNA m6A. This chemical modification has widely been explored in dynamic processes ranging from neurogenesis, memory formation to various pathophysiological processes including cancers [17–19]. We discuss what is known at the m6A/plasticity interface in GBM and finally postulate/propose ways in which epitranscritpomics can function as a predictive or therapeutic tool to affect clinical outcome.

## 2. Cellular plasticity in glioblastoma

GBM exhibits a high degree of intertumoral and intratumoral heterogeneity. Such heterogeneity is sustained by constant, dynamic interconversion between cellular states. Differentiated glioma stem cells (DGCs) undergo spontaneous de-differentiation to primordial states or back to GSCs and vice versa in response to fluctuating microenvironmental cues [20–23]. It is likely that this tumor hijacks highly conserved genetic and epigenetic programming generally associated with stemness multipotency and early embryonic development in order to rapidly adapt to and evade various therapeutic strategies. Therefore, glioma cancer cells leverage such plasticity to maintain an adaptive, shifting cell state population equilibrium

*DOI: http://dx.doi.org/10.5772/intechopen.96792*

that is not amenable to therapy. For example, radiotherapy and temozolamide induce adaptive, spontaneous de-differentiation of DGCs to GSCs, thereby increasing and replenishing the cancer stem pool [24]. Such a shift in cell population distribution towards increased stemness forcibly translates to a more refractory tumor organ.

Recent work shows that GSCs clones are able to readily undergo reversal phenotypic transition between clonal populations [21]. The authors also demonstrated the reversible nature of the cellular equilibria assumed by GSCs in the face of hypoxia as the cells return to a naïve, pre-hypoxia exposure following normoxia [21]. In a fashion reminiscent of the Waddington landscape, GSCs inherently possess a high cellular plasticity potential, thus exist in thermodynamically poise cellular states, and can adaptively differentiate to assume multiple population equilibria in response to external perturbation [21]. These rapid processes entail myriad cellular epigenetic regulatory mechanisms, one of which is the dynamic regulation of m6A.

## 3. The epitranscriptome in glioblastoma

Currently, there are over 170 possible chemical modifications on RNA species [25]. The majority occurs on highly abundant non-coding RNA species such as rRNAs, tRNAs and snRNAs and consequently influence RNA stability and RNA secondary/tertiary structure [26]. Most of these modifications are challenging to study in mRNA due to their sparsity and relatively higher abundance in rRNA and tRNA, hence imposing a detection problem in coding RNA [25, 27]. Conversely, N6-methyladenosine (m6A) is highly enriched in mRNA, but sparse in rRNA and absent in tRNAs. The occurrence of m6A on mRNA and its effector role on mRNA stability were established in the 1970s [28, 29]. Since, a set of complexes responsible for 1) placement of m6A on transcripts (m6A methyltransferases or "writers") 2) removal of m6A (m6A demethylases or "erasers" 3) "interpretation" or effector function of m6A marks (readers) have been identified. Readers include the YTH domain containing YTHDF1-F3 and YTHDC1-C2. YTHDC1 and YTHDC2 bind methylated nuclear transcript, while YTHDF1, YTHDF2 and YTHDF3 bind methylated cytoplasmic transcript [30–35]. Methyltransferase-like 3 (METTL3), methyltransferase-like 14 (METTL14) and Wilm's-tumor-1-associated protein (WTAP) form a multimeric methyltransferase complex responsible for m6A mark transcript placement [36–38]. The removal of m6A is mediated by the fat mass-and-obesity-associated protein (FTO) and alkylation repair homolog protein 5 (ALKBH5) [39, 40]. The discovery of these m6A RNA demethylases implied possible reversibility or dynamism inherent to the epitranscriptome. Once placed on transcripts, m6A has been shown to modulate mRNA stability, splicing and translation and thus ultimately influence gene expression kinetics and outcome [32–34]. Following the refinement of m6A detection techniques, m6A has been widely studied in physiologic processes, such as early development, and in pathophysiologic processes, ranging from psychiatric disorders to cancers. Here, we focus our attention to the glioblastoma/m6A interface as it pertains to plasticity.

### 3.1 m6A writers in glioblastoma

The most common way the m6A code has been probed in GBM is via enzymatic inhibition or transcript level perturbation of the m6A machinery. The majority of works on the role of writers in GBM suggest an oncogenic role for METTL3/METTL14. The methyltransferase METTL3 has been shown to be essential for sustenance of GSCs, radioresistance and GBM oncogenic signaling [41–44]. Yet, METTL3 and

METTL14 have been shown in an overexpression-based study to reduce GSCs tumorigenicity and stemness potential, suggesting a potential tumor suppressive function [45]. The reasons for these discrepancies pertaining to m6A writers are unclear and necessitate additional clarifying studies. Ultimately, these results could possibly reflect GBM heterogeneity/complexity and hence dissuade against generalizations on m6A in GBM.

### 3.2 m6A erasers in glioblastoma

So far, the known m6A erasers exhibit oncogenic tendencies in GBM. Inhibition of FTO demethylase activity has been shown by two independent groups to inhibit stemness propensity in GSCs [45, 46]. In another study, ALKBH5 was shown to be highly expressed in GSCs and functioned to promote tumorigenicity via FOXM1 transcript stabilization [47].

### 3.3 m6A readers in glioblastoma

The functional role of the YTH readers in GBM had been unknown until very recently. Two recent studies show that YTHFD2 promotes GBM aggressiveness, albeit through different proposed mechanisms [48, 49]. One study finds that YTHDF2, though previously shown to destabilize transcripts, does however stabilize *MYC* and *VEGFA* transcripts in GSCs in an m6A-dependent manner [48]. The other study shows that the EGFR/SRC/ERK pathway functions to stabilize YTHDF2 via protein phosphorylation and YTHDF2 consequently destabilizes transcripts implicated in cholesterol dysregulation and invasive GBM growth [49]. Again, these differences may suggest context dependence given GBM's high levels of heterogeneity and plasticity.

Summary of the role of various components of the m6A RNA methylation machinery in glioblastoma is presented in **Figure 1**. Though hinting at plasticity, most of these studies do not explicitly determine m6A dynamics in the context of GBM cell state transition.

### 3.4 Role of m6A in cellular plasticity in glioblastoma

Recent findings in neuroscience pertaining to neurogenesis and gliogenesis emphasize the centrality of m6A in dictating cell fate/state specification and plasticity events during early brain development. Stem cells of the nervous system, known as radial glia cells (RGCs) or neural progenitor cells, which are responsible for neurogenesis and gliogenesis, show m6A dependency [50]. As per one study, conditional KO of *Mettl3/Mettl14* in embryonic mouse brain resulted in premature activation of later stage differentiation specific transcripts that are normally kept low in RGCs [50]. Consequently, m6A depleted RGCs could not undergo appropriate multilineage differentiation and expectedly formed abnormal brain tissue [50]. Another study shows that the process of glial specification relies on m6A [51]. Depletion of Prrc2a, which is a gene coding for the Olig2 stabilizing m6A reader PRRC2A, results in hypomethylation and cognitive defect secondary to Olig2 transcription factor destabilization [51]. These studies demonstrate the key role of the m6A code in driving cell fate specification, differentiation and hence plasticity via transcriptional regulation during neurogenesis. From these data, a corollary can be drawn that GSCs, which are mutated NSCs, could exhibit significant m6A dependence during differentiation, de-differentiation, tumorigenesis and in response to external perturbation such as radiation and chemotherapy. However, this m6A/plasticity axis in GSCs and GBM niche remains poorly understood. Recently, we

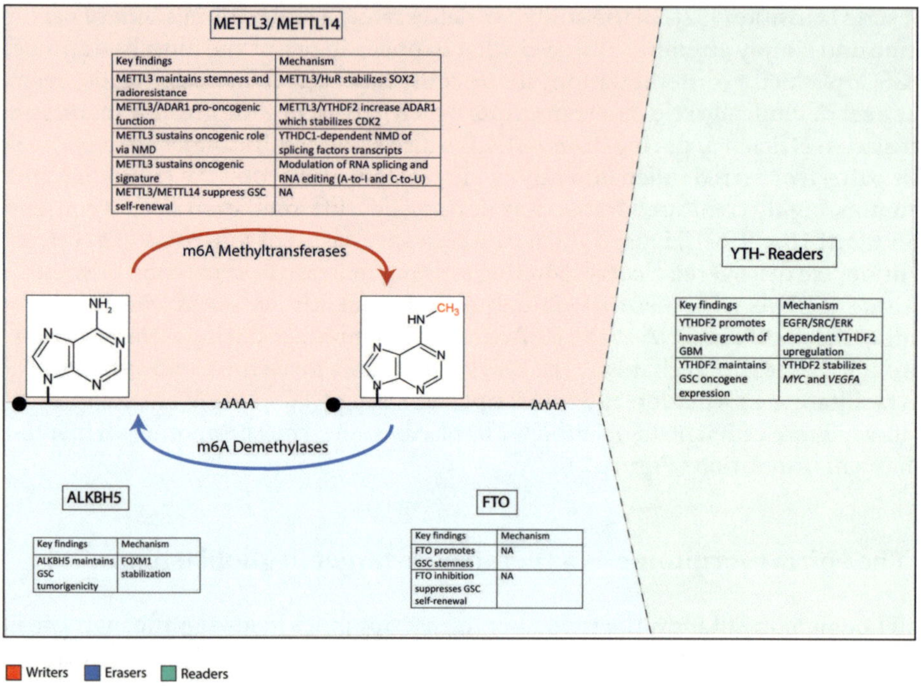


**Figure 1.**
*Summary of key findings for the role of the various components of the m6A machinery in glioblastoma.*

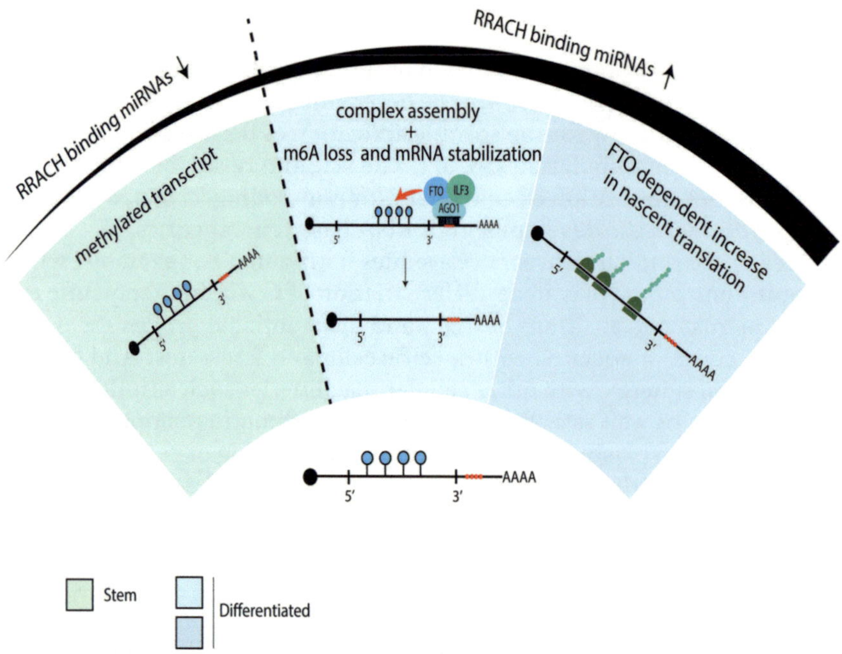


**Figure 2.**
*miRNAs direct FTO/AGO1/ILF3 complex on RRACH m6A motifs to induce RNA demethylation and increase in nascent translation during the transition of GSCs to differentiated progenies.*

performed an integrated whole genome meRIP-seq, RNA-seq and ribo-seq analysis in three patient-derived GSCs and differentiated progenies [52]. This allowed for the interrogation of transcriptional, epitranscriptional and translational kinetics during

cell state transition [52]. In the study, we deliberately avoid m6A machinery perturbation and simply attempt to unravel what happens in one of the most basic process of GSCs plasticity (differentiation) in the context of m6A dynamics. We discovered that a set of clinically relevant transcripts which experience the greatest increase in translation efficiency during differentiation also show significant loss in m6A peaks. This pattern occurred independently of glioblastoma subtypes. We found that these common, highly translated transcripts during GSC differentiation share a consensus m6A motif (the RRACH motif) that overlap a specific set of miRNA sequences. In addition, we discovered a corresponding striking increase in expression of some of these miRNAs with GSC differentiation. Subsequently, we asked whether these findings implicate miRNA at the m6A/translation interface during differentiation. Through a series of mechanistic studies, we propose a mechanism whereby miRNAs can facilitate the formation of a transcript stabilizing FTO-ILF3-AGO1 complex. This results in more efficient association with the ribosome, thus promoting an increase in nascent translation (**Figure 2**).

## 4. The epitranscriptome as a therapeutic target in glioblastoma

Though in its infancy, the field of epitranscriptomics holds significant promise for the development of novel epigenetic therapies against GBM. Currently, strategies for targeting the m6A machinery in glioblastoma are directed at the inhibition of enzymatic activity [45, 46]. Recently, targeting of the m6A erasers as well as YTHDF2 have shown some encouraging results for GBM treatment [48]. Specifically, it was shown that high levels of YTHDF2 correlate with increased sensitivity to Linsitinib, an inhibitor of the YTHDF2 downstream effector IGFBP3 [48].

Another emerging avenue is the fusion of m6A machinery components to RNA targeting CRISPR complexes [53, 54]. The deployment of the m6A machinery-CRISPR complex can allow for the specific activation or deactivation of specific transcripts via m6A manipulation [56, 57]. The safe and reversible target specific stabilization or destabilization of coding and/or non-coding RNA species represents an exciting frontier in the development of RNA based therapeutics.

However, these findings leave more avenues for inquiry. For example, what role does the epitrancriptome play in de-differentiation of GSCs, in therapeutic evasion and in microstate transitions of GSCs and differentiated progenies? Are there specific "m6A codes" associated with specific cellular microstates? And how do m6A processes work in synergy with other cellular machineries such as miRNAs, long non-coding RNAs, or well established GBM tumor promoting/suppressing signaling pathways to maintain plasticity? Are m6A dynamics driving or secondary events in GBM microstate transitions? Evidently, more work needs to be done to probe the m6A/plasticity interface in GSCs in order to aid in the discovery of novel epigenetic therapies targeting GSC plasticity.

## 5. A systems approach towards an epigenetic landscape in glioblastoma

Recent advancements in single cell RNA sequencing, which include integrated single cell multi-omics analysis, as well as the application of novel algorithms such as pseudotime and RNA velocity have allowed for better characterization of the dynamics within the heterogenous GBM tumor niche [21, 55, 56]. Initial single cell analysis demonstrated that GBM cancer cells exist in a cell state continuum

with polarization towards specific fates [55]. Additionally, projection of single cell transcriptomics onto a fetal neurodevelopmental roadmap identified previously unidentified glioma stem cell properties and established GSC at the apex of the glioblastoma tumor hierarchy [21]. These rapidly cycling apical progenitor cancer stem cells were found to have a transcriptional profile that overlapped glial progenitor cells [21]. Furthermore, RNA velocity analysis showed apical stem cell transcriptional adjacency and velocity vector flow towards the more differentiated tumor cell lineages [21]. Collectively, such findings hint at clear plasticity/fluidity within the tumor. The integration of epitranscritpomics with single cell multi-omics technology could help unveil the yet undiscovered mechanism of how dynamic m6A changes play a role in driving plasticity within the tumor niche.

It has been posited that a stem cell may exist at a high or even maximal cellular state of entropy and can readily shift states in the face of perturbation [57]. Our view of the cancer stem cell state in glioblastoma agrees with the theory put forward 20 years ago [58] suggesting that the glioma stem cell is a cellular state or function rather than an entity and this state of maximum cellular entropy is influenced by the constantly adaptable microenvironment of the tumor. In this context, distribution of species would represent heterogeneity, which single cell RNA sequencing adequately captures. Quantum states would equate probability distribution of discrete cell state occupancy bias. In other words, if we looked across a large set of samples and performed, for instance, m6A, ATAC-seq, RNA-seq integrated multi-omics single cell analysis, it is possible to generate cell state probability occupancy distribution and ultimately identify discrete, preferred transcriptomic and epitranscriptomic cell state occupancies or quanta states. This will allow to construct an individualized transcriptomic/epitranscritomic landscape and to find patterns within the seemingly stochastic, chaotic environment that is the tumor.

Can we integrate multiple epigenetic "landscapes" with observed clinical outcomes and use this information on a training predictive model to identify discrete favorable and unfavorable cellular microstates? And ultimately can we target plasticity-based processes to convert the microstate cellular make up of a highly malignant tumor bulk into a less aggressive cellular composition? It is plausible that m6A regulatory processes may represent a key target in this endeavor.

## 6. Conclusion

In this chapter, we introduce GBM in the context of early genetic characterization and suggest that limitations in discrete classification hinted at an inherent cell state fluidity or plasticity. This plasticity may stand as a key function utilized by GSCs and differentiated cancer cells to rapidly and constantly respond to natural and non-natural/therapy induced microenvironmental fluctuations. Epitranscriptomic dynamic changes are explored as a new frontier in epigenetic based adaptation mechanisms. Additionally, single cell multi-omic technology and its yet to occur application to m6A can pave the way for improvement in GBM characterization and patient management. Lastly, we theorize that the integration of multi-omic cell technology and m6A using massive, high dimensional patient data can aid in the characterization of plasticity through the identification of GBM cell states distribution and quantum state occupancy bias. In the future, such works can be used to develop a Waddington like epigenetic landscape predicting favorable cell state distribution and thus help in the development of plasticity-based therapy to convert glioblastoma into a non-adaptable therapeutic target.

## Conflict of interest

"The authors declare no conflict of interest."

## Author details

David Karambizi[1] and Nikos Tapinos[1,2*]

1 Laboratory of Cancer Epigenetics and Plasticity, Brown University, Rhode Island Hospital, Providence, RI, USA

2 Department of Neurosurgery, Brown University, Providence, RI, USA

*Address all correspondence to: nikos_tapinos@brown.edu

## References

[1] Ostrom QT, Gittleman H, Liao P, Vecchione-Koval T, Wolinsky Y, Kruchko C, et al. CBTRUS Statistical Report: Primary brain and other central nervous system tumors diagnosed in the United States in 2010-2014. Neuro-Oncology. 2017;19(suppl_5):v1–v88.

[2] Hanif F, Muzaffar K, Perveen K, Malhi SM, Simjee ShU. Glioblastoma Multiforme: A Review of its Epidemiology and Pathogenesis through Clinical Presentation and Treatment. Asian Pac J Cancer Prev. 2017;18(1):3-9.

[3] Nelson SJ, Cha S. Imaging glioblastoma multiforme. Cancer J. 2003;9(2):134-45.

[4] Phillips HS, Kharbanda S, Chen R, Forrest WF, Soriano RH, Wu TD, et al. Molecular subclasses of high-grade glioma predict prognosis, delineate a pattern of diseaseprogression, and resemble stages in neurogenesis. Cancer Cell. 2006;9(3):157-73.

[5] Cancer Genome Atlas Research Network. Comprehensive genomic characterization defines human glioblastoma genes and core pathways. Nature. 2008;455(7216):1061-8.

[6] Verhaak RGW, Hoadley KA, Purdom E, Wang V, Qi Y, Wilkerson MD, et al. Integrated Genomic Analysis Identifies Clinically Relevant Subtypes of Glioblastoma Characterized by Abnormalities in PDGFRA, IDH1, EGFR, and NF1. Cancer Cell. 2010;17(1):98-110.

[7] Wang Q, Hu X, Hu B, Muller F, Kim H, Squatrito M, et al. Tumor evolution of glioma intrinsic gene expression subtype associates with immunological changes in the microenvironment. 2017;32(1):42-56.

[8] Behnan J, Finocchiaro G, Hanna G. The landscape of the mesenchymal signature in brain tumours. Brain. 2019;142(4):847-66.

[9] Halliday J, Helmy K, Pattwell SS, Pitter KL, LaPlant Q, Ozawa T, et al. In vivo radiation response of proneural glioma characterized by protective p53 transcriptional program and proneural-mesenchymal shift. Proceedings of the National Academy of Sciences. 2014;111(14):5248-53.

[10] Bao S, Wu Q, McLendon RE, Hao Y, Shi Q, Hjelmeland AB, et al. Glioma stem cells promote radioresistance by preferential activation of the DNA damage response. Nature. 2006;444(7120):756-60.

[11] Chen J, Li Y, Yu T-S, McKay RM, Burns DK, Kernie SG, et al. A restricted cell population propagates glioblastoma growth after chemotherapy. Nature. 2012;488(7412):522-6.

[12] Zheng H, Ying H, Yan H, Kimmelman AC, Hiller DJ, Chen A-J, et al. p53 and Pten control neural and glioma stem/progenitor cell renewal and differentiation. Nature. 2008;455(7216):1129-33.

[13] Zhu Z, Khan MA, Weiler M, Blaes J, Jestaedt L, Geibert M, et al. Targeting Self-Renewal in High-Grade Brain Tumors Leads to Loss of Brain Tumor Stem Cells and Prolonged Survival. Cell Stem Cell. 2014;15(2):185-98.

[14] Lee JH, Lee JE, Kahng JY, Kim SH, Park JS, Yoon SJ, et al. Human glioblastoma arises from subventricular zone cells with low-level driver mutations. Nature.2018;560(7717):243-7.

[15] Singh SK, Hawkins C, Clarke ID, Squire JA, Bayani J, Hide T, et al. Identification of human brain tumour initiating cells. Nature. 2004;432(7015):396-401.

[16] Lee J, Kotliarova S, Kotliarov Y, Li A, Su Q, Donin NM, et al. Tumor stem cells derived from glioblastomas cultured in bFGF and EGF more closely mirror the phenotype and genotype of primary tumors than do serum-cultured cell lines. Cancer Cell. 2006;9(5):391-403.

[17] Widagdo J, Zhao QY, Kempen MJ, et al. Experience-Dependent Accumulation of N6-Methyladenosine in the Prefrontal Cortex Is Associated with Memory Processes in Mice. J Neurosci. 2016;36(25):6771-6777.

[18] Widagdo J, Zhao Q-Y, Kempen M-J, Tan MC, Ratnu VS, Wei W, et al. Experience-Dependent Accumulation of N 6 -Methyladenosine in the Prefrontal Cortex Is Associated with Memory Processes in Mice. The Journal of Neuroscience. 2016;36(25):6771-7.

[19] Huo FC, Zhu ZM, Pei DS. $N^6$ -methyladenosine ($m^6$ A) RNA modification in human cancer. Cell Prolif.2020;53(11):e12921.

[20] Dirkse A, Golebiewska A, Buder T, Nazarov PV, Muller A, Poovathingal S, et al. Stem cell-associated heterogeneity in Glioblastoma results from intrinsic tumor plasticity shaped by the microenvironment. Nature Communications. 2019;10(1).

[21] Couturier CP, Ayyadhury S, Le PU, Nadaf J, Monlong J, Riva G, et al. Single-cell RNA-seq reveals that glioblastoma recapitulates a normal neurodevelopmental hierarchy. Nature Communications. 2020;11(1).

[22] Hu B, Wang Q, Wang YA, Hua S, Sauvé C-EG, Ong D, et al. Epigenetic Activation of WNT5A Drives Glioblastoma Stem Cell Differentiation and Invasive Growth. Cell. 2016;167(5).

[23] Bulstrode H, Johnstone E, Marques-Torrejon MA, Ferguson KM, Bressan RB, Blin C, et al. Elevated FOXG1 and SOX2 in glioblastoma enforces neural stem cell identity through transcriptional control of cell cycle and epigenetic regulators. Genes & Development. 2017;31(8):757-73.

[24] Auffinger B, Tobias AL, Han Y, Lee G, Guo D, Dey M, et al. Conversion of differentiated cancer cells into cancer stem-like cells in a glioblastoma model after primary chemotherapy. Cell Death & Differentiation. 2014;21(7):1119-31.

[25] Machnicka MA, Milanowska K, Osman Oglou O, Purta E, Kurkowska M, Olchowik A, et al. MODOMICS: a database of RNA modification pathways—2013 update. NucleicAcids Research. 2012;41(D1).

[26] Pan T. Modifications and functional genomics of human transfer RNA. Cell Research.2018;28(4):395-404.

[27] Legrand C, Tuorto F, Hartmann M, Liebers R, Jacob D, Helm M, et al. Statistically robust methylation calling for whole-transcriptome bisulfite sequencing reveals distinctmethylation patterns for mouse RNAs. Genome Research. 2017;27(9):1589-96.

[28] Perry RP, Kelley DE. Existence of methylated messenger RNA in mouse L cells. Cell.1974;1(1):37-42.

[29] Desrosiers R, Friderici K, Rottman F. Identification of Methylated Nucleosides in Messenger RNA from Novikoff Hepatoma Cells. Proceedings of the National Academyof Sciences. 1974;71(10):3971-5.

[30] Kretschmer J, Rao H, Hackert P, Sloan KE, Höbartner C, Bohnsack MT. The m6A reader protein YTHDC2 interacts with the small ribosomal subunit and the 5′–3′exoribonuclease XRN1. RNA. 2018;24(10): 1339-50.

[31] Roundtree IA, Luo G-Z, Zhang Z, Wang X, Zhou T, Cui Y, et al. Author response: YTHDC1 mediates nuclear

export of N6-methyladenosine methylated mRNAs. 2017;

[32] Xiao W, Adhikari S, Dahal U, Chen Y-S, Hao Y-J, Sun B-F, et al. Nuclear m6A Reader YTHDC1 Regulates mRNA Splicing. Molecular Cell. 2016;61(6):925.

[33] Shi H, Wang X, Lu Z, Zhao BS, Ma H, Hsu PJ, et al. YTHDF3 facilitates translation and decay of N6-methyladenosine-modified RNA. Cell Research. 2017;27(3):315-28.

[34] Wang X, Lu Z, Gomez A, Hon GC, Yue Y, Han D, et al. N6-methyladenosine-dependent regulation of messenger RNA stability. Nature. 2013;505(7481):117-20.

[35] Wang X, Zhao BS, Roundtree IA, Lu Z, Han D, Ma H, et al. N6-methyladenosine. Modulates Messenger RNA Translation Efficiency. Cell. 2015;161(6):1388-99.

[36] Liu J, Yue Y, Han D, Wang X, Fu Y, Zhang L, et al. A METTL3–METTL14 complex mediates mammalian nuclear RNA N6-adenosine methylation. Nature Chemical Biology.2013;10(2):93-5.

[37] Wang X, Feng J, Xue Y, Guan Z, Zhang D, Liu Z, et al. Structural basis of N6-adenosine methylation by the METTL3–METTL14 complex. Nature. 2016;534(7608):575-8.

[38] Schöller E, Weichmann F, Treiber T, Ringle S, Treiber N, Flatley A, et al. Interactions, localization, and phosphorylation of the m6A generating METTL3–METTL14–WTAPcomplex. RNA. 2018;24(4):499-512.

[39] Jia G, Fu Y, Zhao X, Dai Q, Zheng G, Yang Y, et al. N6-Methyladenosine in nuclear RNA is a major substrate of the obesity-associated FTO. Nature Chemical Biology.2011;7(12):885-7.

[40] Zheng G, Dahl JA, Niu Y, Fedorcsak P, Huang C-M, Li CJ, et al. ALKBH5 Is a Mammalian RNA Demethylase that Impacts RNA Metabolism and Mouse Fertility. Molecular Cell. 2013;49(1):18-29.

[41] Visvanathan A, Patil V, Arora A, Hegde AS, Arivazhagan A, Santosh V, et al. Essential role of METTL3-mediated m6A modification in glioma stem-like cells maintenance and radioresistance. Oncogene. 2017;37(4):522-33.

[42] Tassinari V, Cesarini V, Tomaselli S, Ianniello Z, Silvestris DA, Ginistrelli LC, et al. ADAR1 is a new target of METTL3 and plays a pro-oncogenic role in glioblastoma by an editing-independent mechanism. Genome Biology. 2021;22(1).

[43] Li F, Yi Y, Miao Y, Long W, Long T, et al. N6-methyladenosine Modulates Nonsense-mediated mRNA Decay in Human Glioblastoma. 2019;79(22):5785-5798.

[44] Visvanathan A, Patil V, Abdulla S, Hoheisel J, Somasundaram K. N6-Methyladenosine Landscape of Glioma Stem-Like Cells: METTL3 Is Essential for the Expression of Actively Transcribed Genes and Sustenance of the Oncogenic Signaling. Genes. 2019;10(2):141.

[45] Cui Q, Shi H, Ye P, Li L, Qu Q, et al. m6A Methylation Regulates the Self-Renewal and Tumorigenesis of Glioblastoma Stem Cells. Cell Rep. 2012; 18(11):2622-2634.

[46] Huff S, Tiwari SK, Gonzalez GM, Wang Y, Rana TM. m6A-RNA Demethylase FTO Inhibitors Impair Self-Renewal in Glioblastoma Stem Cells. ACS Chemical Biology. 2021;

[47] Zhang S, Zhao BS, Zhou A, Lin K, Zheng S, Lu Z, et al. m6A Demethylase ALKBH5 Maintains Tumorigenicity of Glioblastoma Stem-like Cells by Sustaining FOXM1 Expression and Cell

Proliferation Program. Cancer Cell. 2017;31(4).

[48] Dixit D, Prager BC, Gimple RC, Poh HX, Wang Y, et al. The RNA m6A Reader YTHDF2 Maintains Oncogene Expression and Is a Targetable Dependency in Glioblastoma Stem Cells. 2021;

[49] Fang R, Chen X, Zhang S, Shi H, Ye Y, Shi H, et al. EGFR/SRC/ERK-stabilized YTHDF2 promotes cholesterol dysregulation and invasive growth of glioblastoma.Nature Communications. 2021;12(1).

[50] Yoon KJ, Ringeling FR, Vissers C, Jacob F, Pokrass M, Jimenez-Cyrus D, et al. Temporal Control of Mammalian Cortical Neurogenesis by m6A Methylation. Cell.2017;172(4): 877-889

[51] Wu R, Li A, Sun B, Sun J-G, Zhang J, Zhang T, et al. A novel m6A reader Prrc2a controls oligodendroglial specification and myelination. Cell Research. 2018;29(1):2341.

[52] Zepecki JP, Karambizi D, Fajardo E, Snyder KM, Guetta-Terrier C, Tang O, Chen J-S, Fiser A, Toms SA, Tapinos N. miRNA-mediated loss of m6A increases nascent translation in glioblastoma (PLOS Genet). https://doi.org/10.1371/journal.pgen.1009086.

[53] Liu X-M, Zhou J, Mao Y, Ji Q, Qian S-B. Programmable RNA N6-methyladenosineediting by CRISPR-Cas9 conjugates. Nature Chemical Biology. 2019;15(9):865-71.

[54] Rau K, Rösner L, Rentmeister A. Sequence-specific m6A demethylation in RNA by FTO fused to RCas9. RNA.2019;25(10):1311-23.

[55] Neftel C, Laffy J, Filbin MG, Hara T, Shore ME, et al. An Integrative Model of Cellular States, Plasticity, and Genetics for Glioblastoma. Cell. 2019;178(4):835-849.

[56] La Manno G, Soldatov R, Zeisel A, Braun E, Hochgerner H, et al. RNA velocity of single cells. Nature. 2018;560(7719):494-498.

[57] Prager BC, Bhargava S, Mahadev V, Hubert CG, Rich JN. Glioblastoma Stem Cells: Driving Resilience through Chaos. Trends in Cancer. 2020;6(3):223-35.

[58] Blau HM, Brazelton TR, Weimann JM. The Evolving Concept of a Stem Cell. Cell. 2001;105(7):829-41.

Section 6

# Tumors of the Pituitary and Pineal Regions

Chapter 12

# Pituitary Tumours

*Sumitra Sivakoti, Beatrice Anne, Abhishek J. Arora and Rajesh Alugolu*

## Abstract

The chapter focuses on understanding the latest classification of the pituitary adenomas in light of immuno-histological and molecular signatures as envisaged in the latest WHO classification guidelines. It further looks into evaluating and analysing the symptoms of the adenoma locally and at distant organs. Imaging and hormonal analysis has been discussed in detail for both functional, non-functional and pituitary apoplexy. Further, the therapeutic options- medical, surgical and their outcomes have been highlighted.

**Keywords:** Functional, non-functional, recurrent, approach, outcomes

## 1. Introduction

Pituitary adenoma (PA) is the third most common intracranial neoplasm accounting for approximately 15% of all such tumors and is the commonest one, accounting for 85% of sellar and suprasellar region. These tumors arise from various cells in the pea sized gland, measuring about 0.5 gms, located in a bony cavity of the sphenoid bone called sella turcica (Latin for *Turkish seat*) covered by dura all around, cavernous sinuses laterally and its anterior and posterior intercavernous venous channels [1–4].

## 2. Development and histology

Human pituitary gland is composed of two anatomically and functionally distinct parts: the adenohypophysis (anterior) and the neurohypophysis (posterior). The adenohypophysis develops from an evagination of primitive stomatal ectoderm, Rathke's pouch. The neurohypophysis originates from the infundibular process of the diencephalon [5].

Adenohypophysis is an epithelial gland of endodermal origin and is composed of acini that contain the six specialized hormone- secreting cells within a reticulin -rich stroma. It is controlled by hypothalamic hormones that stimulate or inhibit the release of anterior pituitary hormones. The posterior pituitary is composed of axonal processes of neurons whose cell bodies are located in the supraoptic and paraventricular nuclei of the hypothalamus, and pituicytes (modified glial cells).

Pituitary development is complex and includes a highly spatio-temporally regulated network of integrating extrinsic signaling pathways and homeobox transcriptional factors. Timely activation of signaling molecules is required for

evolution of pituitary gland and to determine cell-specific lineages for hormone production [6].

The factors involved in early organogenesis and maintenance of pituitary primordium are six homeodomain proteins- (1) paired homeodomain proteins like *Prx 1* and *Prx 2*, (2) LIM homeodomain transcription proteins, (3) SOX transcription factors (4) WNT/ beta-catenin and (5) Notch signaling. Transcriptional factors which play main role in lineage determination, cytodifferentiation and hormonal production, that target specific hormonal genes.

## 3. Pituitary specific transcription factors

Three main pathways have been described in cell differentiation in adenohypophysis (**Figure 1**) and have become a part of tumour classification in the most recent WHO 2017 classification [7–9]:

1. Pituitary transcription factor 1 (PIT1): has role in differentiation of somatotroph, thyrotroph, lactotroph, mammosomatotrophs and their respective tumours.

2. Steroidogenic factor 1 (SF1): is responsible for differentiation of gonadotrophs and is expressed in gonadotrophic adenomas.

3. T-box pituitary transcription factor (TPIT): is responsible for transcription of pro-opiomelanocortin, a precursor of adrenocorticotrophic hormone and is expressed in corticotroph adenomas.

## 4. Ancillary IHC markers

1. Low molecular weight cytokeratin (LMWCK): are important in differentiating sparsely vs. densely granulated tumours. In the former, >70% of tumour is occupied with paranuclear cytokeratin positive fibrous body and less of secretory granules.

2. Estrogen receptor alpha (ER): is expressed in lactotroph and gonadotroph adenomas

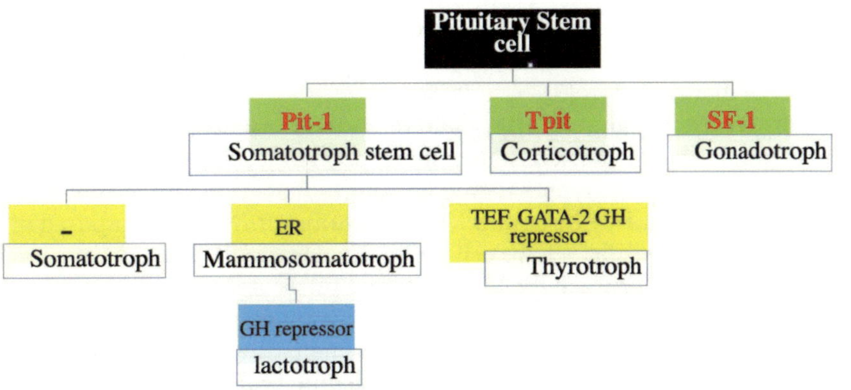


**Figure 1.**
*Factors involved in lineage specific adenohypophysial cells.*

3. GATA transcription factor 2 (GATA2): is expressed in gonadotroph and thyrotroph adenomas.

## 5. Genes associated with pituitary adenomas

Few genes have been identified as causes of pituitary adenomas-

### 5.1 Familial pituitary tumor syndromes

1. Multiple endocrine neoplasia type 1 (MEN 1)- Mutations in the coding for *menin*, reverses functions of tumor suppressor genes. Patients with MEN1 present with anterior pituitary adenomas in approximately 40% of all cases and have been described in children as young as 5 years. Most of the PAs in MEN1 are PRL-secreting (42–62%) or non-functioning tumors (15–42%), but GH- (6.5–9%) and ACTH-secreting (3–4%) adenomas have also been described. PAs in MEN1 have higher chance of co-secreting multiple hormones compared to *MEN1*-negative patients, in up to 39% of cases. PAs in MEN1 are considered more aggressive and at higher risk for resistance to treatment, especially in children with large prolactinomas [10–12].

2. Multiple endocrine neoplasia Type 2 (MEN-2)- are caused by *RET* gene mutations, which codes for a transmembrane receptor with tyrosine kinase activity acting as a proto-oncogene [12–15].

3. Multiple endocrine neoplasia type 4 (MEN 4)- is caused by *CDKN1B* gene mutations, which codes for a cyclin-dependent kinase (p27) that regulates cell cycle and progression from G1 to S phase of mitosis. MEN4 is a rare genetic syndrome, accounting for approximately 1.5–3% of patients clinically classified as MEN1, without genetic defects in *MEN1* gene [16–19].

4. Carney complex (CNC)- Carney complex (CNC) describes the constellation of myxomas, spotty skin pigmentation, and endocrine overactivity due to germline mutations of the *PRKAR1A* gene and are responsible for more than 70% of cases of CNC. *PRKAR1A* codes for the type 1 alpha regulatory subunit of the protein kinase A (PKA) tetramer, inactivation of which leads to dissociation of the regulatory from the catalytic subunit, aberrant activity of PKA and phosphorylation of downstream targets, leading to cell proliferation and tumour formation. Pituitary involvement in CNC is thought to be a progressive disorder with normal pituitary tissue progressing to somato-mammotroph hyperplasia and subsequently, to distinct tumour formation. Thus, multiple adenomas may be present synchronous or metachronous in the same patient [20–23].

5. Familial isolated pituitary adenomas (FIPA)- Familial pituitary tumors that are not associated with MEN 1 and CNC have been united under a new term-FIPA. It is used to describe families with at least two members with pituitary adenomas, with or without other abnormalities. About 15–25% of patients with FIPA harbour mutations in the AIP gene. This reaches up to 75% when families of GH-secreting adenomas are selected. AIP (aryl hydrocarbon receptor- interacting protein, 11q13) acts as tumor suppressor gene and its mutation predisposes to growth hormone secreting adenomas [24–27].

### 5.2 Sporadic pituitary adenomas

These account for 40% of GH adenomas and are due to mutations in Gs alpha gene mutations which results in cAMP/PKA signal transduction pathway leading to neoplastic transformation of somatotroph cells [28].

## 6. Pathology

All somatotrophic adenomas definitely express PIT-1 transcriptional factor and GH hormone. These tumors are broadly classified into pure somatotroph adenoma and Mixed somatotroph adenoma with co-expressing PRL or other hormonal markers. Based on secretary granules of GH, Pure somatotroph adenomas are further divided into two clinically significant and morphologically distinct subtypes: sparsely granulated (SG) and densely granulated (DG) somatotroph adenomas. Mixed SA are further classified into Mammosomatotroph adenomas (MSA), mixed somatotroph-lactotroph adenomas (MSLA) and plurihormonal adenomas.

Similar to other adenomas, SA are soft white to grey macroscopically. MSA are smaller in size with better prognosis compared to MSLA are larger with more invasiveness at the time of presentation.(75) SA are often seen arising from GH expressing pituitary cells in lateral wing of the gland. Extra seller extension of these tumors gives a characteristic shape of snowman (76).

Microscopically, SA share characteristics of other endocrine tumors: colonies of relatively large monomorphic cells with eosinophilic cytoplasm and spherical nuclei. Disruption of dense reticulin meshwork around the nests of cells distinguishes PA from normal pituitary cells (**Figure 2**). Hyperplasia to adenoma progression of SA were observed in some cases with familial isolated pituitary adenoma and X-linked acro-gigantism syndrome. (112) DGSAs are the most common and expresses diffuse cytosolic positively of GH and cytokeratin (CAM 5.2). These are predominantly seen in older age group with slower growth and excellent response to somatostatin treatment. SGSA are less common and behave differently with more aggressive nature like being larger, more invasiveness & proliferation and poor response to somatostatin response. They show co-segregation of cytokeratin and growth hormone granules resulting in characteristic fibrous bodies. These bodies are juxtanuclear keratin aggregates highlighted by cytokeratin immunohistochemical stain (CAM 5.2). MSA are histologically similar to DGSA and ultra-structurally distinct a single cell expressing both GH and PRL granules. MSLA are composed of

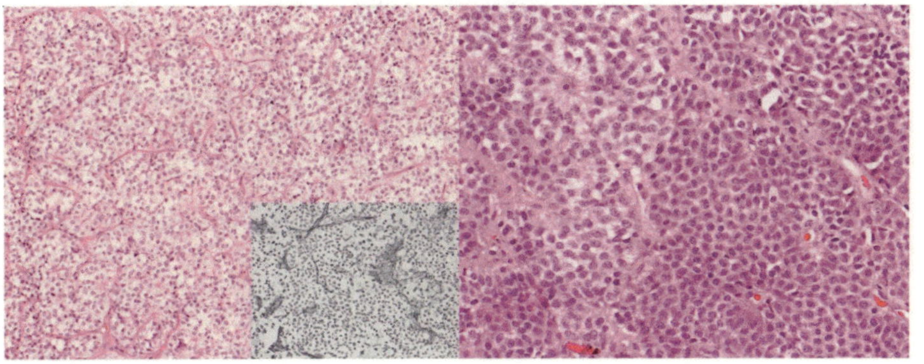

**Figure 2.**
*Histopathological section of pituitary adenoma exhibit colonies of monomorphic round cells with disruption of reticulin meshwork. (H & E 100X, (insert- Reticulin stain) and 200X).*

mixture of two different cells with GH and PRL secreting granules respectively. Either of the cell population can be densely or sparsely granulated with various combinations.

## 7. Radiology of pituitary tumors

'The Pituitary Body and its Disorders' was one of the first books written on the subject of Neuroradiology, based on work done at the Johns Hopkins Hospital, and consisted of detailed explanation of lesions detected on radiographs [29].

Pituitary imaging is indicated in patients, presenting with symptoms secondary to derailed pituitary hormones or symptoms indicating pituitary mass, like visual field deficit or headaches.

The sella turcica, as described earlier in chapter, is located deep within the cranium and can be demonstrated on a number of projections of skull radiographs. A right or left true lateral view of the skull demonstrates a clear profile view of sella and dorsum sellae. In a properly positioned lateral skull supine view, the line extending from the outer canthus of the eye to the external auditory meatus is perpendicular to the table. A caudally angled occipito-frontal projection, or Skull PA Axial (Caldwell View) is taken to demonstrate the floor of sella turcica. In this view, X-rays pass at an angle of 15 degrees from occiput and exit at the nasion, with film kept perpendicular to the orbitomeatal line (OML). For demonstration of dorsum sellae through the foramen magnum, Haas View, another Skull PA Axial view is taken where the central ray is angled 25 degrees cephalad to the orbitomeatal line (OML). The patient sits or stands facing an upright Bucky with the forehead and nose touching the imaging receptor. The neck is flexed to bring the OML perpendicular to the IR. It has been proven that PA axial radiographs add wealth of information pertaining to sella, and is complimentary to the sagittal view [30, 31].

Radiographic signs associated with pathology of pituitary gland and surrounding structures include i) enlargement with associated distortion of shape of the sella turcica, usually associated with empty sella syndrome or pituitary tumors, ii) Erosions in the floor or lateral walls, secondary to aneurysms or chronic increased intracranial pressure, iii) Sclerosis of the tuberculum or clinoid processes due to meningioma involving diaphragm sellae, iv) Sclerosis of sellar floor likely secondary to nasopharyngeal carcinoma or craniopharyngioma, v) Fat or calcifications in the intrasellar, suprasellar or parasellar region indicate presence of germ cell tumors or craniopharyngioma, vi) Eggshell calcification may point towards presence of aneurysms, Rathke's cyst or craniopharyngioma [32–34]. Usually sellar to cranial index of more than 8 is considered as abnormal and indicative of a sellar lesion on lateral skull radiograph [35].

With advent of Computed Tomography (CT) and Magnetic Resonance Imaging (MRI), MRI has become the modality of choice for imaging of pituitary lesions, due to its better soft-tissue contrast details and its ability to demonstrate pituitary gland and parasellar anatomy with increased spatial resolution and without artefacts from surrounding bones. CT is usually reserved for patients with contraindications to MRI and for those undergoing emergent evaluation.

In normal adults, the anterior pituitary is isointense to grey matter on T1- weighted and T2- weighted sequences, while posterior pituitary is inherently hyperintense onT1 weighted sequences, appearing as bright spot, secondary to antidiuretic hormone neurosecretory granules present within the posterior pituitary. In neonates till 2 months of age and in pregnant women, the anterior pituitary may be as hyperintense as the posterior pituitary. On post contrast dynamic

imaging, the enhancement of infundibulum is seen earlier than posterior pituitary, which turn enhances earlier than anterior pituitary [36].

Radiologically, pituitary adenomas are classified by size; microadenomas are 10 mm or less in diameter, and macroadenomas are greater than 10 mm in diameter. Microadenomas usually show signs and symptoms of hormonal excess, and if suspected, previous biochemical analysis for pituitary hormones is helpful in indicating a dynamic pituitary scan for their diagnosis. They could be either, prolactinomas, growth hormone-secreting adenomas or ACTH-secreting tumours. On MRI, microadenomas are iso to hypointense on T1W images and usually appear hyperintense on T2W sequences. Dynamic imaging following bolus injection of contrast, is helpful in depicting differential uptake of contrast between a microadenoma and normal pituitary gland and thus increases the detection rate of microadenomas [37, 38].

Pituitary macroadenomas are twice as common as microadenomas and are the most common suprasellar masses, resulting in visual symptoms. A slow-growing macroadenoma expands the bony sella and extends into the suprasellar cistern, giving "figure of 8" or "snowman" like appearance because the rigid diaphragm sellae. On CT imaging, macroadenomas are isodense to the surrounding brain, however, scalloping/destruction of the surrounding bones is better depicted on CT. On MRI, macroadenoma appears isointense to gray matter on T1- and T2-weighted MR images, and usually demonstrates intense contrast enhancement unless there are areas of necrotic degeneration or hemorrhagic foci within [39].

Invasive macroadenomas are usually prolactin-excreting tumors, and in such cases prolactin levels found are more than 1000 ng/dL [40]. It is difficult to distinguish invasive adenomas from rarer pituitary carcinoma, only on imaging.

Microadenomas may occasionally present with intrapituitary hemorrhage or tumor cyst without discerning solid component on MRI. Such cystic lesions within microadenomas are usually off midline unlike Rathke's cleft cyst, and are sometimes difficult to differentiate. In such cases, temporal growth of the lesion or associated hormonal changes give an indication of tumoral lesion. Intralesional hemorrhage can be picked up as hyperdense focus on CT and show peculiar MRI signal on T1W and T2W sequences based on the age of bleed.

Non adenomatous tumors of pituitary like, pituicytoma, spindle cell oncocytoma or granular cell tumors, are usually suprasellar/infudibular in location and some of them like granular cell tumors appear hyperdense on CT. Pituicytomas show homogeneous vascular enhancement on post contrast studies and are more vascular than adenomas, and their posterior location and increased vascularity makes them amenable for complete resection [41].

## 8. Classifications

Pituitary adenomas are broadly classified as functioning or non-functioning adenomas based on hypersecretion of specific hormones [42–47].

Functioning adenoma account for 2/3 of pituitary adenomas and present with specific clinical sign and symptoms related to excess hormonal secretion. Non-functioning adenomas account for 1/3 of all pituitary tumors, where they present incidentally or with clinical signs and symptoms related to degree of mass effect on adjacent structures with no evidence of hormone excess either clinically or on biochemical analysis. These are considered to be producing inactive peptides/glycoproteins or the hormone secretion was defective. These are further subtyped as-silent adenomas and null cell adenomas.

The definitions and thus the incidence of such adenomas has seen a sea of change with the addition of transcription factors and other IHC markers. Null cell

adenomas are defined as non-functional adenomas that are immune-negative for all hormones and pituitary specific transcription factors and has led to decrease of their incidence from 16.5% to <1% and has also led to the emergence of silent gonadotroph adenomas which were underdiagnosed. Silent adenomas were earlier described on ultrastructural findings on electron microscopy are now defined as tumors with no clinical or biochemical features of hormone excess but are positive for pituitary specific transcription factors. Silent corticotroph adenoma was classically described and subtyped as- I) densely granulated, II) sparsely granulated and III) Subtype 3. The immunoreactivity with PIT1 and inconsistent immunoreactivity to POMC has led to dropping of the word "corticotroph" from subtype 3and has been classified along with plurihormonal PIT1 adenomas (**Table 1**).

The new WHO classification of tumors of pituitary was mainly based on morphology and function of tumor cells (**Table 2**). Diagnostic and prognostic practical aspects included in new WHO are summarized below:

1. Elimination of term 'Atypical Adenoma': This term atypical adenoma was used for invasive tumors with invasiveness with elevated Ki67/MIB-1 and > 3% immunostaining for p53. This has been replaced by "high risk adenomas" and Includes

    a. Sparsely granulated somatotroph adenoma

    b. Lactotroph adenoma in men

    c. Crooke's cell adenoma

    d. Silent corticotroph adenoma

    e. Plurihormonal PIT1 positive adenoma.

2. Deletion of the term Oncocytoma, which is now considered a subset of gonadotroph adenoma.

3. A novel approach for classifying pituitary neuroendocrine tumors according to pituitary adenohypophyseal cell lineage pituitary specific transcription factors.

4. Re-definition of old entities like the null-cell adenoma based on pituitary specific transcription factors.

5. Introduction of new entities like pituitary blastoma, associated with DICER1 mutations, occurring exclusively in infants and children younger than 24 months.

| Transcription factors | IHC | Diagnosis |
|---|---|---|
| SF1 + | FSH+/LH+/ER+ | Gonadotroph |
| SF1 + | FSH-/LH−/ER- | Gonadotroph |
| TPIT1+ | ACTH- | Silent corticotroph |
| TPIT 1+ | ACTH + | Silent corticotroph |
| PIT 1+ | Variable GH/Prl/TSH/ER | Pit-1 lineage, poorly differentiated |
| PIT 1+ | LMWCK+, Variable GH/Prl/TSH/ER | Silent subtype 3 |

**Table 1.**
*Clinically non-functional adenomas.*

| S.No | Adenoma type | Morphological subtypes | Hormonal markers | Transcriptional factors | Cytokeratin (LMWCK) | Prognosis |
|---|---|---|---|---|---|---|
| 1 | Somatotroph adenoid | Densely granulated somatotroph adenoma | GH ± PRL ± α-subunit | PIT-1 | Perinuclear or diffuse positivity | |
| | | Sparsely granulated somatotroph adenoma | GH ± PRL | PIT-1 | Dot-like (fibrous body) | Aggressive |
| | | Mammosomatotroph adenoma | GH ± PRL ± α-subunit | PIT-1, ER-∝ | — | |
| | | Mixed somatotroph-lactotroph adenoma | GH ± PRL (in different cells) ± α-subunit | PIT-1, ER-∝ | — | |
| 2 | Lactotroph adenoid | Densely granulated lactotroph adenoma | PRL | PIT-1, ER-∝ | — | |
| | | Sparsely granulated lactotroph adenoma | PRL | PIT-1, ER-∝ | — | |
| | | Acidophil stem cell adenoma | PRL ± GH, | PIT-1, ER-∝ | Dot-like (fibrous body) | Aggressive<br>LA in men show aggressive behaviour |
| 3 | Thyrotroph adenoid | | b-TSH, α-subunit | PIT-1, GATA2 | — | |
| 4 | Corticotroph adenoid | Densely granulated | ACTH, | T-PIT | Diffuse | |
| | | Sparsely granulated | ACTH, | T-PIT | Diffuse | |
| | | Crooke's cell adenoma | ACTH, | T-PIT | Ring-like | Aggressive<br>Silent CA show aggressive behavior |
| 5 | Gonadotroph adenoid | | b-FSH, b-LH, α-subunit | SF-1, GATA2, ER-∝ | — | |
| 6 | Null cell adenoid | | No markers | None | — | |
| 7 | Plurihormonal adenoid | Plurihormonal PIT-1 positive adenoma (previously called subtype 3 adenoma) | GH, PRL, b-TSH, ± α-subunit | PIT-1 | — | Aggressive |
| | | Adenoma with unusual immunohistochemical combination | various | | — | |

**Table 2.**
*Classification of Pituitary Adenoma. Modified from the 2017 WHO classification of tumors of pituitary gland.*

*DOI: http://dx.doi.org/10.5772/intechopen.98311*

6. Introduction of new entities like plurihormonal tumors based on immunohistochemical combinations.

7. Introduction of double/multiple adenomas that show geographically distinct cell populations.

8. Replacing terminologies like term "hormone producing" has been changed to 'troph' to emphasize the role of transcription factors in cell differentiation and specific regulatory hormones of adenohypophysis.

Significant changes affecting the diagnosis of pituitary adenomas (PA) were introduced, and simultaneously panels of experts have also proposed replacing the term PA for Pituitary neuroendocrine tumour (Pit NET) [42–47].

## 9. Non-functioning pituitary adenomas

Non-functioning pituitary adenomas (NFPAs) are benign pituitary neoplasms that arise from the adenohypophyseal cells and lack clinical or biochemical evidence of hormone excess except for a mild hyperprolactinaemia in some cases, due to stalk effect. They account for 14–54% of pituitary adenomas. These include the silent adenomas and the null cell adenomas. Oncocytomas, which were included as a subset of null cell adenomas are now an obsolete term, and are accepted as phenotype with abundant mitochondria.

Immunohistochemical, secretory studies, in vitro tissue cultures have demonstrated the presence of all adenohypophyseal hormone components in the adenomas, the most common being the gonadotrophs. Even electron microscopic studies have shown that these tumour cells have secretory granules despite having assayable hormones. Chromophobe adenomas have also shown staining for ACTH despite being clinically negative for Cushing's syndrome or elevated cortisol levels.

### 9.1 What makes these tumors non-functional?

Various explanations have been offered to these tumours which have positive transcription factors except null cell adenomas for being hormonally or clinically negative. These are-

1. The glycoprotein hormones like FSH, LH, TSH need a combination of both alpha and beta subunits and these tumours might be producing the uncombined subunits and hence are clinically inactive.

2. Low levels of hormone production resulting in near normal values.

3. Abnormalities is secretion despite normal synthesis.

4. Lack of specific assays for subunit detection [48–52].

### 9.2 Clinical presentation

The clinical spectrum of NFPA varies from being completely asymptomatic to causing significant hypothalamic/ pituitary dysfunction and visual field compromise due to their large size. The absence of clinical symptoms of hormonal hypersecretion causes a delay in diagnosis with a mean time of delay

1.96 ± 2.9 years. Most patients present with symptoms of mass effect, such as headaches, visual field defects, ophthalmoplegias, and hypopituitarism. Other manifestations are hyperprolactinaemia due to pituitary stalk deviation and less frequently pituitary apoplexy (3.7–14.1%) [53, 54].

Headaches have been described with a varying incidence of 19–75% regardless of the size of the tumours. The possible reasons for the headaches are- (a) increased intrasellar pressure and stretching of dural membranes containing pain receptors, (b) activation of trigeminal pain pathways by tumours affecting the cavernous sinus (c) due to apoplexy, or (d) hydrocephalus [55].

Neuroophthalmological symptoms are caused by the pressure effects, ischemia or a combination of both on the on the optic chiasm. The typical visual field defect associated with pituitary tumours is bitemporal hemianopia, occurring when the body of the chiasm (which is comprised of the crossing nasal fibres of each optic nerve) is compressed by the enlarged gland. Variations in the anatomy of the chiasm leads to different patterns of field loss which can be uni-, bilateral or even central. The defect may be complete, involving the whole hemi-field or partial, usually beginning superiorly and progressing inferiorly, depending on the degree of nerve compression. Macular fibres, located in the postero-superior quadrant are more distant and are late to be involved. Chronic compression may lead to primary optic atrophy and may lead to decrease in the visual acuity.

Ophthalmoplegia is caused by pressure on the abducens or oculomotor nerves in the cavernous sinus. The invasion of the cavernous sinus (parasellar expansion) may affect the cranial nerves, causing a varied clinical profile according to the compromised nerve: ptosis (III nerve lesion), deviation of the eyeball superiorly and slightly inward (IV nerve involvement) and convergent strabismus (lesion VI nerve) [56].

Giant tumours, defined as ≥40 mm in one dimension or within 6 mm of Foramen of Monro, may rarely cause obstructive hydrocephalus. Erosion of the sellar floor may lead to CSF rhinorrhoea [57–59].

NFPAs may demonstrate mild elevations in serum prolactin ("disconnection hyperprolactinaemia"), due to blockage of dopamine which inhibits the lactotrophs. However, this value is never beyond 2000 mU/L. Mechanical compression of the normal anterior pituitary gland and/or pituitary stalk may prevent the passage of stimulatory hypothalamic factors resulting partial or complete hypopituitarism. Hypopituitarism develops slowly and often goes undetected. The overall prevalence of partial hypopituitarism in patients with NFPAs ranges from 37 to 85%. Panhypopituitarism occurs in 6–29% of patients and GH axis is affected in 61–100% of patients showing laboratory evidence of GH deficiency [60–62].

Central hypogonadism is noted in 36–96% of patients and adrenal insufficiency is noted in 17–62%. Finally, 8–81% exhibit central hypothyroidism. Presentation with diabetes insipidus is very rare [63].

## 9.3 Investigations

The investigations are aimed at-

1. Detecting the hormonal deficiencies,

2. Find out any hormonal excess especially double dilution to rule out Hook effect in hyperprolactinemia.

3. Imaging, the preferred one is MRI brain to demonstrate the morphology of the tumor, invasion of surrounding structures and assess the targeting routes.

4. Neuro-opthmological evaluation includes visual acuity, field vision and fundus characterisation.

The differential diagnosis of an incidentally discovered sellar mass is broad and includes a large number of entities: anterior pituitary tumours, posterior pituitary tumours (e.g., pituicytoma, granular cell tumours), benign parasellar tumours (e.g., meningioma, craniopharyngioma), malignant tumours (e.g., glioma, germ cell tumour), developmental lesions (e.g.,, Rathke's cleft cysts, dermoid cyst, epidermoid cyst, arachnoid cyst), inflammatory and granulomatous lesions (e.g., lymphocytic hypophysitis, granulomatous hypophysitis, Langerhans cell histiocytosis) and vascular lesions (e.g., aneurysms) [62].

### 9.4 Grading of tumor

1. Based on the size of tumor

   a. Microadenomas- less than 10 mm

   b. Macroadenomas- 10 mm to 40 mm in size

   c. Giant pituitary adenomas- tumors in excess of 40 mm in size, or extending within 6 mm of Foramen of Monro

2. **Hardy's Classification** [64–66]

   The large variation in sellar invasion and suprasellar extension of pituitary adenomas was recognized in the 1970s by Hardy and Vezina and prompted the development of the Hardy classification criteria to better characterize these lesions. Since that time, the Hardy classification system has served as a descriptive tool for pituitary adenomas and is often utilized in research studies. The Hardy classification comprises of two subscales: one describes the integrity of the sellar floor and invasion into the sphenoid sinus (Grades 0–IV), whereas the other describes the degree of suprasellar extension of the tumor (Types A–D). Although these two subscales were described using lateral radiographs and encephalograms, respectively, the Hardy grading scale is still used to classify adenomas based on magnetic resonance imaging (MRI) scans.

| Sellar Invasion | |
|---|---|
| Grade 0 | The enclosed adenoma is described as a tumor that remains within the anatomical confines of the osteo-aponeural sheath of the sella turcica. The floor of the sella is always intact. |
| 1 | The sella turcica is within normal limits in size (less than 16 × 13mm; 208 mm) but shows a lowering of the floor on one side or a bulging of the cortex. |
| 2 | The sella turcica is enlarged to various degrees but the floor remains intact. |
| 3 | The sella is more or less enlarged but there is a local erosion or destruction of the floor. |
| 4 | The entire floor of the sella is diffusely eroded or destroyed, giving a characteristic "phantom sella" with all the boundaries barely visible. |
| Suprasellar extension | |
| Type O | The tumour is entirely confined within the sella turcica. |
| A | The suprasellar expansion bulges into the chiasmatic cistern but does not reach the floor of the anterior third ventricle. |

| | |
|---|---|
| B | The tumour reaches the floor of the third ventricle, giving the image of an inverse cupula of the anterior recesses of the third ventricle. |
| C | A voluminous suprasellar expansion bulges largely into the third ventricle up to the foramen of Monro. |
| D | Rare aberrant expansions occur in temporal or frontal fossa. |

3. Wilson's modification of Hardy's classification [67]

Wilson modified Hardy's classification to distinguish between extrasellar extensions, including extension into the cavernous sinus.

Suprasellar extension

0: none
A: expanding into suprasellar cistern
B: anterior recesses of 3rd ventricle obliterated
C: floor of 3rd ventricle grossly displaced

Parasellar extension

D: intracranial (intradural); specify (1) anterior (2) middle, or (3) posterior fossa
E: into or beneath cavernous sinus (extradural)

Invasion

Floor of sella intact

I: sella normal or focally expanded; tumor <= 10 mm
II: sella enlarged; tumor > = 10 mm

Sphenoid extension

III: localized perforation of sellar floo
IV: diffuse destruction of sellar floor

Distant spread

V: spread via CSF or blood-borne

4. Knosp's grading for invasiveness into cavernous sinus

Knosp et al. introduced a classification of the parasellar extension of PAs based on MRI coronal sections. Three lines (medial, median and lateral), which cross the internal carotid artery (ICA), determine the degree of invasion. They further suggested a subdivision of grade 3 into 3A and 3B: in Grade 3A, the tumor extends laterally in the superior compartment of the cavernous sinus, whereas in Grade 3B the lesion extends laterally, but in the inferior compartment. This finding is clinically and biologically relevant, and is most probably the consequence of better surgical visualization provided by an endoscope [68–70].

| Grade 0 | No involvement of the cavernous sinus (normal condition) |
|---|---|
| 1 | The tumour pushes into the medial wall of the cavernous sinus, but does not go beyond a hypothetical line extending between the centres of the two segments of the internal carotid artery (non-invasive PA) |
| 2 | The tumour goes beyond hypothetical line, but without passing a line tangent to the lateral margins of the artery itself (non-invasive PA) |

| | |
|---|---|
| 3 | The tumour extends laterally to the internal carotid artery within the cavernous sinus (invasive PA) |
| 4 | Total encasement of the intra-cavernous carotid artery (invasive PA) |

### 9.5 Treatment

The primary goal of treatment of these non-functioning adenomas is reduction of the tumour mass and relieve the compressive effects on the optic apparatus, ventricular system, cavernous sinus and adjacent brain parenchyma.

In the absence of visual impairment, the optimal treatment choice is still a matter of debate, especially in patients presenting with hypopituitarism, headache, or tumours close to the chiasma. Surgery may improve pituitary function in up to 30% of patients with pre-existing hypopituitarism, but the risk of new hormone deficiency following surgery is 2–15%. Therefore, hypopituitarism alone is not an indication for surgical treatment. Surgical resection of non-functioning microadenomas is not indicated since tumour growth is rare (3–13%) with less than 5% growing > 1 cm during long-term follow-up.

Surgical excision either through trans-sphenoidal endoscopic or microscopic or trans-cranial route are the mainstay.

Bromocriptine, Octreotide and other agents have been shown to be partially successful in reducing the tumour.

Radiotherapy is indicated in case of inadequate tumour resection, high mitotic index and at recurrence.

Gross total resection is achieved in 60–73% of patients with NFPAs. In a recent meta-analysis on NFPA patients, TSS was associated with 1% mortality. Postoperative complications such as cerebrospinal fluid (CSF) leakage, fistula, meningitis, vascular injury, persistent DI, or new visual field defect occurred in ≤ 5% of patients. Surgical complications are reported to be less frequent with higher-volume surgeons or hospitals. The risk of CSF leakage is increased in patients with large adenomas with suprasellar extension, intraoperative CSF leakage, repeat TSS, and high body mass index.

### 9.6 Outcomes

The visual improvement in acuity and visual fields is seen in 70–80% following gross total or subtotal excision of tumours [71–73].

### 9.7 Residual or recurrent NFPA

The rate of complete excision of these nonfunctional adenoma varies from 60 to 70% depending on the experience of surgeon. Additional use of intra-operative MRI has increased the rate of complete removal to 82%. Factors leading to less than complete removal are- 1) invasion into cavernous sinus, 2) increased diameter, and 3) absence of apoplexy [74].

Recurrences following complete removal of tumour is usually low. Recurrence rates in 10-year follow-up was found to be approximately 5%, 25% and 50% for initial complete removal, suspicious residue and initial incomplete removal, respectively.

Indications for re-surgery for both recurrences or growing remnants are- 1) increasing tumour size, 2) new endocrinological deficits and 3) new ophthalmological symptoms.

Management of recurrence is based on the following factors- 1) time of tumour recurrence, 2) size and location, 3) age, 4) general condition, 5) ophthalmological findings, 6) neurological findings and 7) endocrine findings.

Re-do surgery is recommended for accessible tumours in young and healthy adults. Early recurrences after complete excision are better treated with radiotherapy. Small and asymptomatic recurrences need to be followed up for tumour growth and clinical factors. Elderly with severe systemic diseases is managed conservatively [75–86].

## 10. Lactotroph adenomas or prolactinomas

LA are also derived from PIT-1 lineage adenohypophyseal cells with chief expression of PRL. LA are the most common hormone expressing pituitary adenoma, accounting for 30–50% of all adenomas. The reported prevalence is 35 per 100,000 people. The highest incidence is seen in women of child-bearing age and in patients with MEN 1 [87–90].

### 10.1 Clinical presentation

This endocrinopathy which was classically described as amenorrhea-galactorrhea syndrome was first described to be associated with prolactin hypersecretion by Forbes in 1954. However, the manifestations are quite varied among the genders and in females in relation to their menopausal status. The increased levels of prolactin cause decrease in the levels of gonadotropins resulting in hypogonadism. In females in reproductive ages, they present with- 1) delayed puberty, 2) oligomenorrhea, 3) primary or secondary amenorrhea or 4) regular menstural cycles with infertility. Galactorrhea is seen in 30–80% females in this age group. Post-menopausal women and men, who conspicuously lack these features, present with visual disturbances and subtle symptoms like loss of libido or dyspareunia. Osteoporosis which was earlier considered due to direct effects of prolactin on the bone is correlated to hypogonadism and lack of estrogen in women. Headaches are a common presentation in all. Psychiatric manifestations include hostility, depression, anxiety and weight gain [90–92].

### 10.2 Pathology

Macroscopically, LA are pseudo capsulated and show grey white appearance with firm consistency and gritty on cut. Stromal amyloid deposition and microcalcification are observed in few cases. Some tumors have microscopic invasion and some macroadenoma are widely invasive into adjacent structures. SGLA are distinct from DGLA, as the prolactin staining pattern is paranuclear golgi type. ASLA are composed of abundant vacuolated eosinophilic cytoplasm, so called oncocytic change and occasional fibrous bodies.

Immunohistologically, these tumors are subdivided into sparsely granulated lactotroph adenoma (SGLA), densely granulated lactotroph adenoma and acidophil stem cell adenoma (ASCA). These subtypes have a distinct biological behavior and response to treatment. LA are most common in women and predominantly seen in childhood and adolescents age group. Biological and prognostically distinct differences are observed between males and females. In men, tumor present more aggressively with invasiveness and 80% are larger of them are macroadenoma, whilst size of tumor is small in women. Estrogen plays a significant role in

pathogenesis of tumor. A significant correlation between the estrogen receptor and tumor volume was observed, but mechanism is not known.

### 10.3 Laboratory evaluation

The normal levels of prolactin are <20 ng/ml. Single elevation of >200 ng/ml are almost always due to prolactinomas. However, the values between 20 and 200 ng/ml need careful evaluation of drug, systemic condition and correlation with the size of the tumour to rule out "pseudo-prolactinomas" due to "stalk sectioning effects" [93].

Prolactin may be elevated in other conditions as well. Hence, a careful history especially pertaining to drugs needs to be taken (**Table 3**). Non–prolactin-producing macroadenomas can cause prolactin elevations from disinhibition of prolactin secretion by compressing the pituitary stalk or hypothalamus. Very high prolactin levels seen in macroadenomas can saturate the antibodies in the assays and lead to artifactually low or normal results (the "Hook effect") and prolactin levels should be rerun at 1:100 dilution to exclude this possibility [8].

Two distinct biological profiles of prolactinomas have been observed- 1) benign microadenomas with very little growth potential and 2) aggressive, invasive macroadenomas. Natural history and autopsy studies have shown that not all microadenomas proceed to develop into macroadenomas. The risk of progression of

| | |
|---|---|
| Hypothalamic causes | Craniopharyngiomas<br>Meningiomas<br>Dysgerminomas<br>Sarcoidosis<br>Langerhans cell histiocytosis<br>Vascular<br>Pituitary stalk section |
| Pituitary causes | Prolactinomas<br>Acromegaly<br>Lymphocytic hypophysitis<br>Cushing disease<br>Non secreting adenomas (stalk compression) |
| Medications | Phenothiazines<br>Haloperidol<br>Atypical antipsychotics<br>Monoamine-oxidase inhibitors<br>Tricyclic antidepressants<br>Reserpine<br>Methyldopa<br>Metoclopramide, Levosulpride<br>Verapamil<br>Serotonin reuptake inhibitors<br>Estrogen |
| Neurogenic | Chest wall lesions<br>Spinal cord lesions<br>Nipple stimulation |
| Other | Pregnancy<br>Hypothyroidism<br>Chronic kidney disease<br>Cirrhosis<br>Pseudocyesis |

**Table 3.**
*Causes of hyperprolactinemia.*

microadenomas to macroadenomas is 3–7%. However, the natural history of macroprolactinomas is not known. The risk of macroadenomas enlarging during pregnancy is approximately 15%.

Dopamine agonist therapy is the mainstay of treatment, instituted to lower prolactin levels, decrease tumour size, and restore gonadal function for patients harbouring symptomatic prolactin-secreting microadenomas or macroadenomas.

Bromocriptine, the prototype dopamine agonist was introduced into clinical trials in 1971. It acts by stimulating dopamine receptors on lactotrophs, a potent analogue of dopamine, decreases cAMP activity, reduction in intracellular calcium, and hence decreased synthesis and release of prolactin. It is given in doses of 5-20 mg/day in three divided doses. The cellular and ultra-structural changes noticed after bromocriptine therapy are- 1) loss of cytoplasmic volume, 2) involution of rough endoplasmic reticulum, 3) at subcellular level, decrease in prolactin gene transcription and translation, 4) in vivo PET studies demonstrating reduced metabolic activity and 5) varying degrees of calcification, amyloid deposition, perivascular and interstitial fibrosis. All the above except 5, are reversible especially in macroadenoma. The fibrosis may preclude successful tumour excision. Bromocriptine resistance may be noted in 25% patients, 80% of whom may show response to cabergoline [94, 95].

The long-acting dopamine agonist cabergoline is preferred due to its higher efficacy in normalizing prolactin levels and pituitary adenoma shrinkage [8]. The higher efficacy is probably due to the higher affinity for dopamine receptor binding sites. Control of hyperprolactinemia requires doses of cabergoline ranging from 0.25 to 3 mg/wk.; resistance to cabergoline may be seen in upto 10% patients and may require doses up to 11 mg/wk. [12, 13]. Echocardiograms should be advised yearly in those patients exceeding a weekly dose of 2 mg, to look for valvular regurgitation [96].

Another adverse effect of dopamine agonist, occurring in about 5% of patients, is compulsive behaviour, such as excessive gambling and hypersexuality. Asymptomatic patients harbouring a microprolactinoma may be followed up without treatment. In patients with amenorrhea due to the microadenoma, the clinician can choose between a dopamine agonist or oral contraceptives.

Resistance to therapy is defined by failure to achieve a normal prolactin level and failure to achieve a 50% tumour reduction after maximal conventional doses of DA (Bromocriptine >15 mgs per day or 2 mg/week of cabergoline for at least 3 months). The possible reason for resistance is decreased D2 receptor expression or mutations in post receptor mechanisms.

The alkylating agent, Temozolamide, has been used in patients with malignant prolactinomas.

Patients on medical management should be followed up at regular intervals in the following manner:

a. Serum prolactin levels to be measured at regular intervals, beginning 1 month after the start of treatment in order to guide the clinician for titration of dopamine agonist therapy to achieve normo-prolactinemia/restore eugonadal status.

b. Repeat MRI in 1 yr.

c. Earlier repeat MRI (in 3 months) in patients with macroprolactinoma, if prolactin levels continue to rise while patient is receiving dopaminergic agents, or in the presence of new symptoms, e.g., galactorrhoea, visual disturbances, headaches, or other hormonal disorders.

d. Visual field examinations in patients with macroadenomas at risk of impinging the optic chiasm

e. Evaluation and management of comorbidities, e.g., sex steroid-dependent bone loss, persistent galactorrhoea and pituitary trophic hormone reserve.

### 10.4 Surgical Indications for prolactinomas

1. Pituitary Apoplexy

2. Visual deficits due to compression of the optic apparatus

3. Cystic prolactinomas

4. DARP- Dopamine agonist resistant prolactinomas

5. Women seeking fertility

6. CSF fistulas

7. Recurrent tumors

8. Increasing tumor during pregnancy

9. Macroadenoma in psychiatric patients

Remission rates after surgical excision vary from 30 to 93%. Restarting DA following surgical decompression normalises prolactin levels which can be maintained at lower doses [97–101].

### 10.5 Surgical issues with pregnancy in prolactinomas

The major issue with regards to pregnancy in patients with prolactinomas are

1. Infertility

2. Risk of tumour growth during pregnancy

3. Effects on foetal growth

The risk tumour enlargement is upto 5% for microadenomas while it reaches upto 15% for macroadenomas. However, prior surgery and/or radiotherapy reduces this risk to 4.3%. Both surgery and bromocriptine therapy are equally effective in microadenomas for fertility. However, no such comparison is available for macroadenomas. Bromocriptine needs to be stopped at the first sign of pregnancy [100, 102].

## 11. Somatotroph adenoma

Somatotroph adenoma (SA) is a subtype of pituitary adenoma which are derived from PIT-1 lineage cells with GH expression and with or without co-expression of prolactin (PRL). These tumors account for 10–15% of all pituitary adenoma, and can occur at any age with mean age at diagnosis of 47 years.

## 11.1 Pathology

All somatotrophic adenomas definitely express PIT-1 transcriptional factor and GH hormone. These tumors are broadly classified into pure somatotroph adenoma and Mixed somatotroph adenoma with co-expressing PRL or other hormonal markers. Based on secretary granules of GH, Pure somatotroph adenomas are further divided into two clinically significant and morphologically distinct subtypes: sparsely granulated (SG) and densely granulated (DG) somatotroph adenomas. Mixed SA are further classified into Mammosomatotroph adenomas (MSA), mixed somatotroph-lactotroph adenomas (MSLA) and plurihormonal adenomas.

Similar to other adenomas, SA are soft white to grey macroscopically. MSA are smaller in size with better prognosis compared to MSLA are larger with more invasiveness at the time of presentation.SA are often seen arising from GH expressing pituitary cells in lateral wing of the gland. Extra seller extension of these tumors gives a characteristic shape of snowman.

Microscopically, SA share characteristics of other endocrine tumors: colonies of relatively large monomorphic cells with eosinophilic cytoplasm and spherical nuclei. Disruption of dense reticulin meshwork around the nests of cells distinguishes PA from normal pituitary cells. Hyperplasia to adenoma progression of SA were observed in some cases with familial isolated pituitary adenoma and X-linked acrogigantism syndrome. (WHO 2017) DGSAs are the most common and expresses diffuse cytosolic positively of GH and cytokeratin (CAM 5.2). These are predominantly seen in older age group with slower growth and excellent response to somatostatin treatment. SGSA are less common and behave differently with more aggressive nature like being larger, more invasiveness & proliferation and poor response to somatostatin response. They show co-segregation of cytokeratin and growth hormone granules resulting in characteristic fibrous bodies. These bodies are juxtanuclear keratin aggregates highlighted by cytokeratin immunohistochemical stain (CAM 5.2). MSA are histologically similar to DGSA and ultrastructurally distinct a single cell expressing both GH and PRL granules. MSLA are composed of mixture of two different cells with GH and PRL secreting granules respectively. Either of the cell population can be densely or sparsely granulated with various combinations.

## 11.2 Clinical manifestations

Growth hormone adenomas are commonly seen in 4th and 5th decades with no gender predominance. More than 60% are macroadenomas compared to other hormonally active tumors and hence have predominant local effects apart from systemic effects. Endocrine systemic effects produce gigantism (pre-pubertal) and acromegaly (after apophyseal fusion). Despite widespread changes including in the appearance, the mean interval between the disease onset and diagnosis is 8.7 years [103].

The facial features described as "beetle brow" appearance include the following changes- deeply furrowed scalp, coarse skin, frontal bossing, fleshy nose, prominent nasolabial folds, thick lips, prognathism, maxillary widening, dental malocclusion with increased inter-dental space and macroglossia with tooth marks on the tongue. The voice changes include low pitched deep voice due to laryngeal hypertrophy and enlarged paranasal sinuses. Hypertrophy of sebaceous glands gives oily appearance to the face. Enlargement of sweat glands gives rise to malodors [104, 105]. Sleep apnea syndrome is seen in up to 75% of acromegalics [106–108].

Enlargement of hands which are thick, fleshy and are classically described as "spade like hands". The bony hyperostosis and soft tissue thickening causes entrapment neuropathy like carpel tunnel syndrome.

Periosteal new bone formation leads to osteophyte formation, disc degeneration and spinal stenosis. Arthropathy of weight bearing joints is common. Myopathy is a common feature of acromegaly.

Pachydermoperiostosis is a very rare osteoarthrodermopathic disorder whose clinical and radiographic presentations may mimic those of acromegaly and should be considered as a differential diagnosis [109].

The cardiovascular manifestations include hypertension, concentric biventricular hypertrophy and arrhythmias. These changes in the cardiovascular system are least resistant to reversal [110, 111].

Hypertrophy of internal organs like hepatomegaly and splenomegaly is frequently encountered. Diabetes mellitus and islet cell neoplasms are also noted. Oral glucose tolerance is impaired in 50%, while frank diabetes mellitus is seen in 10% of acromegalics. These metabolic changes are however reversible [111].

Colonic malignancies are also documented in patients with GH adenomas [112–114].

Risk factors for colonic malignancies in Acromegaly

1. Age > 50 years

2. Family history of colonic malignancy

3. >3 skin tags

4. Prior colonic polyps

Reproductive abnormalities have also been observed in patients with GH adenomas. These include menstrual disturbances and galactorrhea in women and decreased libido and impotence in men. These effects are due to hyper prolactinemia with mammosomatotrophs or mixed tumors, stalk effect or decrease FSH, LH secretion.

### 11.3 Endocrine diagnostic criteria

Serum IGF-1 is the initial screening method of choice. The diagnosis is confirmed by the unsuppressed nadir of GH >1 ng/ml and GH > 0.4 ng/ml following 75 gms of OGTT with documented hyperglycemia.

### 11.4 Criteria for cure

The criteria for cure in GH adenomas are-

1. GH < 1 ng/ml

2. OGTT and GH <0.4 ng/ml done at 12 weeks post-surgery

3. Normalization of somatomedin -C levels

Transsphenoidal surgery is recommended as primary therapy. Experienced pituitary neurosurgeons can achieve the therapeutic goals in 80–90% of patients with microadenomas and 40–60% of those with macroadenomas. The 5-year recurrence rate is approximately 2–8%. Repeat IGF-1 levels and growth hormone levels during an oral glucose tolerance test should be obtained about 12 weeks following surgery, along with an MRI to assess the changes in tumour size. The goal

| Drug | Dose | Indication | Side effects |
|---|---|---|---|
| Cabergoline | 0.5–2 mg/ week | modest elevations of serum IGF-1 and mild signs and symptoms of GH excess | Nausea, vomiting, constipation, dizziness, headache, compulsive behavior |
| Octreotide LAR | 10–30 mg/ month | significant disease (ie, with moderate-to-severe signs and symptoms of GH excess and without local mass effects) | Abdominal cramps, flatulence, diarrhea, gall bladder stones and sludge, alopecia |
| Lanreotide depot | 60–120 mg/ month | significant disease | Abdominal cramps, flatulence, diarrhea, gall bladder stones and sludge, alopecia |
| Pasireotide LAR | 20–60 mg/ month | significant disease | Abdominal cramps, flatulence, diarrhea, gall bladder stones and sludge, alopecia, hyperglycemia |
| Pegvisomant | 10–20 mg/ day | significant disease | Hepatotoxicity, nausea, diarrhea |
| *LAR – Long-acting release* | | | |

**Table 4.**
*Drugs used for medical management of GH excess.*

of therapy is to normalize the serum IGF 1 level and reduce the GH levels <1.0 ug/L [115].

Medical management is recommended for patients with persistent disease following surgery. Medical therapy (**Table 4**) may be considered as first line in patients who cannot be cured by surgery, has extensive cavernous sinus invasion, does not have chiasmal compression, or is a poor surgical candidate. If medical therapy is unavailable, unsuccessful, or not tolerated, stereotactic radiotherapy (SRT)/Gamma-knife radiosurgery should be considered unless the technique is not available, there is significant residual tumour burden, or the tumour is too close to the optic chiasm. The response to radiation therapy takes an average of 3.17 years and in the meantime the therapy needs to be bridged with medical management. Remission rates of approximately 60% are observed at 10 years [116].

There is an overall 72% increase in mortality and decrease in 10 years of average life expectancy in patients with acromegaly. Cardiovascular causes are the leading cause accounting for about 25%, while cerebrovascular, malignancies and respiratory diseases are responsible for 15% each. Mortality is 2.4 times higher in females while it is 4.8 times more in males.

Factors associated with increased mortality

1. Older age at diagnosis
2. Male gender
3. Increased disease duration
4. High GH levels [>2.5 ng/ml]
5. Elevated IGF-1 levels
6. Active disease

7. Associated hypopituitarism

8. Associated systemic malignancies

9. Need for radiotherapy for disease control

## 12. Corticotroph adenoma and Cushing's disease

Of all the pituitary adenomas, the corticotroph adenomas are the most difficult ones to diagnose and treat. The diagnosis revolves between Cushing's syndrome and disease wherein the first one is of non-specific etiology and is produced by any cause of glucocorticoid excess while the latter is due to a pituitary adenoma secreting excess ACTH and thus hypercortisolemia. Cushing's disease is seen in up to 10–16% of all surgically resected pituitary adenomas.

Females are more commonly affected than male, with a M:F ration ranging between 1:3 to 1:10. Though can be seen at any age, is commonly found in 3rd and 5th decade [117].

### 12.1 Pathology

Corticotroph adenoma (CA) are derived from TPIT-lineage adenohypophysial cells that express ACTH and proopiomelanocortin-derived peptides. These tumors are subdivided into densely granulated CA, sparsely granulated CA and Crooke cell adenoma (CCA) based on secretary granules and cytokeratin accumulation.

More than 80% of the tumors are microadenomas and the rest are macroadenomas. DGCA is the most common subtype in patients presented with Cushing disease. The staining pattern of ACTH granules in SGCA and DGCA are parallel to staining pattern of GH in pure somatotroph adenoma. SGCA are less frequent than DGCA and usually presented as macroadenoma. CCA are rare subtypes, in which cells have typical Crooke hyaline change. These cells are composed of dense perinuclear deposition of cytokeratin filaments appearing as thick hyaline ring. As a result of this rearrangement of cellular organelles and secretary granules to the periphery noted.

### 12.2 Clinical features

These adenomas are usually microadenomas and seldom cause symptoms of mass effect on the parasellar structures. The main clinical features are due to the hypercortisolemia [118, 119].

1. There is abnormal centripetal fat deposition leading to truncal obesity. The accumulation of fat in the face gives rise to characteristic "moon facies", while the deposition in the supraclavicular area and cervicodorsal region gives rise to "buffalo-hump" appearance.

2. There is thinning of the skin due to atrophy of epidermis and connective tissue. Increased capillary fragility leads to easy bruising and a plethoric face. Purple striae due to stretching of the skin are noted on the abdomen and flanks. Hyperpigmentation and hirsutism are also observed.

3. A multitude of metabolic disturbances are observed in these patients. Hypertension, hyperlipidemia and diabetes mellitus are quite common. Bone

demineralization leading to osteoporosis especially in the vertebral bodies is frequent. Hypocalacemic tetany have also been described. Hypokalemic alkalosis due to mineralocorticoid effect of cortisol on the renal tubules [120].

4. The effects of hypercortisolemia lead to suppression of TSH leading to features of hypothyroidism. Suppression of gonadotropic releasing hormone leads to menstrual disturbances in females, impotence in males and decreased libido in either gender [121–123].

5. Impaired host defences due to hypercortisolaemic effects on the immune system leads to repeated infections ranging from superficial skin infections like tinea versicolor or oral candidiasis to severe life-threatening sepsis [124–126].

6. Psychiatric disturbances range from depression, emotional liability to frank psychosis. Structural changes and cognitive effects have also been observed [127–131].

The case fatality rate in Cushing's disease reaches up to 50% at 5 years, with cardiovascular events leading the cause followed by infections and suicide [118, 132].

### 12.3 Endocrine evaluation

The first step in a suspected case of Cushing's disease is establishment of the fact that there is a state of hypercortisolaemia and that pituitary adenoma is the cause of it before jumping upon radiological investigations as incidentalomas occur in 10% of cases. Further a detailed evaluation of the medications used to rule out exogenous use of steroids is required.

The biochemical evaluation is to rule out exogenous steroid use by ordering a basal serum cortisol [10].

Step1: Establish hypercortisolaemic state: [133].

a. 24 hours urinary cortisol – this is a simple and sensitive screening measure. This is based on the fact that urinary free cortisol raises exponentially for quantum increases in plasma cortisol. With sensitivity (53–97%) and specificity (86–91%), this is highly useful in patients with high cortisol binding globulins.

b. Elevation of basal plasma cortisol at 11 pm

c. Salivary cortisol measurements at 11 pm is another method to detect cortisol excess and alterations in diurnal variations which are the earliest and subtle biochemical changes, with sensitivity and specificity of 92 and 100%, respectively.

d. Low Dose Dexamethasone test: This is based on the principle of suppression of hypothalamic-pitutitary axis and this decrease in ACTH and morning cortisol levels to <5 micogms/dl by dexamethasone. This was conventionally done by giving 0.5 mgs every 6th hourly for 48 hours before 8 am serum cortisol. This has been replaced by single 11 pm dose of 1 mg of dexamethasone and 8 am serum cortisol measurement.

Step 2: Determine if the cortisol excess is ACTH dependent or independent.

ACTH levels are low (<10 pg./ml) if there is autonomous production by the adrenal gland and the levels are elevated (>20 pg./ml) if a pituitary tumor or ectopic ACTH or corticotropin releasing hormone production is the cause. The level of elevations also give a clue to the cause with moderate elevations of 80–200 pgm/ml seen in corticotroph adenomas while values >200 pg./ml are seen in ectopic ACTH lesions.

Step 3: Distinguishing Cushing's disease from ectopic ACTH states.

The secretory activity of corticotroph adenoma, unlike ectopic ACTH is not autonomous and retains negative feedback responsiveness to glucocorticoid, at higher thresholds. This is the basis of high dose dexamethasone test.

2mgs of dexamethasone is given every 6th hourly for 48 hours and the urinary cortisol is measured. A 50% reduction in urinary cortisol secretion is appropriate suppression and is suggestive of pituitary adenoma. Otherwise, 8–32 mgs of single dose dexamethasone is given at 11 pm and serum cortisol is measured at 8 am. A 50% reduction is suggestive of suppressive response. This has a sensitivity, specificity and diagnostic accuracy of 89%, 100% and 91%, respectively [134].

CRH stimulation test:

The corticotroph adenomas have CRH receptors and hence the levels of ACTH increase following intravenous CRH. A positive response of increase in 50% in plasma ACTH or 20% raise in plasma cortisol is observed in corticotrophs adenomas. Negative results are seen in ectopic ACTH producing lesions as the pituitary corticotrophs are chronically suppressed and are resistant to stimulatory effects of CRH. Diagnostic accuracy of this test is approximately 98% [135, 136].

In some cases, to differentiate between a pituitary vs. an ectopic source of ACTH, inferior petrosal sinus sampling is done, in which catheters are threaded up to the petrosal sinuses that drain the pituitary venous system. ACTH levels are measured from each petrosal sinus and peripherally before and after stimulation with corticotropin-releasing hormone. The basal central to peripheral ACTH >2 is suggestive of corticotroph adenoma while a ratio < 1.7 is suggestive of ectopic ACTH lesion. Following CRH stimulation, a ratio of >3 is diagnostic of corticotroph adenoma with sensitivity and specificity of 96–100%.

The ACTH concentration that exceeds the other side by 1.5 times is likely to be the side of adenoma with sensitivity, specificity and diagnostic accuracy for laterality is 96%, 100% and 78%, respectively [135–138].

### 12.4 Radiology

As 80–90% of corticotroph adenomas are microadenomas, dynamic contrast MRI of the pitutitary is needed with sensitivity and specificity of 60 and 87%, respectively. Volume interpolated 3D spoiled gradient echo (VI-SGE) helps in detection of microadenoma with a sensitivity and specificity of 87% and 100%, respectively [139–143].

Trans sphenoidal surgery is the initial treatment for an ACTH secreting pituitary adenoma. The remission rates with surgery are 52–96%. The positive predictors for remission following surgery are- 1. Visualisation of adenoma on imaging, 2. Size and extent of adenoma, with microadenomas and without invasion into cavernous sinus faring better and 3. Histopathological confirmation of adenoma. The recurrence rates vary from 15 to 66%. Radiotherapy is the second line of management for persistent or recurrent disease with conventional radiotherapy faring better than stereotactic radiosurgery.

In case of no cure after surgery, or radiotherapy/ stereotactic radiosurgery, medical therapy (**Table 5**), or bilateral adrenalectomy are the options.

## 13. TSH secreting adenoma

Thyrotroph adenoma (TA) arise from PIT-1 lineage adenohypophyseal cells with chief expression of Thyroid stimulating hormone.

(TSH). These tumors are most infrequent tumors, accounting for less than 2% of all pituitary adenomatous tumors. Excessive secretion of TSH makes thyroid to make excess production of T3 and T4 resulting in hyperthyroidism. An occasional case of TA associated with primary hypothyroidism are reported. The tumor derived from thyroid deficiency are distinct from classical TA clinically, routine microscopy and ultra-structurally.

Patients should be rendered euthyroid with antithyroid drugs like methimazole, propylthiouracil before undertaking transsphenoidal surgery. Patients not cured by surgery can be treated with somatostatin analogues (Octreotide LAR and Lanreotide depot) and by irradiation.

## 14. Gonadotroph adenoma

Gonadotroph adenoma (GA) are most common pituitary adenoma arise from SF-1 lineage adenohypophysial cell with production of FSH and or LH. These tumors account for highest percentage as clinically non-functioning adenomas. GA are usually macroadenomas with often infiltration into suprasellar and parasellar compartments. Incidental detection of these tumors is increasing these days due to widespread use of CT and MRI. There is a male predominance among middle age and older people. These tumors show a prominent pseudo-rosette pattern around blood vessels mimicking a close diagnosis of esthesioneuroblastoma. Usage of SF-1 immunohistochemistry helps in differentiating these two.

## 15. Plurihormonal adenoma

Plurihormonal adenomas are also rare adenohypophysial tumours with two or more hormone expressions. They account for 0.9% of all pituitary adenomas. They are morphologically monomorphous with single type of tumours cells, but functionally mixture of different hormone families. There are two subtypes of plurihormonal adenomas, PIT-1 positive adenoma (previously called subtype 3 adenoma) and Adenoma with unusual immunohistochemical combination. Most common of these are Plurihormonal PIT-1 positive adenomas with unusual combination of GH, PRL and TSH. Adenomas with combination of GH and PRL or FSH and LH are not considered as plurihormonal. Adenoma with unusual immunohistochemical combination is unrelated to single cell lineage. For example, combination of GH or PRL with ACTH.

Double adenoma is different from plurihormonal adenomas, existence of two distinct tumor masses in same gland, representing a collision tumor. They tumours are usually incidental tumours, whereas plurihormonal adenomas are macroadenomas.

Silent adenoma presents clinically as non-functioning adenomas, but the surgical resected samples are immunopositive for hormonal factors and their corresponding transcriptional factors. They account for approximately 30% of all pituitary adenomas. To present clinically early, they lack hormonal function. At the time of presentation, several cases tend to exhibit signs of mass effects and few cases with hypothyroidism due to stalk compression or tissue destruction. The diagnosis of

| Drug | Mechanism of action | Dosage | Adverse effects |
|---|---|---|---|
| Ketoconazole | Inhibits the side-chain cleavage complex (steroidogenic acute regulatory protein [StAR] and 20,22-desmolase [CYP11A1]), CYP11B1 and 17α hydroxylase/17,20-lyase (CYP17) in the adrenal cortex | 200–1200 mg/day | Hepatotoxicity, nausea, dizziness, diarrhea, rash, hypogonadism in men |
| Etomidate | Blocks multiple steps of steroidogenesis, including CYP11B1, CYP17 and cholesterol side-chain cleavage | 0.04–0.05 mg/kg/h | Sedation (avoid overdose [>0.1 mg/kg/h], which will cause apnea and somnolence) |
| Metyrapone | Inhibitor of steroid 11-β-monooxygenase. | 500–4000 mg/day | Hypertension, hirsutism, acne, hypokalemia |
| Mitotane | a. Adrenolytic action caused by lipid accumulation and atrophy of the fascicularis and reticularis regions of the adrenal cortex<br><br>b. inhibition of steroidogenesis enzymes such as side-chain cleavage complex, CYP11B1, CYP11B2 and 3β-hydroxysteroid dehydrogenase (3β-HDS)<br><br>c. increases in cortisol-binding globulin (CBG), reducing free active cortisol | 2–5 g/day | Gastrointestinal disturbances, dizziness, cognitive alterations |
| Osilodrostat (Phase III trial) | potent inhibitor of CYP11B1 Inhibits aldosterone synthase | 2–50 mg twice daily | Nausea, headache, fatigue, hirsutism, hypertension, hypokalemia |
| Levoketoconazole (Phase III trial) | Inhibits side-chain cleavage complex, CYP17, 21-hydroxylase (CYP21A2) and CYP11B1 | 150–600 mg/day | Nausea, headache, edema, liver enzyme increase, adrenal insufficiency |
| Nevanimibe (Phase II trial) | cholesterol acyltransferase 1 inhibitor | Under study | Under study |
| Abiraterone acetate (Phase II trial) | Inhibits CYP17 and CYP21A2 | 250–500 mg twice daily | Hypertension, hypokalemia, adrenal insufficiency |
| Pasireotide | Targets four of five SSTR subtypes, with highest affinity for SSTR5, followed by SSTR2, SSTR3, and SSTR1 and reduces ACTH secretion | 600–900 μg twice daily. LAR: 10–30 mg/month | Diarrhea, nausea, cholelithiasis, hyperglycemia |
| Cabergoline (Off-label) | Dopamine receptor type 2 Agonist Reduces ACTH secretion | 0.5–7 mg/week | Nausea, dizziness, compulsive behaviour |
| Temozolamide (Off-label) | DNA alkylation | 150–200 mg/m2/day for 5 days each month per cycle | Fatigue, hearing loss, liver enzyme increase, cytopenia |

**Table 5.**
*Drugs used in the treatment of Cushing's syndrome.*

silent adenoma is exclusively based on immunohistochemical markers against transcriptional factors and hormones expressed. The morphology of these tumors corresponds to those of their functioning counterparts. The characterization of silent adenoma is important as they determine prognosis. For e.g.: Silent Corticotroph adenoma is associated with aggressive behavior of early recurrence rate when compared to other silent tumors.

Atypical adenoma is defined as tumor cells with extensive nuclear staining for p53, high mitotic index and Ki-67 proliferative index >3%. The prognostic activity related to proliferation of pituitary tumors are extensively studied in the last two decades. But, the significance of proliferation markers or correlation with tumor invasiveness and recurrence could not be established using above classification. Ki67 labelling is not predictive factor for recurrence risk, but could be a useful predictor of progression risk in tumor remnants. Hence, in new classification the term atypical adenomas are no longer used. The best prognosticator still remains the tumor invasiveness hormone produced and subtype of particular adenoma.

## 16. Follow up of patients with pituitary adenoma

The frequency of testing and the criteria for remission/cure for patients undergoing treatment for pituitary adenoma are elaborated in the **Table 6** [144].

| Tumor type | Tests | Timing of tests | Interpretation |
|---|---|---|---|
| Corticotroph adenoma | Morning serum cortisol<br>24 hours urinary free cortisol(UFC) | Within 7 days of surgery | < 5 ug/dL (138 nmol/L)<br>UFC < 28–56 nmol/d (<10–20 ug/d) |
| GH secreting adenoma | Serum IGF 1<br>Random GH<br>GH after oral glucose load<br>MRI | 12 weeks after surgery | IGF 1– normal(remission)<br>serum GH <0.14 ug/L suggests "surgical remission,"<br>serum GH <1 ug/L indicates "control<br>serum GH > 1 ug/L – measure GH nadir after glucose load |
| Prolactinomas | Serum prolactin<br>MRI | After 2 years of therapy | Serum prolactin every 3 months for the first year after completion of therapy and annually thereafter<br>MRI if there is increase in serum prolactin |
| TSH secreting adenoma | TSH<br>T3 suppression test | One week after surgery | Undetectable TSH and positive T3 suppression test with undetectable TSH and no response to TRH (or central hypothyroidism) |

**Table 6.**
*Follow up and remission criteria for patients with pituitary adenoma.*

## 17. Pituitary apoplexy

Pituitary apoplexy, is a clinical syndrome with incidence ranging from 4 to 20%, due to varying defining clinical criteria and presentation, ranging from subclinical to life threatening situation. It is a serious yet rare condition affecting the patients with pituitary lesions. Apoplexy is referred to as acute infarction of pituitary gland with or without haemorrhage. Usually, patients present due to sudden haemorrhage in adenoma and less often with bleed within infarcts or in the cystic lesions like Rathke's cyst. The rapid expansion of sellar contents manifests classically as headache, visual disturbances, and varying features of hypopituitarism [145, 146].

### 17.1 Pathogenesis

Varying pathophysiological mechanisms have been postulated for the occurrence of pituitary apoplexy- (1) rapid growth of the tumour outgrowing the vascular supply, (2) compression of the superior hypophyseal trunk along the stalk, (3) intrinsic vasculopathy with incomplete maturation of the basal membrane and (4) overexpressed VEGF leading to risk of haemorrhage.

### 17.2 Precipitating factors

Though most often pituitary apoplexy occurs without any external precipitating events, few events like a head injury, coughing/sneezing, idiopathic thrombocytopenic purpura, spinal anaesthesia, radiotherapy, pregnancy have been implicated. Medications like anti-platelet drugs, anti-coagulants, clomiphene, leuprolide, goserlin and oestrogen have been implicated. Bromocriptine and cabergoline administered for prolactinomas have also been reported to have precipitated pituitary apoplexy.

### 17.3 Grading of pituitary apoplexy

The first grading of pituitary apoplexy was suggested by Rajashekaran et al., in their seminal work of guidelines suggested a scoring system from 0 to 10, which included level of consciousness (0–4), visual acuity (0–2), visual field defects (0–2) and ocular palsies (0–2). They proposed such objective scoring system to monitor conservatively managed patients and assess the effect of surgical intervention, with a long-term aim of a randomised control trial for validation of management [147]. Giritharan et al. (2016) applied this scoring system retrospectively to their database of cases with apoplexy and observed that lower PAS grades could be managed conservatively while higher grades required immediate surgical intervention [148].

Jho et al. (2014) [149] proposed a severity grading system based on clinical and imaging features into a 5-grades: (1) Grade 1- asymptomatic (subclinical); (2) Grade 2- only endocrine symptoms; (3) Grade 3- presence of headache; (4) Grade 4- ocular palsies; (5) Grade 5- Visual deficits or altered consciousness not allowing testing for visual deficits. They had further 3 clinical subgroups or modifiers (p, r, s) wherein the presence of prolactinoma(p), Rathke's cyst (r) with haemorrhage and co-morbidities/sick (s) were preferentially managed medically. They reviewed their database of over 20 years and proposed algorthimic based treatment with immediate surgery for higher grades and conservative/medical management for lower grades.

### 17.4 Imaging in pituitary apoplexy

MRI of the brain is the current modality of choice for pituitary apoplexy. MRI is much superior to CT in the diagnosis of pituitary apoplexy with a sensitivity ranging from 88–90% [145, 150]. The signal intensity changes depend upon the changes in the haemoglobin or in turn the age of the bleed.

Fluid–fluid level sign can be seen in old bleeds with supernatant T1W hyperintense upper/anterior fluid level corresponds to extracellular met Hb, while the lower/posterior iso to hypo intense area is related to sedimented blood products [151].

Thickening of mucosa in pituitary apoplexy was demonstrated by Arita et al. [150] in 9 of their 11 patients at 7 days, which was predominantly in the compartment below the sella and was postulated to be due to venous congestion.

Histopathological examination of the mucosa in those who underwent transsphenoidal resection swollen subepithelial layer of mucosa. In others, a repeat MRI showed complete resolution without any treatment. Mucosal thickening does not preclude a transsphenoidal surgical approach.

Sheehan syndrome refers to postpartum apoplexy and usually occurs in women having suffered postpartum hemorrhage and hypovolemia. It is hypothesized that hypertrophied pituitary gland is more susceptible to infarction from hypovolemia.

## 18. Recurrent pituitary apoplexy

Recurrent pituitary apoplexy, is a rare event described by several authors as few case reports. The prominent one is by Houseman et al. (2019) wherein they retrospectively analysed their data of 798 surgically treated patients over a period of 27 years and found that apoplexy was noted in 76 patients. There were only 4 patients (5.3%) who had recurrent episodes of apoplexy. These haemorrhagic recurrences were noticed when the Knosp's score was more than 4, implying complete encasement of ICA and hence incomplete tumor resection (8%) in the cavernous sinus (23.5%). Brown et al. (2020) described a single case of multiple episodes of pituitary apoplexy over 11 years, which interestingly has varying phenotypes changing from silent gonadotropic to silent corticotroph adenoma. The MIB-1 index was however, consistently high at 10%. Teasdale et al. (2015) described recurrent pituitary apoplexy following development of a neoplasm adjacent to the sella. Tumour residue or recurrence are the major factors responsible for recurrent pituitary apoplexy and need a close follow-up. The management is similar to any other pituitary apoplexy which includes stabilisation of general and hormonal status. Surgical decompression of the hematoma and the residual tumour is the treatment of choice, followed closely by hormone replacements. Follow-up imaging to look for residual/recurrent tumour and radiotherapy. A further look into the molecular markers predisposing to recurrent haemorrhages to be looked in future [152–160].

## 19. Conclusion

- Pituitary neoplasms are common intracranial tumours accounting for approx. 15% of all intracranial tumours.

- The pituitary neoplasms are believed to originate due to aberration in the normal growth and differentiation of pituitary stem cells. The detection of the pituitary specific transcription is now the basis of the recent most WHO classification.

- The clinical manifestations of such tumours are due to- hormone excess, deficiency of other pituitary hormones, pressure effects on optic pathways, surrounding brain parenchyma, ventricular system, paranasal sinuses and systemic.

- The diagnosis and management require a close collaboration between endocrinologist, radiologist, neurosurgeon, pathologist and radiation oncologist.

- The goals of therapy include- hormonal remission, decompression of neural elements, restoration/replacement of deficient hormones, maximising tumour remission.

## Author details

Sumitra Sivakoti[1], Beatrice Anne[2], Abhishek J. Arora[3] and Rajesh Alugolu[4]*

1 Department of Pathology, All India Institute of Medical Sciences, Hyderabad, Telangana, India

2 Department of Endocrinology, Nizam's Institute of Medical Sciences, Hyderabad, India

3 Department of Radio-Diagnosis, All India Institute of Medical Sciences, Hyderabad, India

4 Department of Neurosurgery, Nizam's Institute of Medical Sciences, Punjagutta, Hyderabad, Telangana, India

*Address all correspondence to: drarajesh1306@gmail.com

## References


[1] Saeger W, Lüdecke DK, Buchfelder M, Fahlbusch R, Quabbe HJ, Petersenn S. Pathohistological classification of pituitary tumors: 10 years of experience with the German Pituitary Tumor Registry. Eur J Endocrinol. 2007 Feb;156(2):203-216.

[2] Scheithauer BW, Gaffey TA, Lloyd RV, Sebo TJ, Kovacs KT, Horvath E,

[3] Yapicier O, Young WF Jr, Meyer FB, Kuroki T, Riehle DL, Laws ER Jr. Pathobiology of pituitary adenomas and carcinomas. Neurosurgery. 2006 Aug;59 (2):341-353; discussion 341-53.

[4] Ostrom QT, Gittleman H, Liao P, Vecchione-Koval T, Wolinsky Y, Kruchko C, et al. CBTRUS Statistical Report: Primary brain and other central. *Neuro Oncol*. 2016. 6;19(suppl_5):v1-v88.

[5] Shaid M, Korbonits M. Genetics of pituitary adenoma. Neurol India 2017; 65:577-587

[6] Watanabe YG. Effects of brain and mesenchyme upon the cytogenesis of rat adenohypophysis in vitro. I. Differentiation of adrenocorticotropes. Cell Tissue Res 1982; 227:257-266.

[7] Scully KM, Rosenfeld MG. Pituitary development: regulatory codes in mammalian organogenesis. *Science* 2002; **295**: 2231–5. Asa SL, Ezzat S. Molecular determinants of pituitary cytodifferentiation. Pituitary 1999; **1**: 159–168.

[8] Jastania RA, Alsaad KO, Al Shraim M, *et al.* Double adenomas of the pituitary: transcription factors Pit-1, T-pit, and SF-1 identify cytogenesis and differentiation. Endocr Pathol 2005; **16**: 187–194.

[9] Asa SL, Puy LA, Lew AM, *et al.* Cell type-specific expression of the pituitary transcription activator Pit-1 in the human pituitary and pituitary adenomas. J Clin Endocrinol Metab 1993; *77*: 1275–1280.

[10] Villa C, Vasiljevic A, Jaffrain-Rea ML, Ansorge O, Asioli S, Barresi V, et al,. A standardised diagnostic approach to pituitary neuroendocrine tumours (PitNETs): a European Pituitary Pathology Group (EPPG) proposal. Virchows Arch. 2019 Dec;475 (6):687-692.

[11] De Laat J.M., Dekkers O.M., Pieterman C.R., Kluijfhout W.P., Hermus A.R., et al. Long-Term Natural Course of Pituitary Tumors in Patients With MEN1: Results From the DutchMEN1 Study Group (DMSG) *J.* Clin. Endocrinol. Metab. 2015;100:3288–3296.

[12] Verges B., Boureille F., Goudet P., Murat A., Beckers A., Sassolas G., et al. Pituitary disease in MEN type 1 (MEN1): Data from the France-Belgium MEN1 multicenter study. J. Clin. Endocrinol. Metab. 2002;87:457–465.

[13] Mulligan L.M., Kwok J.B., Healey C. S., Elsdon M.J., Eng C., Gardner E., et al. Germ-line mutations of the RET proto-oncogene in multiple endocrine neoplasia type 2A. Nature. 1993;363: 458–460.

[14] Saito T., Miura D., Taguchi M., Takeshita A., Miyakawa M., Takeuchi Y. Coincidence of multiple endocrine neoplasia type 2A with acromegaly. Am. J. Med. Sci. 2010;340:329–331

[15] Heinlen J.E., Buethe D.D., Culkin D. J., Slobodov G. Multiple endocrine neoplasia 2a presenting with pheochromocytoma and pituitary macroadenoma. ISRN Oncol. 2011;2011: 732452.

[16] Ezzat T., Paramesawaran R., Phillips B., Sadler G. MEN 2 syndrome

masquerading as MEN 1. Ann. R Coll. Surg. Engl. 2012;94:e206–e207.

[17] Sherr C.J., Roberts J.M. CDK inhibitors: Positive and negative regulators of G1-phase progression. Genes Dev. 1999;13:1501–1512.

[18] Agarwal S.K., Mateo C.M., Marx S.J. Rare germline mutations in cyclin-dependent kinase inhibitor genes in multiple endocrine neoplasia type 1 and related states. J. Clin. Endocrinol. Metab. 2009;94:1826–1834.

[19] Georgitsi M., Raitila A., Karhu A., van der Luijt R.B., Aalfs C.M., Sane T., Vierimaa O., Makinen M.J., Tuppurainen K., Paschke R., et al. Germline CDKN1B/p27Kip1 mutation in multiple endocrine neoplasia. J. Clin. Endocrinol. Metab. 2007;92: 3321–3325.

[20] Trouillas J., Labat-Moleur F., Sturm N., Kujas M., Heymann M.F., Figarella-Branger D., Patey M., Mazucca M., Decullier E., Verges B., et al. Pituitary tumors and hyperplasia in multiple endocrine neoplasia type 1 syndrome (MEN1): A case-control study in a series of 77 patients versus 2509 non-MEN1 patients. Am. J. Surg. Pathol. 2008;32:534–543.

[21] Stratakis C.A. Carney complex: A familial lentiginosis predisposing to a variety of tumors. Rev. Endocr. Metab. Disord. 2016;17:367–371.

[22] Salpea P., Stratakis C.A. Carney complex and McCune Albright syndrome: An overview of clinical manifestations and human molecular genetics. Mol. Cell. Endocrinol. 2014; 386:85–91.

[23] Boikos S.A., Stratakis C.A. Pituitary pathology in patients with Carney Complex: Growth-hormone producing hyperplasia or tumors and their association with other abnormalities. Pituitary. 2006;9:203–209.

[24] Lonser R.R., Mehta G.U., Kindzelski B.A., Ray-Chaudhury A., Vortmeyer A.O., Dickerman R., Oldfield E.H. Surgical Management of Carney Complex-Associated Pituitary Pathology. Neurosurgery. 2017;80:780–786.

[25] Vasilev V, Daly AF, Petrossians P, Zacharieva S, Beckers A. Familial pituitary tumor syndromes. Endocr Pract. 2011 Jul-Aug;17 Suppl 3:41-46.

[26] Stiles C.E., Korbonits M. Familial Isolated Pituitary Adenoma. In: Feingold K.R., Anawalt B., Boyce A., Chrousos G., Dungan K., Grossman A., Hershman J.M., Kaltsas G., Koch C., Kopp P., et al., editors. *Endotext.* South Dartmouth; Dartmouth, MA, USA: 2000.

[27] Vierimaa O, Georgitsi M, Lehtonen R, Vahteristo P, Kokko A, Raitila A, Tuppurainen K, Ebeling TM, Salmela PI, Paschke R, Gündogdu S, De Menis E, Mäkinen MJ, Launonen V, Karhu A, Aaltonen LA. Pituitary adenoma predisposition caused by germline mutations in the AIP gene. Science. 2006 May 26;312(5777): 1228-1230.

[28] Daly A.F., Vanbellinghen J.F., Khoo S.K., Jaffrain-Rea M.L., Naves L. A., Guitelman M.A., Murat A., Emy P., Gimenez-Roqueplo A.P., Tamburrano G., et al. Aryl hydrocarbon receptor-interacting protein gene mutations in familial isolated pituitary adenomas: Analysis in 73 families. J. Clin. Endocrinol. Metab. 2007;92:1891–1896.

[29] Ronchi CL, Peverelli E, Herterich S, Weigand I, Mantovani G, Schwarzmayr T, Sbiera S, Allolio B, Honegger J, Appenzeller S, Lania AG, Reincke M, Calebiro D, Spada A, Buchfelder M, Flitsch J, Strom TM, Fassnacht M. Landscape of somatic mutations in sporadic GH-secreting pituitary adenomas. Eur J Endocrinol.

2016 Mar;174(3):363-372. doi: 10.1530/EJE-15-1064.

[30] Cushing H. The Pituitary Body and Its Disorders: Clinical States Produced by Disorders of the Hypophysis Cerebri. JB Lippincott; 1912. Luger A. Some features of roentgenographic changes in pituitary diseases. JAMA 1913;61:752–754

[31] FariÑas PL. The value of the X-ray examination of the sella turcica in the sagittal positions. Radiology. 1939 Apr; 32(4):411-415.

[32] Long B, Smith B, Merrill V. Merrill's atlas of radiographic positioning & procedures. 6th ed. Mosby;Vol.3: 1003-8.

[33] de Herder WW, Lamberts SW. Imaging of pituitary tumours. Bailliere's clinical endocrinology and metabolism. 1995 Apr 1;9(2):367-389.

[34] Wolpert SM. The radiology of pituitary adenomas. Endocrinology and metabolism clinics of North America. 1987 Sep 1;16(3):553-584.

[35] Pisaneschi M, Kapoor G. Imaging the sella and parasellar region. Neuroimaging Clin North Am 2005; 15: 203–219

[36] Martinez-Farinas LO. The sellar-cranial index. Radiology. 1967 Feb;88 (2):264-267.

[37] Roppolo HM, Latchaw RE. Normal pituitary gland: 2. Microscopic anatomy-CT correlation. AJNR Am J Neuroradiol 1983;4:937–944.

[38] Lundin P, Nyman R, Burman P, et al. MRI of pituitary macroadenomas with reference to hormonal activity. Neuroradiology 1992;34:43–51.

[39] Bartynski WS, Lin L. Dynamic and conventional spin-echo MR of pituitary microlesions. AJNR Am J Neuroradiol 1997;18:965–972.

[40] Osborn AG. Diagnostic neuroradiology. St. Louis (MO) 7 Mosby-YearBook; 1994.

[41] Cottier JP, Destrieux C, Brunereau L, et al. Cavernous sinus invasion by pituitary adenoma: MR imaging. Radiology 2000;215:463–469.

[42] Covington MF, Chin SS, Osborn AG. Pituicytoma, spindle cell oncocytoma, and granular cell tumor: clar- ification and meta-analysis of the world literature since 1893. AJNR Am J Neuroradiol 2011;32:2067–2072.

[43] Lopes MBS. The 2017 World Health Organization classification of tumors of the pituitary gland: a summary. Acta Neuropathol. 2017 Oct;134(4):521-535.

[44] Dai C, Kang J, Liu X, Yao Y, Wang H, Wang R. How to Classify and Define Pituitary Tumors: Recent Advances and Current Controversies. Front Endocrinol. 2021;12:604644.

[45] Mete O, Lopes MB. Overview of the 2017 WHO Classification of Pituitary Tumors. Endocr Pathol. 2017 Sep;28(3): 228–243.

[46] Lloyd RV, Kovacs K, Young Jr WF, Farrell WE, Asa SL. Pituitary tumors: Introduction. DeLellis RA, Lloyd RV, Heitz PU, Eng C, editors In: WHO Classification of tumors. Pathology and Genetics. Tumors of Endocrine Organs. 3rd ed. Lyon:IARC Publications;2004

[47] Liloyd RV, Osamura RY, Kloppel G, Rosai J, editors. WHO Classification of tumors of endocrine. 4th ed. Lyon:IARC Publications; 2017.

[48] Sathyakumar R, Chacko G. Newer Concepts in the Classification of Pituitary Adenomas. Neurol India. 2020 May-Jun;68(Supplement):S7-S12.

[49] Asa SL, Gerrie BM, Singer W, Horvath E, Kovacs K, Smyth HS. Gonadotropin secretion in vitro by

human pituitary null cell adenomas and oncocytomas. J Clin Endocrinol Metab. 1986 May;62(5):1011-1019.

[50] Lamberts SW, Verleun T, Oosterom R, Hofland L, van Ginkel LA, Loeber JG, van Vroonhoven CC, Stefanko SZ, de Jong FH. The effects of bromocriptine, thyrotropin-releasing hormone, and gonadotropin-releasing hormone on hormone secretion by gonadotropin-secreting pituitary adenomas in vivo and in vitro. J Clin Endocrinol Metab. 1987 Mar;64(3): 524-530.

[51] Surmont DW, Winslow CL, Loizou M, White MC, Adams EF, Mashiter K. Gonadotrophin and alpha subunit secretion by human 'functionless' pituitary adenomas in cell culture: long term effects of luteinizing hormone releasing hormone and thyrotrophin releasing hormone. Clin Endocrinol (Oxf). 1983 Sep;19(3):325-336.

[52] Yamada S, Asa SL, Kovacs K, Muller P, Smyth HS. Analysis of hormone secretion by clinically nonfunctioning human pituitary adenomas using the reverse hemolytic plaque assay. J Clin Endocrinol Metab. 1989 Jan;68(1):73-80.

[53] Horvath E, Kovacs K, Killinger DW, Smyth HS, Platts ME, Singer W. Silent corticotropic adenomas of the human pituitary gland: a histologic, immunocytologic, and ultrastructural study. Am J Pathol. 1980 Mar;98(3): 617-638

[54] Greenman Y, Stern N (2009) Non-functioning pituitary adenomas. Best Pract Res Clin Endocrinol Metab 23(5): 625–638

[55] Ferrante E, Ferraroni M, Castrignanò T et al (2006) Non-functioning pituitary adenoma database: a useful resource to improve the clinical management of pituitary tumors. Eur J Endocrinol 155(6):823–829

[56] Ntali G, Capatina C, Fazal-Sanderson V, Byrne JV, Cudlip S, Grossman AB, Wass JA, Karavitaki N. Mortality in patients with non-functioning pituitary adenoma is increased: systematic analysis of 546 cases with long follow-up. Eur J Endocrinol. 2016 Feb;174(2):137-145.

[57] Kim SH, Lee KC, Kim SH. Cranial nerve palsies accompanying pituitary tumour. J Clin Neurosci. 2007 Dec;14 (12):1158-1162.

[58] Verhelst J, Berwaerts J, Abs R, Dua G, Van Den Weyngaert D, Mahler C. Obstructive hydrocephalus as complication of a giant nonfunctioning pituitary adenoma: therapeutical approach. Acta Clin Belg. 1998 Feb;53 (1):47-52.

[59] Baumann F, Schmid C, Bernays RL. Intraoperative magnetic resonance imaging-guided transsphenoidal surgery for giant pituitary adenomas. Neurosurg Rev. 2010 Jan;33(1):83-90.

[60] Landeiro JA, Fonseca EO, Monnerat AL, Taboada GF, Cabral GA, Antunes F. Nonfunctioning giant pituitary adenomas: Invasiveness and recurrence. Surg Neurol Int. 2015 Nov 26;6:179.

[61] Dekkers OM, Pereira AM, Roelfsema F, Voormolen JH, Neelis KJ, Schroijen MA, Smit JW, Romijn JA. Observation alone after transsphenoidal surgery for nonfunctioning pituitary macroadenoma. J Clin Endocrinol Metab. 2006 May;91(5):1796-1801.

[62] Arafah BM. Reversible hypopituitarism in patients with large nonfunctioning pituitary adenomas. J Clin Endocrinol Metab. 1986 Jun;62(6): 1173-1179.

[63] Cury ML, Fernandes JC, Machado HR, Elias LL, Moreira AC, Castro Md. Non-functioning pituitary adenomas: clinical feature, laboratorial

and imaging assessment, therapeutic management and outcome. Arq Bras Endocrinol Metabol. 2009 Feb;53(1): 31-39.

[64] Greenman Y, Tordjman K, Kisch E, Razon N, Ouaknine G, Stern N. Relative sparing of anterior pituitary function in patients with growth hormone-secreting macroadenomas: comparison with nonfunctioning macroadenomas. J Clin Endocrinol Metab. 1995 May;80(5): 1577-1583.

[65] Hardy J, Vezina J L. Transsphenoidal neurosurgery of intracranial neoplasm. Adv Neurol. 1976;15:261–273.

[66] Hardy J. New York, NY: Igaku-Shoin Medical Publishers; 1991. Atlas of Transsphenoidal Microsurgery in Pituitary Tumors.

[67] Hardy J. New York: Raven Press; 1979. Transsphenoidal Microsurgical Treatment of Pituitary Tumors.

[68] Wilson C. B. Neurosurgical management of large and invasive pituitary tumors. In: Tindall G. T., editor. *Clinical management of pituitary disorders.* New York, NY, USA: Raven; 1979. pp. 335–342.

[69] Knosp E., Steiner E., Kitz K., Matula C. Pituitary adenomas with invasion of the cavernous sinus space: A magnetic resonance imaging classification compared with surgical findings. Neurosurgery. 1993;33: 610–618

[70] Micko A.S.G., Wöhrer A., Wolfsberger S., Knosp E. Invasion of the cavernous sinus space in pituitary adenomas: Endoscopic verification and its correlation with an MRI-based classification. J. Neurosurg. 2015;122: 803–811.

[71] Micko A., Oberndorfer J., Weninger W.J., Vila G., Hoftberger R., Wolfsberger S., Knosp E. Challenging Knosp high-grade pituitary adenomas. J. Neurosurg. 2019;1:1–8.

[72] Losa M, Mortini P, Barzaghi R, Ribotto P, Terreni MR, Marzoli SB, Pieralli S, Giovanelli M. Early results of surgery in patients with nonfunctioning pituitary adenoma and analysis of the risk of tumor recurrence. J Neurosurg. 2008 Mar;108(3):525-532.

[73] Chang EF, Zada G, Kim S, Lamborn KR, Quinones-Hinojosa A, Tyrrell JB, Wilson CB, Kunwar S. Long-term recurrence and mortality after surgery and adjuvant radiotherapy for nonfunctional pituitary adenomas. J Neurosurg. 2008 Apr;108(4):736-745.

[74] Marazuela M, Astigarraga B, Vicente A et al (1994) Recovery of visual and endocrine function following transsphenoidal surgery of large nonfunctioning pituitary adenomas. J Endocrinol Investig 17(9):703–707

[75] Brochier S, Galland F, Kujas M et al (2010) Factors predicting relapse of nonfunctioning pituitary macroadenomas after neurosurgery: a study of 142 patients. Eur J Endocrinol 163(2):193–200 31.

[76] Sheehan J, Lee CC, Bodach ME, Tumialan LM, Oyesiku NM, Patil CG, Litvack Z, Zada G, Aghi MK. Congress of Neurological Surgeons Systematic Review and Evidence-Based Guideline for the Management of Patients With Residual or Recurrent Nonfunctioning Pituitary Adenomas. Neurosurgery. 2016 Oct;79(4):E539-E540.

[77] Kasper G, Samuel N, Alkins R, Khan OH. Practice patterns in the management of recurrent and residual non-functioning pituitary adenomas: Results from a Canada-wide survey. eNeurologicalSci. 2021 Jan 22;22:100317.

[78] Lasio G, Ferroli P, Felisati G, Broggi G. Image-guided endoscopic

transnasal removal of recurrent pituitary adenomas. Neurosurgery. 2002 Jul;51(1):132-136; discussion 136-7

[79] Nimsky C, Ganslandt O, von Keller B, Fahlbusch R. Intraoperative high-field MRI: anatomical and functional imaging. Acta Neurochir Suppl. 2006;98:87-95.

[80] Ciric I, Rosenblatt S, Kerr W Jr, Lamarca F, Pierce D, Baumgartner C. Perspective in pituitary adenomas: an end of the century review of tumorigenesis, diagnosis, and treatment. Clin Neurosurg. 2000;47: 99-111.

[81] Nomikos P, Ladar C, Fahlbusch R, Buchfelder M. Impact of primary surgery on pituitary function in patients with non-functioning pituitary adenomas – a study on 721 patients. Acta Neurochir (Wien). 2004 Jan;146(1): 27-35.

[82] Brada M, Ajithkumar TV, Minniti G. Radiosurgery for pituitary adenomas. Clin Endocrinol (Oxf). 2004 Nov;61(5): 531-543.

[83] Brada M, Rajan B, Traish D, Ashley S, Holmes-Sellors PJ, Nussey S, Uttley D. The long-term efficacy of conservative surgery and radiotherapy in the control of pituitary adenomas. Clin Endocrinol (Oxf). 1993 Jun;38(6): 571-578.

[84] Ajithkumar T, Brada M. Stereotactic linear accelerator radiotherapy for pituitary tumors. Treat Endocrinol. 2004;3(4):211-216.

[85] Ntali G, Wass JA. Epidemiology, clinical presentation and diagnosis of non-functioning pituitary adenomas. Pituitary. 2018 Apr;21(2):111-118.

[86] Drange MR, Fram NR, Herman-Bonert V et al (2000) Pituitary tumor registry: a novel clinical resource. J Clin Endocrinol Metab 85(1):168–174

[87] Robenshtok E, Benbassat CA, Hirsch D et al (2014) Clinical course and outcome of nonfunctioning pituitary adenomas in the elderly compared with younger age groups. Endocr Pract 20(2): 159–164

[88] Casanueva FF, Molitch ME, Schlechte JA, Abs R, Bonert V, Bronstein MD, *et al*. Guidelines of the Pituitary Society for the diagnosis and management of prolactinomas. Clin Endocrinol (Oxf) 2006;65:265-273.

[89] Gruppetta M, Mercieca C, Vassallo J. Prevalence and incidence of pituitary adenomas: A population based study in Malta. Pituitary 2013;16: 545-553.

[90] Raappana A, Koivukangas J, Ebeling T, Pirila T. Incidence of pituitary adenomas in Northern Finland in 1992-2007. J Clin Endocrinol Metab 2010;95:4268-4275.

[91] Tjornstrand A, Gunnarsson K, Evert M, Holmberg E, Ragnarsson O, Rosén T, *et al*. The incidence rate of pituitary adenomas in western Sweden for the period 2001-2011. Eur J Endocrinol 2014;171:519-526.

[92] FORBES AP, HENNEMAN PH, GRISWOLD GC, ALBRIGHT F. Syndrome characterized by galactorrhea, amenorrhea and low urinary FSH: comparison with acromegaly and normal lactation. J Clin Endocrinol Metab. 1954 Mar;14(3): 265–271.

[93] Kleinberg DL, Noel GL, Frantz AG. Galactorrhea: a study of 235 cases, including 48 with pituitary tumors. N Engl J Med. 1977 Mar 17;296(11): 589-600.

[94] Huang Y, Ding C, Zhang F, Xiao D, Zhao L, Wang S. Role of prolactin/adenoma maximum diameter and prolactin/adenoma volume in the differential diagnosis of prolactinomas

and other types of pituitary adenomas. Oncol Lett 2018;15:2010-2016.

[95] Kovacs K, Stefaneanu L, Horvath E, Lloyd RV, Lancranjan I, Buchfelder M, Fahlbusch R. Effect of dopamine agonist medication on prolactin producing pituitary adenomas. A morphological study including immunocytochemistry, electron microscopy and in situ hybridization. Virchows Arch A Pathol Anat Histopathol. 1991;418(5):439-446.

[96] Verhelst J, Abs R, Maiter D, Van Den Bruel A, Vandeweghe M, Velkeniers B, *et al*. Cabergoline in the treatment of hyperprolactinemia: A study in 455 patients. J Clin Endocrinol Metab 1999;84:2518-2522.

[97] Ono M, Miki N, Kawamata T, Makino R, Amano K, Seki T, *et al*. Prospective study of high-dose cabergoline treatment of prolactinomas in 150 patients. J Clin Endocrinol Metab 2008;93:4721-4727.

[98] Klibanski A. Prolactinomas. *N* Engl J Med 2010;362:1219-1226.

[99] Primeau V, Raftopoulos C, Maiter D. Outcomes of transsphenoidal surgery in prolactinomas: Improvement of hormonal control in dopamine agonist-resistant patients. Eur J Endocrinol 2012;166:779-786.

[100] Molitch ME. Management of medically refractory prolactinoma. J Neurooncol 2014;117:421-428.

[101] Molitch ME. Pregnancy and the hyperprolactinemic woman. N Engl J Med. 1985 May 23;312(21):1364-1370.

[102] Glezer A, Bronstein MD. Prolactinomas, cabergoline, and pregnancy. Endocrine. 2014 Sep;47(1): 64-69.

[103] Molitch ME, Elton RL, Blackwell RE, Caldwell B, Chang RJ, Jaffe R, Joplin G, Robbins RJ, Tyson J, Thorner MO. Bromocriptine as primary therapy for prolactin-secreting macroadenomas: results of a prospective multicenter study. J Clin Endocrinol Metab. 1985 Apr;60(4):698-705.

[104] Molitch ME. Clinical manifestations of acromegaly. Endocrinol Metab Clin North Am. 1992 Sep;21(3):597-614.

[105] Vilar L, Vilar CF, Lyra R, Lyra R, Naves LA. Acromegaly: clinical features at diagnosis. Pituitary. 2017 Feb;20(1): 22-32.

[106] Kuan EC, Peng KA, Kita AE, Bergsneider M, Wang MB. Acromegaly: otolaryngic manifestations following pituitary surgery. Am J Otolaryngol. 2015 Jul-Aug;36(4):521-525.

[107] Wennberg A, Lorusso R, Dassie F, Benavides-Varela S, Parolin M, De Carlo E, Fallo F, Mioni R, Vettor R, Semenza C, Maffei P. Sleep disorders and cognitive dysfunction in acromegaly. Endocrine. 2019 Dec;66(3): 634-641.

[108] Turan O, Akinci B, Ikiz AO, Itil O, Oztura I, Ada E, Akdeniz B, Yener S, Kaya M, Gedik A, Comlekci A. Airway and sleep disorders in patients with acromegaly. Clin Respir J. 2018 Mar;12 (3):1003-1010.

[109] Parolin M, Dassie F, Alessio L, Wennberg A, Rossato M, Vettor R, Maffei P, Pagano C. Obstructive Sleep Apnea in Acromegaly and the Effect of Treatment: A Systematic Review and Meta-Analysis. J Clin Endocrinol Metab. 2020 Mar 1;105(3):dgz116.

[110] Abdullah NRA, Jason WLC, Nasruddin AB. Pachydermoperiostosis: a rare mimicker of acromegaly. Endocrinol Diabetes Metab Case Rep. 2017 May 16;2017:17-0029.

[111] Briet C, Ilie MD, Kuhn E, Maione L, Brailly-Tabard S, Salenave S, Cariou B,

Chanson P. Changes in metabolic parameters and cardiovascular risk factors after therapeutic control of acromegaly vary with the treatment modality. Data from the Bicêtre cohort, and review of the literature. Endocrine. 2019 Feb;63(2):348-360.

[112] Pivonello R, Auriemma RS, Grasso LF, Pivonello C, Simeoli C, Patalano R, Galdiero M, Colao A. Complications of acromegaly: cardiovascular, respiratory and metabolic comorbidities. Pituitary. 2017

[113] Dworakowska D, Grossman AB. Colonic Cancer and Acromegaly. Front Endocrinol (Lausanne). 2019 Jun 21;10: 390.

[114] Iliaz R, Dogansen SC, Tanrikulu S, Yalin GY, Cavus B, Gulluoglu M, Akyuz F, Yarman S. Predictors of colonic pathologies in active acromegaly: single tertiary center experience. Wien Klin Wochenschr. 2018 Sep;130(17–18):511-516.

[115] Ochiai Y, Inoshita N, Iizuka T, Nishioka H, Yamada S, Kitagawa M, Hoteya S. Clinicopathological features of colorectal polyps and risk of colorectal cancer in acromegaly. Eur J Endocrinol. 2020 Mar;182(3):313-318.

[116] Katznelson L, Laws ER Jr, Melmed S, et al. Acromegaly. J Clin Endocrinol Metab. 2014;99(11): 3933-3951.

[117] Ding D, Mehta GU, Patibandla MR, Lee CC, Liscak R, Kano H, Pai FY, Kosak M, Sisterson ND, Martinez-Alvarez R, Martinez-Moreno N, Mathieu D, Grills IS, Blas K, Lee K, Cifarelli CP, Katsevman GA, Lee JYK, McShane B, Kondziolka D, Lunsford LD, Vance ML, Sheehan JP. Stereotactic Radiosurgery for Acromegaly: An International Multicenter Retrospective Cohort Study. Neurosurgery. 2019 Mar 1;84(3): 717-725.

[118] Jane JA Jr, Laws ER Jr. The surgical management of pituitary adenomas in a series of 3,093 patients. J Am Coll Surg. 2001 Dec;193(6):651-659.

[119] Pivonello R, De Martino MC, De Leo M, Simeoli C, Colao A. Cushing's disease: the burden of illness. Endocrine. 2017 Apr;56(1):10-18.

[120] Pivonello R, De Martino MC, Iacuaniello D, Simeoli C, Muscogiuri G, Carlomagno F, De Leo M, Cozzolino A, Colao A. Metabolic Alterations and Cardiovascular Outcomes of Cortisol Excess. Front Horm Res. 2016;46:54-65.

[121] Goyal A, Gupta U, Kandasamy D, Khadgawat R. Severe Hypercortisolism with Hypokalemic Alkalosis Mimicking Ectopic Cushing Syndrome in a Patient with Cushing Disease Due to Pituitary Microadenoma. Indian J Endocrinol Metab. 2018 Nov-Dec;22(6):860-863.

[122] Paragliola RM, Corsello A, Papi G, Pontecorvi A, Corsello SM. Cushing's Syndrome Effects on the Thyroid. Int J Mol Sci. 2021 Mar 19;22 (6):3131.

[123] Orth DN. The old and the new in Cushing's syndrome. N Engl J Med. 1984 Mar 8;310(10):649-651.

[124] Ross EJ, Linch DC. Cushing's syndrome–killing disease: discriminatory value of signs and symptoms aiding early diagnosis. Lancet. 1982 Sep 18;2(8299):646-649.

[125] Gupta A, Gupta RK, Banerjee D, Bhatia E. Magnetic resonance image detection of coincidental sphenoid sinus aspergillosis and pituitary microadenoma: a potential surgical disaster. Australas Radiol. 1998 May;42 (2):128-129.

[126] Nieman LK. Cushing's syndrome: update on signs, symptoms and biochemical screening. Eur J Endocrinol. 2015 Oct;173(4):M33-M38.

[127] Pivonello R, Isidori AM, De Martino MC, Newell-Price J, Biller BM, Colao A. Complications of Cushing's syndrome: state of the art. Lancet Diabetes Endocrinol. 2016 Jul;4(7):611-629.

[128] Buliman A, Tataranu LG, Paun DL, Mirica A, Dumitrache C. Cushing's disease: a multidisciplinary overview of the clinical features, diagnosis, and treatment. J Med Life. 2016 Jan-Mar;9 (1):12-18.

[129] Chen YF, Li YF, Chen X, Sun QF. Neuropsychiatric disorders and cognitive dysfunction in patients with Cushing's disease. Chin Med J (Engl). 2013 Aug;126(16):3156-3160.

[130] Tiemensma J, Kokshoorn NE, Biermasz NR, Keijser BJ, Wassenaar MJ, Middelkoop HA, Pereira AM, Romijn JA. Subtle cognitive impairments in patients with long-term cure of Cushing's disease. J Clin Endocrinol Metab. 2010 Jun;95(6): 2699-2714.

[131] Patil CG, Lad SP, Katznelson L, Laws ER Jr. Brain atrophy and cognitive deficits in Cushing's disease. Neurosurg Focus. 2007;23(3):E11.

[132] Andela CD, van der Werff SJ, Pannekoek JN, van den Berg SM, Meijer OC, van Buchem MA, Rombouts SA, van der Mast RC, Romijn JA, Tiemensma J, Biermasz NR, van der Wee NJ, Pereira AM. Smaller grey matter volumes in the anterior cingulate cortex and greater cerebellar volumes in patients with long-term remission of Cushing's disease: a case-control study. Eur J Endocrinol. 2013 Oct 21;169(6):811-819.

[133] Li D, El Kawkgi OM, Henriquez AF, Bancos I. Cardiovascular risk and mortality in patients with active and treated hypercortisolism. Gland Surg. 2020 Feb;9(1):43-58.

[134] Corcuff JB, Tabarin A, Rashedi M, Duclos M, Roger P, Ducassou D. Overnight urinary free cortisol determination: a screening test for the diagnosis of Cushing's syndrome. Clin Endocrinol (Oxf). 1998 Apr;48(4): 503-508.

[135] al-Saadi N, Diederich S, Oelkers W. A very high dose dexamethasone suppression test for differential diagnosis of Cushing's syndrome. Clin Endocrinol (Oxf). 1998 Jan;48(1): 45-51.

[136] Findling JW, Raff H. Cushing's Syndrome: important issues in diagnosis and management. J Clin Endocrinol Metab. 2006 Oct;91(10):3746-3753.

[137] Findling JW, Raff H. DIAGNOSIS OF ENDOCRINE DISEASE: Differentiation of pathologic/neoplastic hypercortisolism (Cushing's syndrome) from physiologic/non-neoplastic hypercortisolism (formerly known as pseudo-Cushing's syndrome). Eur J Endocrinol. 2017 May;176(5):R205-R216.

[138] Mengden T, Hubmann P, Müller J, Greminger P, Vetter W. Urinary free cortisol versus 17-hydroxycorticosteroids: a comparative study of their diagnostic value in Cushing's syndrome. Clin Investig. 1992 Jul;70(7):545-548.

[139] Oldfield EH, Doppman JL, Nieman LK, Chrousos GP, Miller DL, Katz DA, Cutler GB Jr, Loriaux DL. Petrosal sinus sampling with and without corticotropin-releasing hormone for the differential diagnosis of Cushing's syndrome. N Engl J Med. 1991 Sep 26;325(13):897-905.

[140] Sahdev A, Reznek RH, Evanson J, Grossman AB. Imaging in Cushing's syndrome. Arq Bras Endocrinol Metabol. 2007 Nov;51(8):1319-1328

[141] Klibanski A, Zervas NT. Diagnosis and management of hormone-secreting pituitary adenomas. N Engl J Med. 1991 Mar 21;324(12):822-831.

[142] Ross EJ, Marshall-Jones P, Friedman M. Cushing's syndrome: diagnostic criteria. Q J Med. 1966 Apr; 35(138):149-192.

[143] Tabarin A, Laurent F, Catargi B, Olivier-Puel F, Lescene R, Berge J, Galli FS, Drouillard J, Roger P, Guerin J. Comparative evaluation of conventional and dynamic magnetic resonance imaging of the pituitary gland for the diagnosis of Cushing's disease. Clin Endocrinol (Oxf). 1998 Sep;49(3): 293-300.

[144] Grober Y, Grober H, Wintermark M, Jane JA, Oldfield EH. Comparison of MRI techniques for detecting microadenomas in Cushing's disease. J Neurosurg. 2018 Apr;128(4): 1051-1057.

[145] Losa M, Giovanelli M, Persani L, Mortini P, Faglia G, Beck-Peccoz P. Criteria of cure and follow-up of central hyperthyroidism due to thyrotropin-secreting pituitary adenomas. J Clin Endocrinol Metab. 1996;81:3086–3090.

[146] Semple PL, Jane JA, Lopes MB, Laws ER. Pituitary apoplexy: correlation between magnetic resonance imaging and histopathological results. J Neurosurg. 2008 May;108(5):909-915

[147] Semple P, Webb M, de Villiers J, et al. Pituitary apoplexy. Neurosurgery 2005;56(1):65.

[148] Rajasekaran S, Vanderpump M, Baldeweg S, Drake W, Reddy N, Lanyon M, Markey A, Plant G, Powell M, Sinha S, Wass J. UK guidelines for the management of pituitary apoplexy. Clin Endocrinol (Oxf). 2011 Jan;74(1):9-20.

[149] Giritharan S, Gnanalingham K, Kearney T. Pituitary apoplexy - bespoke patient management allows good clinical outcome. Clin Endocrinol (Oxf). 2016 Sep;85(3):415-422.

[150] Jho DH, Biller BM, Agarwalla PK, Swearingen B. Pituitary apoplexy: large surgical series with grading system. World Neurosurg. 2014 Nov;82(5): 781-790.

[151] Arita K, Kurisu K, Tominaga A, Sugiyama K, Ikawa F, Yoshioka H, Sumida M, Kanou Y, Yajin K, Ogawa R. Thickening of sphenoid sinus mucosa during the acute stage of pituitary apoplexy. J Neurosurg. 2001 Nov;95(5): 897-901.

[152] Piotin M, Tampieri D, Rüfenacht DA, Mohr G, Garant M, Del Carpio R, Robert F, Delavelle J, Melanson D. The various MRI patterns of pituitary apoplexy. Eur Radiol. 1999;9 (5):918-923.

[153] Hosmann A, Micko A, Frischer JM, Roetzer T, Vila G, Wolfsberger S, Knosp E. Multiple Pituitary Apoplexy-Cavernous Sinus Invasion as Major Risk Factor for Recurrent Hemorrhage. World Neurosurg. 2019 Jun;126:e723-e730.

[154] Brown TV, Cheesman KC, Post KD. RECURRENT PITUITARY APOPLEXY IN AN ADENOMA WITH SWITCHING PHENOTYPES. AACE Clin Case Rep. 2020 Sep 21;6(5):e221-e224.

[155] Teasdale S, Hashem F, Olson S, Ong B, Inder WJ. Recurrent pituitary apoplexy due to two successive neoplasms presenting with ocular paresis and epistaxis. Endocrinol Diabetes Metab Case Rep. 2015;2015: 140088.

[156] UIHLEIN A, BALFOUR WM, DONOVAN PF. Acute hemorrhage into pituitary adenomas. J Neurosurg. 1957 Mar;14(2):140-151.

[157] Weisberg LA. Pituitary apoplexy. Association of degenerative change in pituitary adenoma with radiotherapy and detection by cerebral computed

tomography. Am J Med. 1977 Jul;63(1): 109-115.

[158] Randeva HS, Schoebel J, Byrne J, Esiri M, Adams CB, Wass JA. Classical pituitary apoplexy: clinical features, management and outcome. Clin Endocrinol (Oxf). 1999 Aug;51(2): 181-188.

[159] Ayuk J, McGregor EJ, Mitchell RD, Gittoes NJ. Acute management of pituitary apoplexy–surgery or conservative management? Clin Endocrinol (Oxf). 2004 Dec;61(6): 747-752.

[160] Rovit RL, Fein JM. Pituitary apoplexy: a review and reappraisal. J Neurosurg. 1972 Sep;37(3):280-288.

Chapter 13

# Pineal Region Tumors

*Nu Thien Nhat Tran*


## Abstract

The pineal gland is a small endocrine gland located in the brains of vertebrates near the brain center that helps regulate circadian rhythms. Pineal tumors are tumors located in this region including tumors of the pineal gland and tumors of the components and structures of this region. Pineal tumors can compress the third ventricle, squeeze the cerebral drain causing hydrocephalus, compress the brain stem, compress the cerebellum, compress the posterior fossa ... causing various disorders. The pineal gland has a rather complicated anatomy, deep in the brain parenchyma, surrounded by many blood vessels and other important structures, so surgery to approach this area is still a challenge for many surgeons. Because these cancers are so rare, it has always been difficult to collect a large number of cases to study and compare. This chapter will describe the features of pineal tumor from the information collected so far.


**Keywords:** pineal tumors, pineocyte, Parinaud syndrome, germinomas, teratomas

## 1. Introduction

The pineal gland is a small endocrine gland located in the brains of vertebrates near the brain center that helps regulate circadian rhythms.

Pineal tumors are tumors located in this region including tumors of the pineal gland and tumors of the components and structures of this region. Pineal tumors can compress the third ventricle, squeeze the cerebral drain causing hydrocephalus, compress the brain stem, compress the cerebellum, compress the posterior fossa, ... causing various disorders.

The pineal gland has a rather complicated anatomy, deep in the brain parenchyma, surrounded by many blood vessels and other important structures, so surgery to approach this area is still a challenge for many surgeons.

Because these cancers are so rare, it has always been difficult to collect a large number of cases to study and compare. This chapter will describe the features of pineal tumors from the information collected so far.

## 2. Epidemiology

According to many studies, pineal region tumors are rare, accounting for less than 1% of brain tumors in adults, 5–10% in children. In particular, 95% of pineal region tumors are found in patients <35 years old.

Gender distribution of pineal region tumors showed a high incidence in male, with a male: female ratio of 3:1 [1].

Geographically, this tumor is found in many Asian and American people, of which Japan accounts for 16% of the total pineal tumors [2–4]. There is no known reason for this difference.

## 3. Etiology and screening

Located near the center of the brain, the pineal gland is a tiny organ shaped like a pine cone. It is seen as a mysterious organ because in the endocrine glands, its function is discovered in the end [5, 6]. Researchers claim that it produces and regulates a number of hormones including melatonin. Melatonin (a hormone derived from serotonin) is best known for its role in regulating sleep - maintaining circadian rhythms, and in regulating fertility hormones [7, 8].

Until now, the cause of pineal region tumors has not been clarified. Several studies have noted an association between this tumor and retinoblastoma or rarely with Klinefelter's syndrome [9, 10]. In addition, no specific genetic mutations have been associated with pineal region tumors.

## 4. Classification

Tumors of the pineal region have a varied histology that generally can be divided into germ cell and non–germ cell derivatives.

Germ cell tumors are the most common of pineal region tumors. These tumors are classified into two subtypes: germinomas and a group of nongerminomatous germ cell tumors (NGGCTs) which include teratoma, embryonal carcinoma, yolk sac tumor and choriocarcinoma. These tumors arise from pluripotential germ cells, which usually do not reside in the pineal gland. Theoretically, these germ cells mistakenly migrate to the pineal gland during embryogenesis. It's still not clear why that happened.

The second most common form is pineal parenchymal tumors. Pineal parenchymal cell is a pinocyte. WHO classified it as pineocytoma, pineoblastoma and mixed pineocytoma-pineoblastoma tumors (or PPT of intermediate differentiation).

The pinocyte is surrounded by a stroma of fibrillary astrocytes, which interact with adjoining blood vessels to form part of the blood-pial barrier. These abnormally grown glial cells also become one of the types of pineal region tumors.

Other tumors which located around the pineal gland, are also pineal region tumors. These tumors include papillary tumor of the pineal region, meningioma or metastasis tumor. Papillary tumors of the pineal region are a new classification believed to be derived from specialized ependymocytes. These tumors are so rare that there is very little data available on them.

| | | |
|---|---|---|
| Germ cell tumors (GCTs) | | 50% -75% |
| Pineal parenchymal tumors (PPTs) | | 14% - 27% |
| | Pineocytoma (14% - 60%) | |
| | PPT of intermediate differentiation (10%) | |
| | Pineoblastoma (45%) | |
| Gliomas | | 5–26% |
| Papillary tumors of the pineal region | | |
| Other tumors | | |

**Table 1.**
*The classification and frequency of pineal region tumors.*

The table above shows the classification and frequency of pineal region tumors (**Table 1**).

## 5. Diagnostic

Despite their general anatomic location and similar imaging findings, pineal tumors are extremely heterogeneous in histopathology, natural history, and response to treatment. Diagnosis of pineal region tumors is based on clinical manifestations, imaging and pathological results.

Pathological outcomes are the gold standard in diagnosing pineal tumors. However, because the pineal gland is located deep in the brain, so tissue sampling becomes difficult. Consequently, noninvasive diagnosis become useful. Biological markers in serum and cerebrospinal fluid (CSF) provide additional data prior to invasive procedures.

Specific serum and cerebrospinal biological markers combined with clinical evidence and radiographs of pineal mass can guide diagnosis and treatment without the tissue biopsy.

### 5.1 Clinical presentation

Pineal tumor symptoms usually progress slowly from weeks to years. In the case of rapidly growing tumor may cause acute and severe symptoms [11]. These tumors remain localized to this region where they may compress adjacent structures including the cerebral aqueduct, brain stem, and cerebellum. Signs and symptoms therefore vary and relate to obstructive hydrocephalus, increased intracranial pressure, visual problems, Parinaud syndrome, changes in mental status, and ataxia.

The clinical presentation of these tumors depends on many factors, such as tumor location, its size and extend or patient age. Although the two most common tumor subtypes, GCTs and PPTs, occurred predominantly in children, the third most common, gliomas, were more common in adults. From there, if you encounter pineal region tumors in children, you can think of CGTs or PPTs more than gliomas. The opposite in adults.

One of the most common syndromes is obstructive hydrocephalus. Its presentations are headache (worse in morning), nausea and vomiting. This condition is usually caused by a tumor compressing the Sylvian aqueduct. If left untreated, it may lead to lethargy and death.

Another syndrome is visual problems. Pineal gland is very close to the pretectum so eye symptoms are common. Symptoms of pretectum compression leading to Parinaud's syndrome, which was first described by the French ophthalmologist Henri Parinaud in the late 1800s. This syndrome includes paralysis of vertical gaze, convergence retraction nystagmus, loss of pupillary light reflexes, loss of convergence upper eyelid retraction (Collier's "tucked lid" sign) and "setting sun" sign.

Rarely are symptoms related to the cerebellum. These symptoms include gait abnormality, instability, and frequent falls. The cause is thought to be caused by pressure on the cerebellum from large tumors.

Children with pineal region tumors can present with endocrine malfunction. Some specific endocrine syndromes can arise from secretion of hormones by germ cell tumors. Some of the endocrine disorders that can be mentioned are diabetes insipidus, pseudoprecocious puberty, amenorrhea and growth arrest.

Intracranial hemorrhage is rare but should be considered in pineal adenomas. Firstly, bleeding can cause pineal abscesses or subarachnoid hemorrhage. This

aggravates the symptoms of the disease. Secondly, since this is also one of the complications of surgery, this should be assessed before surgical treatment.

### 5.2 Imaging

#### *5.2.1 Computer tomography*

CT Scan is often used in the emergency, to help diagnose ventricular dilatation caused by pineal region tumor, determine calcification in the tumor and have a role in diagnosing the location, size, density of the tumor [12]. It is worth noting that CT scans are not recommended in children, especially young children. In general, CT Scan is not used to identify or classify pineal tumors.

#### *5.2.2 Cranial magnetic resonance imaging*

High-resolution MRI with gadolinium is necessary in the evaluation of pineal region lesions. On MRI, pineal neoplasms appear as solid, lobulated tumors. It allows to clearly identify the location, vascularity, morphology, and structure of the tumor as well as the anatomic relationship with surrounding structures in order to select surgical access routes. Irregular tumor borders may suggest a malignant tumor and surrounding invasion [12].

Although the exact type of tumor cannot be determined, some features can be used to guide a diagnosis. Most germinomas are readily visible on MR, and tend to be of considerable size by the time of presentation. These tumors are isointense on T1-weighted MRI images, are slightly hyperintense on T2, and have strong homogenous enhancement. Marked contrast enhancement is the rule for germinomas. In addition, in case of suspected germinomas, a MRI of the entire spine is required to assess the metastasis according to cerebrospinal fluid.

Unlike germinomas, teratomas typically have heterogeneous MRI signals. Most have evidence of fat or calcification.

Both pineocytomas and pineoblastomas typically are hypointense to isointense on T1-weighted images, have increased signal on T2, and demonstrate homogeneous enhancement after administration of gadolinium. It is rarely possible to distinguish between pineocytomas and pineoblastomas with MRI.

In addition to MRI, angiography is sometimes used in cases of suspected vascular anomalies.

### 5.3 Pathology

Tumor cells are removed and sent to a laboratory for examination. This is done to find out the type and grade of the tumor. Since the pineal gland is deep in the brain, there is almost no way to obtain tissue samples without invasive procedures. Consequently, there is usually only a pathological outcome after biopsy or surgery. What's more, not all tumors can perform invasive procedures. In facts., about 11% of biopsies are either undiagnosed or misdiagnosed, showing difficulty in obtaining enough tissue for an accurate diagnosis [13] (**Table 2**).

### 5.4 Biomarker

Although pineal cells are the only place to secrete melatonin in the body, numerous reports describe an association between melatonin secretion and pineal parenchymal tumors, indicating that very few pineal parenchymal tumors are disturbed melatonin secretion disorders lead to sleep disturbances [15–18]. Therefore,

| Tumors of the pineal region | Grade I | Grade II | Grade III | Grade IV |
|---|---|---|---|---|
| Germ cell tumors | | x | x | x |
| Pineocytoma | x | | | |
| Pineal parenchymal tumor of intermediate differentiation | | x | x | |
| Pineoblastoma | | | | x |
| Gliomas | | x | x | x |
| Papillary tumor of the pineal region | | x | x | |
| Other tumors | | | | |

**Table 2.**
*Pathology of tumors of the pineal region [14].*

| Tumor subtype | Beta Human Chorionic Gonadotropin | Alpha – Fetoprotein | Placental Alkaline Phosphatase |
|---|---|---|---|
| Germinoma | +/− | — | + |
| Teratoma | — | + | |
| Choriocarcinoma | + | — | |
| Embryonal carcinoma | + | +/− | |

**Table 3.**
*Biomarkers of germ cell tumors.*

melatonin analysis is presently believed to have little clinical use in diagnosing and monitoring response to treatment in pineal parenchymal tumors.

Germ cell tumors are groups capable of increasing the biological markers involved in germ cells. While germinomas and choriocarcinomas can cause an increase in β-hCG, embryonal carcinomas, immature teratomas, and endodermal sinus tumors can cause an elevated alpha-fetoprotein in the serum or CSF. Germinomas are also associated with elevated lactate dehydrogenase and placental alkaline phosphatase.

Biomarkers of germ cell tumors are summarized in **Table 3**.

As described above, these markers can be somewhat helpful for diagnosis, but they are more useful for monitoring response to treatment.

## 6. Prognosis

Pineal region tumors treatment results depend on the type of tissue, the location and size of the lesion as well as age of patient. In general, patients with germinomas have an excellent prognosis because of the radiosensitivity of these tumors.

A study of incidence, survival and treatment modalities was done based on the SEER data (The Surveillance, Epidemiology, and End Results) on 633 patient diagnosed pineal tumors during the period 1973–2005. The 5-year overall survival (OS) was 65% ± 2.1%. Among them, the best survival was germ cell tumors (OS = 78.9% ± 2.3%), followed by glioma (OS = 61% ± 9.3%) and pineal parenchymal tumors (OS = 47.2% ± 4.2%) [1].

Recurrent germ cell tumors have been shown to respond to chemotherapy, as have some pineal cell tumors, although to a lesser degree. No conventional approach

is designed for managing recurrence. Chemotherapy, radiotherapy, or radiosurgery can be applied if maximal doses have not already been administered.

## 7. Treatment

Due to pineal tumor's rarity, there is no consensus to date on optimal treatment. Some suggested that, complete surgical resection is the mainstay therapy for low-grade tumors, whereas a multimodality approach of surgery, radiotherapy, and chemotherapy is the preferred treatment in high-grade tumors. Some another authors encourage that the first treatment for pineal region tumors is surgery, if possible, followed with irradiation and chemotherapy or clinical trials. Clinical trials, with new chemotherapy, targeted therapy, or immunotherapy drugs, may also be available and can be a possible treatment option [13]. So that, treatments are decided by the physician, based on the patient 's factors, for example: the age at diagnosis, symptoms, remaining tumor after surgery, tumor type, and tumor location.

Notably, germinomas are exceptional. Germinomas, which are exquisitely radiosensitive, can be cured by conventional radiation therapy alone (40 Gy + 15 Gy boost). Craniospinal radiotherapy is indicated if CFS seeding is found. Therefore, diagnosis of germinomas by MRI and biomarkers becomes particularly important.

### 7.1 Surgery

The authors support an aggressive surgical approach to pineal region tumors to provide a definitive histological diagnosis. This strategy is based on their surgical experience in 160 operations for pineal region tumors in which operative mortality was 4% with 3% permanent major morbidity.

There are 2 types of surgery corresponding to 2 different purposes.

Firstly, for the treatment of ventricular dilation, there are two commonly mentioned techniques: ventriculoperitoneal shunt and endoscopic third ventriculostomy. Recently an endoscopic third ventriculostomy has been selected. Because this therapy not only drains cerebrospinal fluid but also may take tissue tumor for testing or pathology.

Another therapy is surgery to remove the pineal region tumors. In the past, surgical exploration of the pineal gland was very hazardous. Given recent advances, this surgical approach is typically performed endoscopically using a high-definition operating microscope and stereotactic techniques through a small bony opening at the back of the head, direct approach to these tumors has become relatively safe. The goal of surgery is to obtain tissue to determine the tumor type and to remove as much tumor as possible without causing more symptoms for the person. Evidence suggests that surgical debulking may improve the response to postoperative adjuvant therapy [19].

In summary, patients with hydrocephalus have evidence of pineal region malignancies on MRI may be treated with either third ventriculostomy or ventriculoperitoneal (VP) shunt prior to biopsy or removed.

Complications after surgery cannot be ignored. The most devastating complication of pineal tumor surgery, regardless of the approach, is postoperative hemorrhage. The bleeding can be early or slow for a few days and is often associated with vascular tumors. This is truly a disaster and a great challenge for all surgeons. Some common complications are extraocular movement dysfunction, ataxia, altered mental status as well as seizures, or hemiparesis. Some factors increased incidence of surgical complications include prior radiation treatment, severe preoperative neurologic symptoms, malignant tumor pathology, and invasive tumor characteristics.

### 7.2 Radiotherapy

Depending on each case, it is possible to have postoperative radiotherapy, concurrent postoperative chemotherapy, or only radiation therapy. There are a number of projection fields that can be applied, for example: whole brain (for multifocal metastatic cancers), tumor region and tumor margins (for large tumors that cannot be removed). The dose of radiation therapy depends on the type of histopathology, tumor location, age, physical condition, malignancy. Some potential complications of radiation therapy are hypothalamic and endocrine dysfunction, cerebral necrosis, dementia. They need careful evaluation and monitoring.

As mentioned above, germinomas are among the most radiosensitive tumors, therefore these tumors can be cured by conventional radiation therapy alone [20]. However, these patients should be carefully monitored with serial MRI to evaluate tumor recurrence or progression.

Remember, radiation therapy is only available for children 5 years of age and older. It has been noted that even low radiation doses can have significant long-term effects on children's cognitive development.

### 7.3 Systemic therapy

Chemotherapy is a supportive treatment that enhances the effectiveness of surgery and radiation therapy [21, 22]. Treatment regimens have included various combinations of vincristine, lomustine, cisplatin, etoposide, cyclophosphamide, actinomycin D, and methotrexate.

Chemotherapy is usually given after surgery, after, or simultaneously with radiation therapy. Using chemotherapy as the first step in the treatment of pineal tumors has only been shown to be effective in certain cases. The success of radiotherapy in the treatment of germ tumors has discouraged the use of chemotherapy as the primary treatment. Chemotherapy should be considered the first line of treatment in young children, especially children younger than 5 years.

## 8. Follow up

After treatment for pineal tumors there are many chronic health problems to be aware of and to screen for in long-term survivors. Lifelong follow-up of children with pineal region tumors is required. MRI scans and biomarkers should be obtained on a periodic basis, even if the result were not abnormal. Patients should be evaluated by an endocrinologist and ophthalmologist every 1–2 years.

## Author details

Nu Thien Nhat Tran
Thu Duc City Hospital, Ho Chi Minh City, Vietnam

*Address all correspondence to: trannuthiennhat24.10@gmail.com

## References

[1] Al-Hussaini M, Sultan I, Abuirmileh N, et al. Pineal gland tumors: experience from the SEER database. Journal of neuro-oncology. 2009;94:351–8. DOI: 10.1007/s11060-009-9881-9.

[2] Dolecek TA, Propp JM, Stroup NE, et al. CBTRUS statistical report: primary brain and central nervous system tumors diagnosed in the United States in 2005–2009. Neuro-oncology. 2012;14: v1-v49. DOI.

[3] Nomura K. Epidemiology of germ cell tumors in Asia of pineal region tumor. Journal of neuro-oncology. 2001; 54:211–7. DOI: 10.1023/a:1012771204732.

[4] Rickert CH, Paulus W. Epidemiology of central nervous system tumors in childhood and adolescence based on the new WHO classification. Child's Nervous System. 2001;17:503–11. DOI: 10.1007/s003810100496.

[5] Reiter RJ. Comparative physiology: pineal gland. Annual review of physiology. 1973;35:305–28. DOI: 10.1146/annurev.ph.35.030173.001513.

[6] Reiter RJ. The mammalian pineal gland: structure and function. American Journal of Anatomy. 1981;162:287–313. DOI: 10.1002/aja.1001620402.

[7] Zisapel N. New perspectives on the role of melatonin in human sleep, circadian rhythms and their regulation. British journal of pharmacology. 2018; 175:3190–9. DOI.

[8] Brzezinski A. Melatonin in humans. New England journal of medicine. 1997; 336:186–95. DOI: 10.1056/NEJM199701163360306.

[9] Hasle H, Mellemgaard A, Nielsen J, et al. Cancer incidence in men with Klinefelter syndrome. British journal of cancer. 1995;71:416–20. DOI: 10.1093/jnci/dji240.

[10] Jakobiec FA, Tso MO, Zimmerman LE, et al. Retinoblastoma and intracranial malignancy. Cancer. 1977;39:2048–58. DOI: 10.1002/1097-0142(197705)39:5<2048::aid-cncr2820390522>3.0.co;2–9.

[11] Gaillard F, Jones J. Masses of the pineal region: clinical presentation and radiographic features. Postgraduate medical journal. 2010;86:597–607. DOI: 10.1136/pgmj.2009.087460.

[12] Deiana G, Mottolese C, Hermier M, et al. Imagery of pineal tumors. Neurochirurgie. 2015;61:113–22. DOI: 10.1016/j.neuchi.2014.10.111.

[13] Konovalov AN, Pitskhelauri DI. Principles of treatment of the pineal region tumors. Surgical neurology. 2003;59:252–70. DOI: 10.1016/s0090-3019(03)00080-6.

[14] Louis DN, Perry A, Reifenberger G, et al. The 2016 World Health Organization classification of tumors of the central nervous system: a summary. Acta neuropathologica. 2016;131:803–20. DOI: 10.1007/s00401-016-1545-1.

[15] Leston J, Mottolese C, Champier J, et al. Contribution of the daily melatonin profile to diagnosis of tumors of the pineal region. Journal of neuro-oncology. 2009;93:387–94. DOI: 10.1007/s11060-008-9792-1.

[16] Grimoldi N, Tomei G, Stankov B, et al. Neuroendocrine, immunohistochemical, and ultrastructural study of pineal region tumors. Journal of pineal research. 1998; 25:147–58. DOI: 10.1111/j.1600-079x.1998.tb00553.x.

[17] Barber S, Smith J, Hughes R. Melatonin as a tumour marker in a

patient with pineal tumour. British medical journal. 1978;2:328. DOI: 10.1136/bmj.2.6133.328.

[18] Kennaway D, McCulloch G, Matthews C, et al. Plasma melatonin, luteinizing hormone, follicle-stimulating hormone, prolactin, and corticoids in two patients with pinealoma. The Journal of Clinical Endocrinology & Metabolism. 1979;49: 144–5. DOI: 10.1210/jcem-49-1-144.

[19] Bruce J, Stein B. Surgical management of pineal region tumors. Acta neurochirurgica. 1995;134:130–5. DOI: 10.1007/BF01417679.

[20] SUN W, YANG W, ZHANG B. Clinical treatment of intracranial germinoma. CHINESE JOURNAL OF MINIMALLY INVASIVE NEUROSARGERY. 2000. DOI.

[21] Jakacki RI, Zeltzer PM, Boyett JM, et al. Survival and prognostic factors following radiation and/or chemotherapy for primitive neuroectodermal tumors of the pineal region in infants and children: a report of the Childrens Cancer Group. Journal of clinical oncology. 1995;13:1377–83. DOI: 10.1200/JCO.1995.13.6.1377.

[22] Cho B-K, Wang K-C, Nam D-H, et al. Pineal tumors: experience with 48 cases over 10 years. Child's Nervous System. 1998;14:53–8. DOI: 10.1007/s003810050175.

Section 7

# Challenges in the Imaging and Mangement of Primary and Metastatic CNS Tumors

Chapter 14

# Diagnosis and Management of Radiation Necrosis in Patients with Brain Metastases and Primary Tumors

*Juan Esteban Garcia-Robledo, Alejandro Ruíz-Patiño, Carolina Sotelo, Álvaro Muñoz, Oscar Arrieta, Lucia Zatarain-Barrón, Camila Ordoñez, Christian Rolfo and Andrés F. Cardona*

## Abstract

The incidence of radiation necrosis has increased secondary to combined modality therapy for brain tumors and stereotactic radiosurgery. The pathology of progressive brain radiation necrosis (RN) primarily includes inflammation and angiogenesis in which cytokines, chemokines, and vascular endothelial growth factors are upregulated. Combined multiparametric imaging, including lesional metabolism, spectroscopy, and blood flow, could enhance diagnostic accuracy compared with a single imaging study. Nevertheless, a substantial risk of bias restricts firm conclusions about the best imaging technique for diagnosing brain RN. Bevacizumab shows promising results of improving radiographic edema and post-gadolinium enhancement with associated symptomatic improvement. However, this was based on small double-blinded randomized controlled trials, which introduces a high risk of bias due to the small sample size despite the high-quality trial design. Edaravone combined with corticosteroids also resulted in a more significant reduction in radiographic edema than corticosteroids alone but had no impact on reducing the enhancing lesion. There is a great need for further prospective randomized controlled trials (RCTs) to treat brain RN.

**Keywords:** radiation necrosis, brain metastases, brain tumors, gliomas, brain injury

## 1. Introduction

For years, radiation therapy (RT) has played a critical role in the treatment of primary brain tumors (PBT) and brain metastases (BM). Different techniques can be used depending on the clinical setting, including brachytherapy, fractionated stereotactic radiotherapy, and stereotactic radiosurgery. The use of RT in brain tumors has been related to improved progression-free survival as well as overall survival, especially in patients with high-risk low-grade gliomas [1]. As with different cytotoxic treatment approaches, the use of cranial irradiation comes with

the possibility of specific side effects known as radiation toxicity that can be acute (early toxicity) or late. Usually, early toxicity symptoms are reversible and treatable with proper supportive care; these symptoms include fatigue, headache, alopecia, dermatitis, nausea, and vomiting. Radiation necrosis (RN) is one of the leading late toxicity clinical manifestations. It usually occurs between 1–3 years after RT in the location that received the most radiation (tumor location) or a nearby area.

Clinical manifestations of RN will depend on the location of its development [2]. Signs and symptoms of focal neurologic deficits might occur, seizures are also present in approximately 20% of patients [3]. Depending on the region of the brain that is affected, different sets of symptoms might be present, including but not limited to motor deficits (2.9%), sensory deficits (1.3%), cognitive deficits (1%), speech deficits (1.3%), visual disturbances (0.6%), ataxia (1.6%) and general symptoms like headache (5%), nausea (1%) and hemorrhage (5%) [4]. This chapter will discuss the epidemiological features of RN, its risk factors, its pathophysiology, its diagnosis, and treatment.

## 2. Incidence of radiation necrosis

The current true incidence of RN is hard to estimate. According to Vellayappan *et al.*, the incidence of this kind of toxicity might vary between 5–25% [5]. This broad range is mainly explained, but the different methodologies used in epidemiological studies of RN in which its definition is not homogenous and only some studies have required histological confirmation, the studies' follow-up can also provide different results. The kind of RT provided, the dosing, and the fractionation of radiation might also impact the incidence of RN [6].

In a study made by Kohutek *et al.*, the evidence of RN (including asymptomatic cases) was 25.8%, with a progressive increase in actuarial incidence regarding the time of evaluation as follows: 5.2% at six months after RT, 17.2% at 12 months, 23% at 18 months and 34% at 24 months. The median time to the first diagnosis of RN was 10.7 months. In this study, the incidence of symptomatic RN was 11.8% at 12 months. Significant variability in diagnostic methods used in this study was seen, with some patients being diagnosed histologically, some via FDG-PET and others by MRI alone [7]. Another study conducted by Blonigen *et al.* analyzed RN in metastatic lesions after stereotactic surgery; a total of 63 patients with 173 lesions were studied. 14% of the lesions presented with RN, 10% were symptomatic. The individual factor related to a higher risk for RN, whether symptomatic or asymptomatic, was an increased dose of radiation. The location of the lesion was not related to the development of RN of any kind [8].

Studies where pathological confirmation of RN was done reported the least incidence, a clear example is an investigation made by Chin *et al* in which the reported incidence was only 7% [9]. This can be explained by a better sensitivity for histopathological diagnosis and a greater rate of false positives in imaging techniques, as some other pathological mechanisms could resemble RN, including pseudoprogression, radiation-induced neoplasms, and vascular thrombotic events [10].

## 3. Pathophysiology of radiation necrosis

Vascular and white matter (myelinated tissue) injury have been stated as the genesis of RN. Since the second half of the 20th century, anecdotal clinical literature argued about the existence of delayed radiation-induced necrosis of the brain; however, scarce evidence was available regarding the exact mechanisms

of disease [11]. In the 1970s and 1980s, two main pathogenetic theories were formulated. The first one was the glial cell theory, in which radiation injury was presumed to induce damage of glial cells, specifically of oligodendrocytes, which will induce a cascade of events that will end in tissue necrosis [12]. The other theory stated that endothelial cell injury induced by radiation was the only cause explaining ischemia and further tissue necrosis. Different experimental studies performed in rats and dogs found data that supported both theories, and today we consider that RN arises as a multifactorial process in which glial cells, endothelial cells, and other cell types result injured by radiation generating different inflammatory and scarring processes that end in tissue necrosis [13–15].

Both theories are currently accepted as part of one single process in which vascular injury precedes glial cell damage. After brain tissue is exposed to radiation, avascular insult occurs within the first 24 hours, followed by parenchymal brain injury [16]. Reactive oxygen species develop because of ionizing radiation, leading to single- and double-stranded DNA damage. Regulatory cell mechanisms are activated and will drive the endothelium to cell cycle arrest and further apoptosis [17]. Ionizing radiation of more than 8 Gy will also induce activation of acid sphingomyelinase in endothelial cells [18, 19], leading to ceramide synthesis and ceramide-induced apoptosis [20]. The injured tissue will also induce inflammation, producing the release of TNF-alpha [21], a molecule that has been shown to disrupt the blood–brain barrier (BBB) in multiple physiological and pathological situations [22–24]. Increased expression of VEGF and ICAM-1 has also been shown [25, 26]. The result of this inflammatory cascades is the development of intravascular thrombi and fibrinoid necrosis, leading to vessel lumen narrowing and further ischemia and necrosis and disrupting, even more, the BBB homeostasis [27], leading to cerebral edema and further demyelination [28]. Thus, vascular injury induces oligodendrocyte injury, but at the same time, the initial ionizing radiation can also directly damage glial cells, generating inflammation and gliosis. In the early-delayed phase of this process, edema might resemble tumor progression or pseudoprogression on imaging findings [29]. Research has also shown that ischemia-induced hypoxia in the perilesional area can induce HIF-α, which also induces VEGF expression generating angiogenesis of weak, leaky capillaries that aggravate edema, necrosis, and demyelination. **Figure 1** shows the pathophysiological characteristics for the development of the RN.

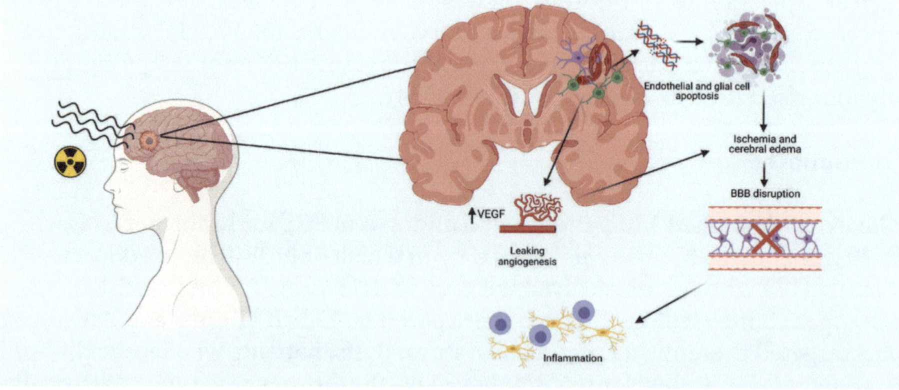


**Figure 1.**
*An illustration depicting RN pathophysiology is shown. When a patient receives radiation over a tumoral lesion, DNA damage occurs in glial and endothelial cells which will further lead to cell apoptosis. Vascular apoptosis leads to tissue ischemia and subsequent cerebral edema, processes that will facilitate BBB disruption with the further recruitment of inflammatory cells mediated by microglia. At the same time, increased expression of VEGF in response to hypoxia generates fragile neovessels that would leak plasma and would increase cerebral edema and BBB permeability.*

## 4. Risk factors related to radiation necrosis

As a result of different epidemiological, clinical, and genomic studies related to radiation-associated brain injury, different risk factors for RN have been identified.

### 4.1 Dose-volume interplay

The incidence of RN increases as dose and volume increase. Different studies have tried to find the ideal dose for different tumor diameters. Lesions of 20 mm or less can be safely treated with 24 Gy, 21–30 mm lesions with 18 Gy, and lesions between 31–40 with 15 Gy. The cumulative incidence of RN at 12 months for these measurements is 8% [30]. In the case of SRS, it has been demonstrated that the brain parenchyma that is irradiated with >10–12 Gy has a greater risk of developing RN. This risk is even higher when $V10 > 10.5\ cm^3$ or $V12 > 7.9\ cm^3$ [8].

### 4.2 Prior radiation exposure

Another essential risk factor for RN is prior radiation exposure, whether as whole-brain radiation therapy (WBRT) or SRS. A study performed by Sneed *et al.* showed that the risk of developing RN after SRS in a patient with prior SRS in the same lesion was 20% at one year, 4% when WBRT was the primary modality, and 8% when concurrent WBRT. When no history of prior irradiation, the risk was only 3% [31]. Andruska *et al.* studied the incidence of symptomatic RN in 75 patients with brain metastases that received different doses in five fractions. With a median follow-up of 8 months, 14 patients were diagnosed with symptomatic RN; half of them were not previously exposed to brain radiation. However, in a subgroup analysis by dose received, patients with a history of prior intracranial irradiation only developed RN after 30 Gy, with the highest incidence when the dose was over 35 Gy [32].

### 4.3 Chemotherapy

Radiosensitization with cytotoxic agents is a common practice in the treatment of different tumors and metastatic diseases [33]. In the same study by Sneed *et al.*, the use of capecitabine +5-fluorouracil was related to a higher incidence of RN [31]. Ruben *et al.* studied 426 patients who underwent intracranial RT for glioma treatment; they found that patients who received subsequent chemotherapy significantly increased the risk of RN ($p = 0.001$) [34].

### 4.4 Immunotherapy

Colaco *et al.* studied 180 patients who underwent SRS for brain metastases. Only 39 developed RN from this cohort, from which only 35% received immunotherapy (IT) (the agents received were anti-CD137, anti-CTLA4, anti-PD-1, interferon, and interleukin-2), from these patients, 12 had IT only, and 2 received IT plus targeted therapy. In the multivariate analysis, patients who received IT only were at higher risk of developing RN; however, the difference was not statistically significant ($p = 0.06$). Statistical significance was evidenced in the univariate analysis ($p = 0.03$) [35]. Another study by Martin *et al.* included 480 patients that underwent SRS for BMs. They found that the receipt of IT was associated with symptomatic RN ($p = 0.04$), with the association being robust in melanoma patients ($p = 0.03$) and being even more substantial in melanoma patients receiving

Ipilimumab ($p = 0.01$). As it is widely known, checkpoint inhibitors are pro-inflammatory. Therefore, it is biologically plausible that its use can exacerbate the myriad of pathological mechanisms underlying RN [36].

### 4.5 Tyrosine-kinase inhibitors

Juloori *et al.* performed a study of 326 patients with 912 renal cell carcinoma with BM that underwent SRS. The cumulative incidence of RN at 12 months was 8%. It was found that the use of TKIs within 30 days from SRS was associated with a significantly increased 12-month cumulative incidence of RN (10.9% vs. 6.4%, $p = 0.04$) [37].

### 4.6 Brain location

Even though most studies did not find a correlation between brain location and RN risk, some observations by Flickinger *et al.* in arteriovenous malformations (AVMs) suggest that the frontal cortex is at higher risk of RN and that the brainstem seems to be more resistant to radiation. Superficial lesions might also be at less risk of RN than the deeper ones [38].

### 4.7 Histology

Specific histological subtypes of tumors might be related to an increased risk of RN. Miller *et al.* at the Cleveland Clinic studied 1979 patients with metastatic lesions that received intracranial irradiation. From this pool, 15% of patients presented with RN. Analysis by histological subgroups revealed that HER2-amplified status ($p = 0.02$), BRAF V600E mutational status ($p = 0.04$), lung adenocarcinoma histology ($p = 0.02$) and ALK rearrangements presence ($p < 0.01$) were associated with a greater risk of RN [39].

### 4.8 Planning target volume (PTV) margin

A higher PTV might be related to an RN's increased risk. A study by Kirkpatrick *et al.* evaluated the risk of RN in 49 patients with 80 BMs. Patients were randomized to receive a 1 mm or 3 mm expansion of their gross tumor volume. Patients with the greater PTV (3 mm) had the highest risk of RN ($p = 0.1$); however, statistical significance was not reached as only six patients developed RN [40].

### 4.9 Intrinsic radiosensitivity

A possible genetic radiosensitivity might also underly some of the risk burdens of some patients that develop RN. One *in vitro* study evaluated the radiosensitivity of fibroblasts extracted from 5 patients with AVMs that did not develop RN compared to those extracted from 2 patients that developed RN. The researchers found an increased sensitivity in the fibroblasts from the patients that had RN [41]. A recent genome-wide association study from China found that the RN of the temporal lobe was related to the presence of a particular single-nucleotide polymorphism in the CEP128 gene promoter related to radionecrotic temporal lobe injury. CEP128 gene encodes the centrosomal protein 128 kDa, which interacts with multiple radiation-resistant genes and plays a crucial role in functional cilia. When this exact mutation is replicated in a glioblastoma cell line (U87), cell survival is considerably decreased under radiation.

## 5. Radiation necrosis imaging

The pathology of progressive brain RN primarily includes inflammation and angiogenesis in which cytokines, chemokines, and vascular endothelial growth factors are upregulated [12, 15, 42, 43]. Distinguishing between RN and tumor progression is somewhat challenging on conventional imaging. Besides, obtaining tissue samples is invasive even in stereotactic biopsies, although pathological diagnosis remains the gold standard. Moreover, needle biopsy poses a risk of misdiagnosis because RN is typically a heterogeneous lesion with coexisting radiation necrosis and tumor cells [44]. Currently, RN is diagnosed by relatively less-invasive radiological examinations that evaluate the whole lesion, compared with needle biopsy. Strategies can be divided into two categories, the use of conventional radiological imaging [computed tomography (CT) and magnetic resonance imaging (MRI)], and nuclear medicine studies [single photon emission CT (SPECT) and positron emission tomography (PET)] [45].

Brain RN may occur during therapy (acute injury), a few weeks to 3 months after therapy (early-delayed injury), or more than three months after treatment (late injury). After conventional radiotherapy, RN typically involves large areas of the brain and may not be amenable to surgery [46]. On the contrary, the injury secondary to radiosurgery tends to be restricted to the site of treatment and, consequently, may respond well to surgical resection [47]. Computed tomography was found to be unreliable in this regard quite early [46, 48, 49]. The most cited MRI features are necrotic foci, contrast enhancement, and perilesional edema [50, 51]; Changes are most evident in T2-weighted and fluid-attenuated inversion recovery sequences. Unfortunately, these features are commonly present with recurrent tumors as well. Some MRI features have been thought to suggest radiation necrosis in previous reports: contrast enhancement with ill-defined borders and little or no mass effect and a "Swiss cheese" or "soap bubble" pattern ("cut green pepper"). On the other hand, Dequesada *et al.* noted that gyriform lesions and edema with marginal or solid enhancement suggested at least some viable tumor, adding that a lesion quotient (LQ) (which is the ratio of the nodule on T2 sequence to the total enhancing area on T1 sequence) of >0.6 was suggestive of tumor recurrence, while an LQ of <0.3 favored radiation necrosis alone [52]. Other authors however found this feature to be only 8% sensitive.

Years ago, some suggested that advanced imaging modalities might prove to be more reliable than MRI in the differential diagnosis of tumor versus necrosis. Taylor et al. [53] found that magnetic resonance spectroscopy (MRS) reliably identified 5 of 7 patients with active tumor and 4 of 5 patients with radiation necrosis. Others have found that MRS reliably distinguished pure tumor from pure necrosis but that no values could distinguish mixed specimens [54, 55].

Almost two decades ago, Tsuyuguchi *et al.* found that methionine positron emission tomography had a sensitivity of 78% and a specificity of 100% for detecting recurrent tumor versus RN [56]. Subsequently, Belohlávek *et al.* found fluorodeoxyglucose PET to be insensitive but specific [57].

Since then, the use of MRS, MR perfusion, and PET has been consolidated as effective techniques to help increase diagnostic confidence. These techniques are discussed below.

### 5.1 MR perfusion

Viable tumor has intact vasculature and thus higher perfusion and blood volume than necrotic tissue. An increased relative cerebral blood volume (rCBV) based on dynamic susceptibility-weighted MRI has been used for differentiating tumor from necrosis [58]. Sugahara *et al.* prospectively studied 20 patients with

enhancing lesions after irradiation using gradient-echo dynamic susceptibility perfusion MRI and reported that a normalized rCBV value greater than 2.6 or less than 0.6 was always indicative of tumor recurrence and radiation necrosis, respectively [59]. Later, Hu *et al.* reported rCBV of <0.71 as 92% sensitivity and 100% specificity for radiation necrosis, while another suggested an rCBV cutoff of <2.1 (100% sensitivity and specificity) [58].

However, much of the published information is retrospective and inconsistent. Barajas *et al.* reported significant overlap in rCBV values and proposed using the percentage of signal-intensity recovery (PSR) [60]. Furthermore, rCBV values vary between machines, depend on the acquisition methods, and are confounded by signal-intensity pileup artifacts and susceptibility artifacts from blood and contrast pooling within the lesions. Intravoxel incoherent motion (IVIM) is another method that provides quantitative diffusion and perfusion measurements based on a diffusion-weighted imaging (DWI) MR acquisition. Compared with the combination of normalized CBV and ADC, adding IVIM to rCBV substantially improved the diagnostic accuracy for differentiating recurrent tumor and RN from 86% to 93% [61]. This data has been validated against gold standard histopathology [62].

### 5.2 MRS

MRS provides additional information on the metabolic composition within an area of tissue by comparing several metabolites' relative concentrations. Ando *et al.* retrospectively studied 20 patients and found that a 1.5 threshold of choline-to-creatine (Cho/Cr) ratio had a sensitivity of 64% (95% CI, 35–87%), and a specificity of 83% (95% CI, 36–100%) for the detection of glioma recurrence [63]. Traber *et al.* reported a series of 43 patients, with an increased choline peak (50% higher than contralateral tissue) which implies a sensitivity of 72% (95% CI, 53–86%), and a specificity of 82% (95% CI, 48–98%) to distinguish tumor from RN; however, not in all patients there was a histopathological verification [64].

Besides, Lichy *et al.* tested multivoxel spectroscopy in a cohort of 24 patients with recurrent tumor suspicion and found that a Cho/Cr threshold ratio of 2.0 had 87% sensitivity and 89% specificity for the detection of tumor recurrence in contrast to RN [65]. Furthermore, Plotkin *et al.* assessed prospectively 25 patients with suspected recurrent glioma versus radiation injury by single-voxel MRS at 3 Tesla. They reported that a combined diagnostic threshold of choline-to N-acetyl aspartate (NAA) of 1.17 and Cho/Cr of 1.11 resulted in 89% sensitivity and 83% specificity for differentiating tumor against radiotherapy-induced chronic changes [66].

Zeng *et al.* also explored the diagnostic effectiveness of MRS with DWI on the evaluation of recurrent contrast-enhancing areas at the site of treated gliomas. The authors found that the Cho/NAA (1.71) and Cho/Cr ratios were significantly higher in recurrent tumors than in regions of radiation injury, and ADC ratios were significantly higher in radiation injury regions than in recurrent tumors. The results showed that the sensitivity, specificity, and diagnostic accuracy were 94.1%, 100%, and 96.2%, respectively [67]. In contrast, an elevated lipid-lactate peak and generalized decrease in other metabolites supported radiation necrosis [68]. MRS is limited by voxel size, often requiring the lesion to be larger than 1 cm [3] and is also affected by sampling errors within heterogeneous tumors and the proximity to the skull base.

Recently, Chuang *et al.* presented the results of a systematic review that included 397 patients included in 13 studies designed to differentiate tumor recurrence versus radiotherapy changes. The pooled difference in means (2.18, 95% CI 0.85–3.50) indicated that the average rCBV in a contrast-enhancing lesion was significantly higher in tumor recurrence than radiation injury ($p = 0.001$). Based

on a fixed-effect model of analysis encompassing the six studies which used Cho / Cr ratios for evaluation, the pooled difference in means (0.77, 95% CI 0.57–0.98) of the average Cho/Cr ratio was significantly higher in tumor recurrence than in RN ($p = 0.001$). In the same direction, there was a significant difference in ratios of Cho to NAA between recurrent tumor and necrosis (1.02, 95% CI 0.03–2.00, $p = 0.044$) [69]. At least two additional integrative studies demonstrated that MRS alone has moderate diagnostic performance in differentiating glioma recurrence from radiation necrosis using metabolite ratios like Cho/Cr and Cho/NAA ratio [70, 71]. **Figure 2** shows the main imaging characteristics in conventional MRI (contrasted T1 phase), MR perfusion and MRS.

### 5.3 PET

Impaired BBB is considered the leading diagnostic indicator of brain tumors and metastases on contrast-enhanced MRI and CT. Similarly, many PET tracers that can identify tumor cells at various sites in the body would only reach the brain if the BBB is disrupted. Therefore, the development of specific tracers that do not depend on BBB damage, such as fluorodeoxyglucose (18F-FDG) and labeled amino acids (aa) that are transferred by specific transporters across the intact BBB was introduced. Different studies showed that 18F-FDG is unhelpful in differentiating tumor progression from RN. Even though 18F-FDG alone has a low sensitivity (43%), its combination with other imaging techniques like MRI might increase its diagnostic usefulness [72]. The fact that tumoral or highly inflamed tissue might have an increased uptake of amino acids [73], and the relatively low uptake of normal brain tissue would provide a considerable tissue contrast. Compared to 201Tl, 18F-FDG is more specific but less sensitive to detect tumor recurrence since the former, before its uptake through the Na+-K+ ATPase pump, has a non-specific accumulation due to BBB breakdown. The latter lacks sensitivity because of the physiological uptake

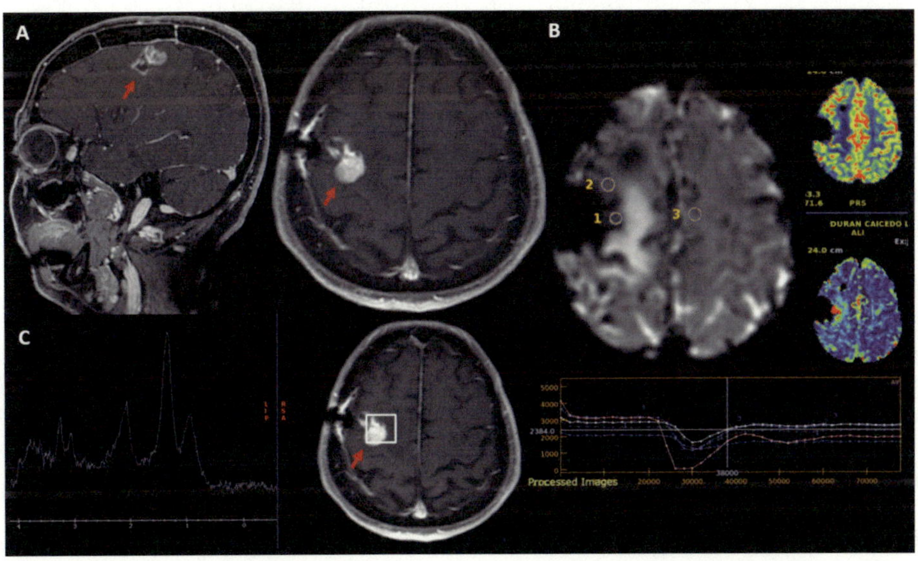


**Figure 2.**
*(A) Post-surgical right parietal changes due to resection of a metastatic lesion adjacent to the precentral sulcus with enhancement in the contrasted T1 sequence after SRS execution (compatible with RN). The lesion has an irregular morphology and measures 18x13x16.7 mm. (B) Decrease in all metabolites compared to the healthy zone, without evidence of Cho/NAA ratios greater than 2.0. There is also an increase in the peak of lactate-lipids, indicating that it corresponds to RN. (C) In the postsurgical cavity and in the nodular lesion that is enhanced with contrast medium, there are low values of rCBV.*

of normal brain [74]. More specifically, in the differentiation of tumor recurrence and RN, 18F-FDG also has low specificity, ranging from 40 to 94%, mainly during the first few weeks post-therapy, with a study that showed a sensitivity of 81–86%. Therefore, it is recommended to perform 18F-FDG PET no less than 3 months after the end of RT, also because it can cause inflammatory changes that can last up to 6 months after therapy but slowly decreases over time, for example, in the lung parenchyma, which will take up FDG and make it difficult to differentiate from the recurrent tumor [75].

Other amino acids have been studied, including fluoro-1-thymidine, fluoro-ethyltyrosine (18F-FET), 3,4-Dihydroxy-6-18F-fluoro- l -phenylalanine (FDOPA), l-[Methyl- 11 C] methionine (11C-MET), 3-Deoxy-30-18F-fluorothymidine (18F-FLT) and carbon-11 choline. Floeth *et al.* compared 18F-FET performance with MRI and MR spectroscopy in 50 patients, showing in 34 tumoral lesions a mean tumor/non-tumor ratio (T/NT) of FET uptake of 2.4 ± 0.9, thus significantly higher than non-neoplastic lesions (16 lesions; $p < 0.001$), with the area of significant 18F-FET uptake that was always included within the area of MR signal abnormality, which means that the latter could often be overestimating the extension of disease. More 30 out of 34 gliomas demonstrated an increased 18F-FET uptake (T/NT ratio > 1.6), with an overall sensitivity and specificity for the distinction of tumors from non-neoplastic tissues of 88% and 88%, respectively [76]. Concerning RN, studies have shown the absence of 18F-FET uptake in a case of RN in contrast to 18F-FDG; this could be due to the absence of 18F-FET uptake from macrophages, which are a common inflammatory mediator usually present in such cases. Recently, a study performed by Radinger *et al.* evaluated 36 patients with a glioma diagnosis. They used 18F-FET vs. MRS to differentiate tumor progression from RN correctly. In this study, pathological assessment and clinical manifestations were used as confirmatory variables. A specificity of 93% and a sensitivity of 100% was calculated for 18F-FET after suspicion of the recurrent tumor revealed by MRI (this highlights the importance of combining techniques for better analysis) [77].

18F-FDOPA is an amino acid tracer that has been used at the beginning for the evaluation of movement disorders by assessing the integrity of the striatal dopamine pathway. Recently, 18F-FDOPA it is studied in the imaging of brain tumors. In this scenario, one of the main pros of 18F-FDOPA lays in the crossing of the BBB thanks to a specific neutral amino acid transporter, which grants a better uptake ratio also because tracer accumulation does not depend on BBB breakdown [78]. In a non-conventional meta-analysis, Yu *et al.* evaluated the accuracy of 18F-FDOPA and compared it to 18F-FET for differentiating RN from brain tumor recurrence going through 48 separate studies (18F-FDOPA, n = 21; 18F-FET, n = 27), in which both tracer showed comparable results in terms of pooled sensitivity (85%), specificity (82%) and diagnostic odds ratio (21.7); in particular, 18F-FDOPA showed better diagnostic accuracy in patients with glioma compared with patients with brain metastases and proved to be better than 18F-FET in diagnosing glioma recurrence. In any case, larger cohorts of patients will be needed to support these preliminary findings [79].

11C-MET is a PET amino acid isotope characterized by a relatively short half-life that in tumors determine the high density and activity of amino acid transporters. Instead, it can accumulate due to active transport and cell proliferation, but in RN, passive diffusion via BBB damage is the most probable uptake mechanism [80]. Therefore, the difference in terms of accumulation mechanisms could be a way to distinguish the two clinical settings. Concerning its role in the differentiation of recurrence from RN, Hustinx *et al.* explain the potential role of 11C-MET to differentiate either low-grade or high-grade gliomas. 11C-MET uptake was directly

related to prognosis and survival in low-grade gliomas since it is increased in the absence of BBB breakdown, thus determining a significant advantage over CT, MRI, or even 18F-FDG PET.

Moreover, in the case of high-grade gliomas, 11C-MET uptake is higher than in low-grade tumors; therefore, it could be used for monitoring purposes to assess anaplastic transformation [81]. In a recent study of 18 lesions from 15 patients with metastatic brain tumors who underwent gamma knife radiosurgery, the authors showed that 11C-MET was superior in terms of both sensitivity and specificity as an imaging technique for differentiating RN and recurrent metastatic tumors after gamma-knife compared with diffusion-weighted imaging (DWI), MR permeability imaging and 18F-FDG. However, it is not widely available yet for clinical use due to its physical limitations [82]. Another study showed that 11C-MET could differentiate recurrence from RN based on the PET/Gd volume ratio and the PET/Gd overlap ratio as these ratios were significantly lower in patients with RN than in patients with glioblastoma recurrence ($p < 0.05$) (analysis were done based on a pathological assessment) [83].

18F-FLT is a radiolabeled analog that has been used to indicate tumor proliferation since thymidine is a nucleoside encountered only in DNA; therefore, it reflects tissue proliferation rate. 18F-FLT transport is mediated mainly by active $Na^+$ −dependent carriers through nucleoside transporters (salvage thymidine pathway) and passive diffusion. Enslow *et al.* made a tracer comparison taking in consideration 18F-FLT kinetic parameters (18F-FLT Kimax) rather than simple SUV max values [18F-FLT Kimax ≥0.0165 (sensitivity 91%, specificity 75%); 18F-FLT SUV max ≥1.34 (sensitivity 73%, specificity 75%)] and although there was no statistically significant difference both 18F-FDG and 18F-FLT proved to be accurate in the differentiation between recurrent glioma and radiation necrosis [84]. Unfortunately, even if dynamic kinetic modeling of 18F − FLT-PET has proven to be crucial and its superiority could not be demonstrated only for the small number of patients included in the study, due to the complexity of the procedure, it is unlikely that it will be broadly accepted in clinical practice. No single technique of PET and other imaging techniques has been shown to be able to differentiate recurrence from RN by itself. Based on the limitations of each modality, a multi-modal approach is currently used. **Figure 3** shows the differences between different PET tracers for the diagnosis of RN versus conventional MRI and the perfusion sequence.

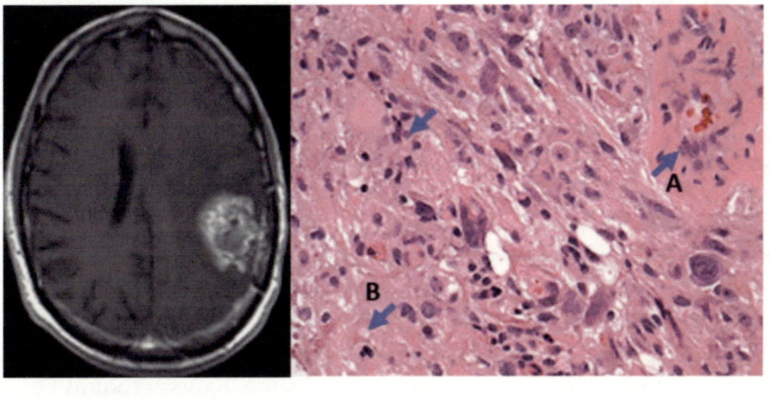


**Figure 3.**
*A. Fibrinoid necrosis or hyalinization, fibrosis of blood vessels, dystrophic calcification and an inflammatory infiltrate consisting predominantly of macrophages. B. Radiation induced cytologic atypia.*

## 6. Pathological assessment

Histopathology is currently the gold standard to diagnose tumor recurrence or RN. A significant difference in histologic findings exists between these two conditions. Macroscopically, RN shows as a firm-like mass or sometimes as a soft cystic lesion. A yellow-to-brown necrotic core is usually accompanied by significant hemorrhage, gliosis, and tissue atrophy [85]. In the case of RN, fibrinoid necrosis, hemorrhage, hyalinization and, blood vessel thrombosis can be seen, with a visible hypoxic injury of the surrounding tissue [5]. The necrotic area is usually paucicellular, characterized by the presence of inflammatory ghost cells and focal perivascular lymphocytes, and surrounded by gliotic brain tissue corresponding mainly to GFAP-reactive astrocytes (reactive gliosis) [86]. Inside the lesion, other cell types like foamy macrophages and hemosiderophages can be seen. A low nuclei-cytoplasmic ratio is characteristic. On the other hand, tumor recurrence shows a high cellularity with a

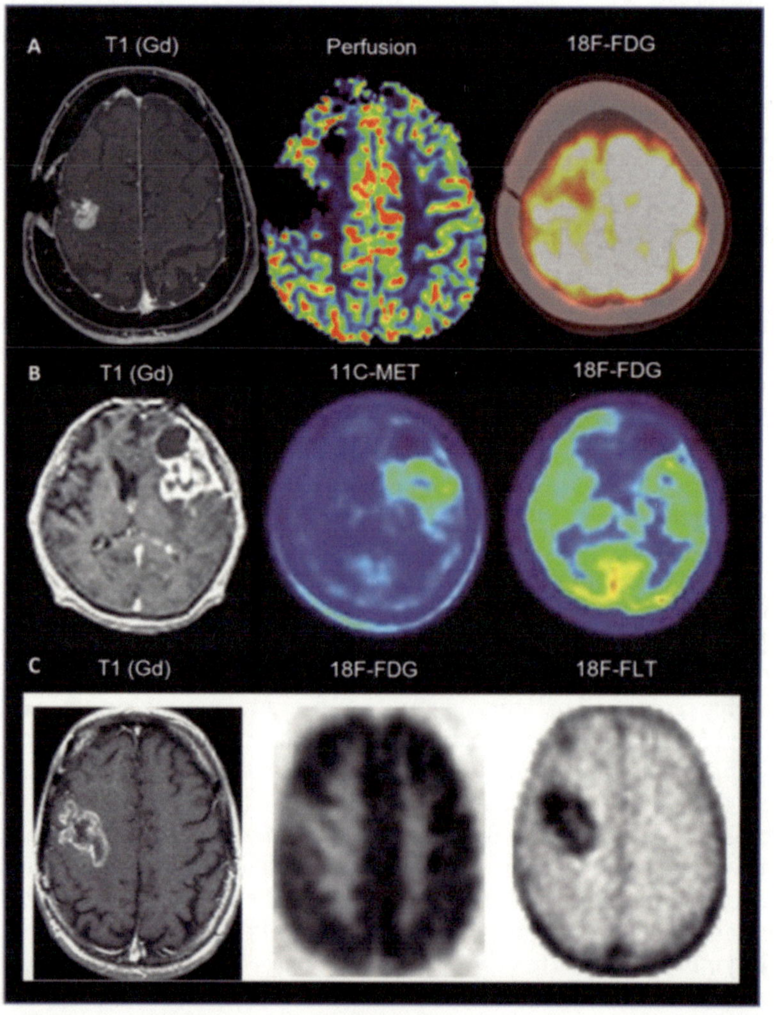


**Figure 4.**
*Representative PET and MRI images of radiation necrosis (RN). (A) Example of an RN area by SRS performed in a postsurgical cavity due to metastasis of a lung adenocarcinoma located in the right precentral sulcus. (B) Variations between 11C-MET and 18F-FDG PET in a large area of left frontal RN after resecting a high-grade glioma treated with IMRT. (C) FLT-PET study from the progression of a recurrent glioblastoma multiforme. MRI T1 Gd shows a large right frontal contrast-enhancing lesion versus FLT- PET and FDG-PET scans.*

ghost cell outline, demonstrating a high nuclei-cytoplasmic ratio. In brain metastases, careful examination of the blood vessels is essential as residual tumor cells might be seen around the Virchow Robin spaces. An immunohistochemistry panel will reveal the usual immunophenotype of the suspected tumor recurrence according to the patient's history. Histopathological assessment is not routinely performed unless an invasive approach to the lesions is needed for other purposes like therapeutic interventions. **Figure 4** shows the main pathological features of radiation injury, including cytological atypia, fibrinoid necrosis, and the marked inflammatory infiltrate.

## 7. Management of radiation necrosis

### 7.1 Observation

Since the 1970s, RN can be controlled with advanced images and left under observation. Wang *et al.* described a series of 124 patients who had radiation for nasopharyngeal carcinoma and developed severe imaging changes in the temporal lobe; among them, 28% of white matter lesions, 39% of contrast-enhanced lesions, and 7% of cysts regressed or resolved [87]. Since RN is not always symptomatic and evolutionary, it is considered that about half of the cases could be managed with observation, especially if the lesions are small and are located in non-eloquent areas.

### 7.2 Steroids

For patients with symptomatic brain RN, steroids are typically the first-line treatment, as they effectively reduce symptoms associated with brain edema and also inhibit the pro-inflammatory cascade involved in radiation injury. However, withdrawal of corticosteroids may result in a rebound of the edema and related symptoms and prolonged use of corticosteroids can be associated with significant toxicity including steroid myopathy, iatrogenic Cushing's syndrome and glucose intolerance [88].

### 7.3 Bevacizumab

There have been several recent reviews addressing the use of bevacizumab for brain RN [89, 90] that included data from both retrospective and prospective studies. Lubelski *et al.* reported on 30 patients included in seven studies of bevacizumab for patients with brain RN following treatment for high-grade glioma. Similar to this review, all patients demonstrated a radiographic response on T1 and T2-weighted MRI. Out of the 23 patients for which clinical data were reported, 16 (70%) showed an improvement. A subsequent broader review that included 71 patients treated with bevacizumab for brain RN after treatment of any brain tumor across 16 studies reported radiographic improvement in 97% of patients and improvement in performance status in 79% of patients [89]. Therefore, these reviews agree around information suggesting that the radiographic response rate to bevacizumab is high for patients with brain RN, and this response may be associated with symptomatic or functional improvement.

A recent systemic review found only three clinical trials with pharmacological interventions to reduce the clinical and radiological features of brain RN [91]. The first one is a randomized, double-blind, placebo-controlled trial of bevacizumab 7.5 mg/kg every three weeks for 2 cycles versus placebo tested in adults treated with radiotherapy for the brain or head and neck neoplasm and with radiological diagnosis of brain RN based on MRI criteria. Included patients were allowed to be taking corticosteroids before study participation, but they were required to be using a stable dose

for at least one week before receiving study treatment. The primary endpoint was the radiological response, defined as at least a 25% reduction in brain edema at six weeks of treatment compared with pre-treatment; this was measured as the volume of hyperintensity on T2-FLAIR MR images [92]. This trial reported that 100% (7/7) of participants on bevacizumab had a reduction in brain edema (T2 hyperintense volume) by at least 25% and a reduction in post-gadolinium enhancement.

In contrast, all those receiving placebo had clinical and/or radiological progression (five participants in the placebo arm experienced progressive clinical symptoms while two patients had radiological progression without progressive symptoms). Three severe adverse events were noted with bevacizumab which included aspiration pneumonia, pulmonary embolus, and superior sagittal sinus thrombosis [92].

The second was an open-label trial of patients treated with methylprednisolone 500 mg intravenously for three days followed by prednisone orally on a tapering schedule over 30 days, as tolerated, with or without the addition of edaravone 30 mg orally twice daily for 14 days. Eligible patients were adults (> 18 years old) treated with radiotherapy at least six months before study enrollment with radiographic evidence of RN based on MRI features. This trial also defined response as at least 25% reduction in the volume of T2-hyperintensity, and the primary endpoint was evaluated at three months following the start of treatment [93]. This study demonstrated a more significant reduction in brain edema in the edaravone plus corticosteroid group than in the corticosteroid alone group (mean difference was 3.03, 95%CI 0.14–5.92), although the result approached borderline significance ($p = 0.04$). There was no evidence of any critical difference in the reduction in post-gadolinium enhancement between arms (mean difference 0.47, 95% CI -0.80-1.74). Similarly, the participants who received the combination treatment were noted to have significantly greater clinical improvement than corticosteroids alone measured using the Late Effects Normal Tissue Task Force-Subjective, Objective, Management, Analytic (LENT-SOMA) scale (OR 2.51, 95%CI 1.26–5.01). No differences in treatment toxicities were observed between arms, and no severe adverse events were reported.

Besides, one prospective non-randomized study allowed patients to choose between vitamin E 1000 IU twice daily for one year or no active treatment. Eligible cases were adults treated with radiotherapy for nasopharyngeal carcinoma with no evidence of recurrence for at least five years who have developed radiological evidence of unilateral or bilateral temporal lobe necrosis without mental impairment. Unlike the two randomized studies, serial imaging was not evaluated in this study. Patients were assessed at baseline and one year using a battery of in-house and more widely utilized neuropsychological tests, including the Cantonese version of the Mini-Mental Status Examination (CMMSE), Hong Kong List Learning Test (HKLLT), Visual Reproduction subtest of the Wechsler Memory Scale III (WMS-III VR), Category Fluency Test (CFT) and computerized Cognitive Flexibility Test [94]. Evaluating cognitive function in patients at baseline and after one year of treatment, a 5.3% improvement in global cognitive function on CMMSE was seen in patients who received vitamin E compared with no improvement in the control group ($P = 0.007$). Assessment of verbal learning using the Hong Kong List Learning Test (HKLLT) demonstrated that the treatment group had a 27.2% improvement at one year versus no improvement in the control group.

Similarly, improvements were seen for visual memory and recall for the group treated with vitamin E. There was no difference in attention, language, or executive function between the two groups at baseline or at one year. Corticosteroid requirements and adverse events to treatment were not reported in this study [94].

Another integrative study gathered the information from two prospective, seven retrospective, and three case report studies involving 89 patients with RN treated with bevacizumab [95]. In total, 93% of patients had a recorded radiographic

response to antiangiogenic therapy, and 6.7% had experienced RN progression. Seven studies (n = 73) reported mean volume reductions on gadolinium-enhanced T1 (mean 47%, +/– 24) and T2-weighted fluid-attenuated inversion recovery (FLAIR) MRI images (mean 62%, +/– 23). Pooling together the T1 and T2 MRI reduction rates revealed a mean of 48 (95% CI 38–59) for T1 reduction rate and 62 (95% CI 52–72) for T2W imaging studies. Eighty-five patients presented with neurological symptoms at bevacizumab exposure, since when nine (10%) had stable symptoms, 39 (48%) had improved, and 34 (40%) patients had complete resolution of their clinical impairment. Similarly, dexamethasone discontinuation or reduction in dosage was observed in 97% of patients who had recorded dosage before and after bevacizumab treatment [95].

Considering the use of alternative ways for the administration of bevacizumab in patients with RN, Dashti *et al.* described two pediatric patients with cerebral arteriovenous malformations (AVM), who presented with medically intractable radiation injury following stereotactic radiosurgery. They received a single intraarterial infusion of 2.5 mg/kg bevacizumab after hyperosmotic BBB disruption. At a mean follow-up duration of 8.5 months, the patients had a significant and durable clinical and radiographic response. Both cases experienced resolution of their previously intractable headaches and reversal of cushingoid features as they were successfully weaned off steroids. One of the patients regained significant motor strength, and there was an associated greater than 70% reduction in cerebral edema [96].

Baroni *et al.* described pediatric patients' experience from five referral centers that treated 26 cases of symptomatic radiation necrosis with bevacizumab. The mean age at diagnosis of radiation necrosis was 10.7 years, with a median time between the last dose of radiation and the presentation of radiation necrosis of 3.8 months (range, 0.6–110 months). Overall, 50% of patients had an objective clinical improvement, with only one suffering from significant hypertension. Radiological benefit, defined as reduced T2/fluid-attenuated inversion recovery signal and mass effect, was observed in 50% of cases; however, this did not completely overlap with clinical response. Both early and late radiation necrosis responded equally well to bevacizumab therapy, and overall the monoclonal antibody was well tolerated, allowing the reduction of corticosteroid dose and/or duration [97].

## 7.4 Surgery

Although surgery is frequently used in clinical practice to address progressive resectable RN lesions, no prospective trials of surgical resection for brain RN were identified in this review. A retrospective series of 24 adult patients who underwent craniotomy and resection of contrast-enhancing lesions in the temporal lobes (16 unilateral and eight bilateral) following radiotherapy for nasopharyngeal carcinoma reported a reduction in the extent of brain edema observed on either CT or MRI (in those cases who had serial imaging). Only one patient required a repeat resection for recurrent necrosis [98]. In patients who were treated with radiosurgery, a retrospective series of 15 patients treated with surgical resection for RN reported improvement in brain edema resulting in either a partial or complete taper off corticosteroids as well as symptom improvement in the majority of patients [99].

## 7.5 Pentoxifylline and vitamin E

Pentoxifylline (PTX) is a methylxanthine derivative that decreases blood viscosity, increasing blood circulation and tissue oxygenation. Vitamin E (or tocopherol) acts as a free-radical scavenger. In a small retrospective study of 11 patients with

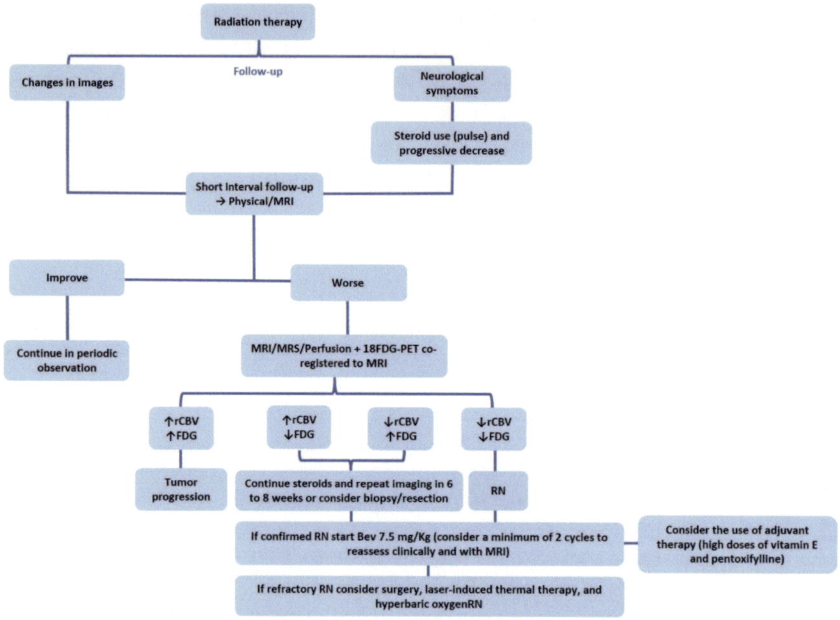


**Figure 5.**
*Diagnostic and therapeutic algorithm for brain RN (modified from: Chao et al. [103]).*

brain RN following radiotherapy for brain metastases, meningioma, and AVMs, the combination of PTX and vitamin E resulted in radiological improvement in all but one patient, who was eventually confirmed to have tumor recurrence [100].

### 7.6 Hyperbaric oxygen

There are limited small retrospective case reports and case studies reporting the outcomes of Hyperbaric oxygen (HBO) therapy for brain RN. Pasquier *et al.* reported limited retrospective reports of HBO as part of a more extensive review of HBO therapy for radiation injury to all body sites. These retrospective reports suggested favorable responses to HBO therapy to some patients; however, no prospective data is available [101]. Only one single-arm study evaluating HBO's impact on clinical improvement and reduction of edema in patients who develop cerebral radiation necrosis following gamma knife radiosurgery (GKS) (NCT02714465) was on-going.

### 7.7 Laser-induced thermal therapy (LITT)

Only one single-arm study of a LITT reported promising local control of 75.8% (13 of 15 lesions) and dramatic reductions in lesion volume to less than 10% of the pre-treated volume in seven of the treated lesions [102]. However, as this was a single-arm study with a limited number of patients, a further prospective investigation is required to compare this treatment's effectiveness against current management approaches. **Figure 5** shows a proposed algorithm for the diagnostic and therapeutic approach of NR.

## 8. Conclusions

Despite the rising incidence of RN because of increased utilization of stereotactic radiosurgery and reirradiation, there remain significant challenges in diagnosing

this complex brain injury. To date, there is no established standard to diagnose RN noninvasively. Over the past few years, there are, however, more treatment options, particularly with bevacizumab. More studies are needed to define who is at risk and how to minimize these risks; to diagnose radiation necrosis more accurately with imaging, blood tests, or other noninvasive techniques; and to treat these patients quickly before neurological signs and symptoms develop and progress.

## Disclaimer

None.

## Author details

Juan Esteban Garcia-Robledo[1], Alejandro Ruíz-Patiño[2,3], Carolina Sotelo[2,3], Álvaro Muñoz[4], Oscar Arrieta[5], Lucia Zatarain-Barrón[5], Camila Ordoñez[2], Christian Rolfo[6] and Andrés F. Cardona[2,3,7]*

1 Division of Hematology/Oncology, Mayo Clinic, Scottsdale, USA

2 Foundation for Clinical and Applied Cancer Research—FICMAC, Bogotá, Colombia

3 Molecular Oncology and Biology Systems Research Group (Fox-G), Universidad El Bosque, Bogotá, Colombia

4 Radiation Oncology Department, Carlos Ardila Lülle Cancer Institute—ICCAL, Fundación Santa Fe de Bogotá, Bogotá, Colombia

5 Thoracic Oncology Unit and Personalized Oncology Laboratory, National Cancer Institute (INCan), México City, México

6 Marlene and Stewart Greenebaum Comprehensive Cancer Center, University of Maryland School of Medicine, Baltimore, Maryland, USA

7 Clinical and Traslational Oncology Group, Clínica del Country, Bogotá Colombia

*Address all correspondence to: andres.cardona@clinicadelcountry.com; a_cardonaz@yahoo.com

## References

[1] Perkins,A. Liu, G. Primary Brain Tumors in Adults: Diagnosis and Treatment-American Family Physician. Am. Fam. Physician **93**, 211-218 (2016).

[2] Patel, U., Patel, A., Cobb, C., Benkers, T. & Vermeulen, S. The management of brain necrosis as a result of SRS treatment for intra-cranial tumor. Translational Cancer Research vol. 3 373-382 (2014).

[3] Huang, X. *et al.* A nomogram to predict symptomatic epilepsy in patients with radiation-induced brain necrosis. Neurology **95**, e1392–e1403 (2020).

[4] Minniti, G. *et al.* Stereotactic radiosurgery for brain metastases: Analysis of outcome and risk of brain radionecrosis. Radiat. Oncol. **6**, 48 (2011).

[5] Vellayappan, B. *et al.* Diagnosis and Management of Radiation Necrosis in Patients With Brain Metastases. Frontiers in Oncology vol. 8 395 (2018).

[6] Donovan, E. K., Parpia, S. & Greenspoon, J. N. Incidence of radionecrosis in single-fraction radiosurgery compared with fractionated radiotherapy in the treatment of brain metastasis. Curr. Oncol. **26**, e328–e333 (2019).

[7] Kohutek, Z. A. *et al.* Long-term risk of radionecrosis and imaging changes after stereotactic radiosurgery for brain metastases. J. Neurooncol. **125**, 149-156 (2015).

[8] Blonigen, B. J. *et al.* Irradiated Volume as a Predictor of Brain Radionecrosis After Linear Accelerator Stereotactic Radiosurgery. Int. J. Radiat. Oncol. Biol. Phys. **77**, 996-1001 (2010).

[9] Chin, L. S., Ma, L. & DiBiase, S. Radiation necrosis following gamma knife surgery: A case-controlled comparison of treatment parameters and long-term clinical follow up. J. Neurosurg. **94**, 899-904 (2001).

[10] Hettal, L. *et al.* Radiomics Method for the Differential Diagnosis of Radionecrosis Versus Progression after Fractionated Stereotactic Body Radiotherapy for Brain Oligometastasis. Radiat. Res. **193**, 471-480 (2020).

[11] Sheline, G. E., Wara, W. M. & Smith, V. Therapeutic irradiation and brain injury. Int. J. Radiat. Oncol. Biol. Phys. **6**, 1215-1228 (1980).

[12] Calvo, W., Hopewell, J. W., Reinhold, H. S. & Yeung, T. K. Time- and dose-related changes in the white matter of the rat brain after single doses of X rays. Br. J. Radiol. **61**, 1043-1052 (1988).

[13] Hopewell, J. W. & Wright, E. A. The nature of latent cerebral irradiation damage and its modification by hypertension. Br. J. Radiol. **43**, 161-167 (1970).

[14] Hopewell, J. W. Late radiation damage to the central nervous system: A radiobiological interpretation. Neuropathology and Applied Neurobiology vol. 5 329-343 (1979).

[15] Van Der Kogel, A. J. Radiation-induced damage in the central nervous system: An interpretation of target cell responses. Br. J. Cancer **53**, 207-217 (1986).

[16] Ali, F. S. *et al.* Cerebral Radiation Necrosis: Incidence, Pathogenesis, Diagnostic Challenges, and Future Opportunities. Current Oncology Reports vol. 21 66 (2019).

[17] Rahmathulla, G., Marko, N. F. & Weil, R. J. Cerebral radiation necrosis: A review of the pathobiology, diagnosis

and management considerations. Journal of Clinical Neuroscience vol. 20 485-502 (2013).

[18] Moeller, B. J. *et al.* Pleiotropic effects of HIF-1 blockade on tumor radiosensitivity. Cancer Cell **8**, 99-110 (2005).

[19] Fuks, Z. & Kolesnick, R. Engaging the vascular component of the tumor response. Cancer Cell vol. 8 89-91 (2005).

[20] Kolesnick, R. & Fuks, Z. Radiation and ceramide-induced apoptosis. Oncogene vol. 22 5897-5906 (2003).

[21] Daigle, J. L., Hong, J.-H., Chiang, C.-S. & McBride, W. H. The Role of Tumor Necrosis Factor Signaling Pathways in the Response of Murine Brain to Irradiation. *Cancer Res.* **61**, 8859 LP – 8865 (2001).

[22] Varatharaj, A. & Galea, I. The blood-brain barrier in systemic inflammation. Brain, Behavior, and Immunity vol. 60 1-12 (2017).

[23] Małkiewicz, M. A. *et al.* Blood-brain barrier permeability and physical exercise. Journal of Neuroinflammation vol. 16 1-16 (2019).

[24] Cheng, Y. *et al.* TNFα disrupts blood brain barrier integrity to maintain prolonged depressive-like behavior in mice. Brain. Behav. Immun. **69**, 556-567 (2018).

[25] Nordal, R. A., Nagy, A., Pintilie, M. & Wong, C. S. Hypoxia and hypoxia-inducible factor-1 target genes in central nervous system radiation injury: A role for vascular endothelial growth factor. Clin. Cancer Res. **10**, 3342-3353 (2004).

[26] Nordal, R. A. & Wong, C. S. Intercellular adhesion molecule-1 and blood-spinal cord barrier disruption in central nervous system radiation injury. J. Neuropathol. Exp. Neurol. **63**, 474-483 (2004).

[27] Remler, M. P., Marcussen, W. H. & Tiller-Borsich, J. The late effects of radiation on the blood brain barrier. Int. J. Radiat. Oncol. Biol. Phys. **12**, 1965-1969 (1986).

[28] Barz, H., Schreiber, A. & Barz, U. Demyelinating diseases as a result of cerebral edema? Med. Hypotheses **104**, 10-14 (2017).

[29] Abdulla, S., Saada, J., Johnson, G., Jefferies, S. & Ajithkumar, T. Tumour progression or pseudoprogression? A review of post-treatment radiological appearances of glioblastoma. *Clinical Radiology* vol. 70 1299-1312 (2015).

[30] Lawrence, Y. R. *et al.* Radiation Dose-Volume Effects in the Brain. Int. J. Radiat. Oncol. Biol. Phys. **76**, S20 (2010).

[31] Sneed, P. K. *et al.* Adverse radiation effect after stereotactic radiosurgery for brain metastases: Incidence, time course, and risk factors. J. Neurosurg. **123**, 373-386 (2015).

[32] Andruska, N. *et al.* Risk Factors Associated with Radiation Necrosis Among Brain Metastasis Patients Undergoing Fractionated Stereotactic Radiosurgery for CNS Brain Metastases. Int. J. Radiat. Oncol. **105**, E70 (2019).

[33] Caffo, O. Radiosensitization with chemotherapeutic agents. in *Lung Cancer* vol. 34 81-90 (Elsevier Ireland Ltd, 2001).

[34] Ruben, J. D. *et al.* Cerebral radiation necrosis: Incidence, outcomes, and risk factors with emphasis on radiation parameters and chemotherapy. Int. J. Radiat. Oncol. Biol. Phys. **65**, 499-508 (2006).

[35] Colaco, R. J., Martin, P., Kluger, H. M., Yu, J. B. & Chiang, V. L. Does

immunotherapy increase the rate of radiation necrosis after radiosurgical treatment of brain metastases? J. Neurosurg. **125**, 17-23 (2016).

[36] Martin, A. M. *et al.* Immunotherapy and symptomatic radiation necrosis in patients with brain metastases treated with stereotactic radiation. JAMA Oncology vol. 4 1123-1124 (2018).

[37] Juloori, A. *et al.* Overall survival and response to radiation and targeted therapies among patients with renal cell carcinoma brain metastases. J. Neurosurg. **132**, 188-196 (2020).

[38] Ohtakara, K. *et al.* Significance of target location relative to the depth from the brain surface and high-dose irradiated volume in the development of brain radionecrosis after micromultileaf collimator-based stereotactic radiosurgery for brain metastases. J. Neurooncol. **108**, 201-209 (2012).

[39] Miller, J. A. *et al.* Association Between Radiation Necrosis and Tumor Biology After Stereotactic Radiosurgery for Brain Metastasis. Int. J. Radiat. Oncol. Biol. Phys. **96**, 1060-1069 (2016).

[40] Kirkpatrick, J. P. *et al.* Defining the optimal planning target volume in image-guided stereotactic radiosurgery of brain metastases: Results of a randomized trial. Int. J. Radiat. Oncol. Biol. Phys. **91**, 100-108 (2015).

[41] Raaphorst, G. P. *et al.* Skin fibroblasts in vitro radiosensitivity can predict for late complications following AVM radiosurgery. Radiother. Oncol. **64**, 153-156 (2002).

[42] Miyata, T. *et al.* The roles of platelet-derived growth factors and their receptors in brain radiation necrosis. Radiat. Oncol. **9**, (2014).

[43] Li, Y. Q., Ballinger, J. R., Nordal, R. A., Su, Z. F. & Wong, C. S. Hypoxia in radiation-induced blood-spinal cord barrier breakdown. Cancer Res. **61**, 3348-3354 (2001).

[44] Ehrenfeld, C. E., Maschke, M., Dörfler, A., Reinhardt, V. & Koeppen, S. Is stereotactic biopsy a reliable method to differentiate tumor from radiation necrosis? Clin. Neuropathol. **21**, 9-12 (2002).

[45] Furuse, M. *et al.* Radiological diagnosis of brain radiation necrosis after cranial irradiation for brain tumor: a systematic review. Radiat. Oncol. **14**, 28 (2019).

[46] Constine, L. S., Konski, A., Ekholm, S., McDonald, S. & Rubin, P. Adverse effects of brain irradiation correlated with MR and CT imaging. Int. J. Radiat. Oncol. Biol. Phys. **15**, 319-330 (1988).

[47] Sundaresan, N., Galicich, J. H., Deck, M. D. F. & Tomita, T. Radiation necrosis after treatment of solitary intracranial metastases. Neurosurgery **8**, 329-333 (1981).

[48] Kingsley, D. P. E. & Kendall, B. E. CT of the adverse effects of therapeutic radiation of the central nervous system. Am. J. Neuroradiol. **2**, 453-460 (1981).

[49] van Dellen, J. R. & Danziger, A. Failure of computerized tomography to differentiate between radiation necrosis and cerebral tumour. S. Afr. Med. J. **53**, 171-172 (1978).

[50] Van Tassel, P. *et al.* MR of toxic effects of accelerated fractionation radiation therapy and carboplatin chemotherapy for malignant gliomas. AJNR. Am. J. Neuroradiol. **16**, 715-726 (1995).

[51] Valk, P. E. & Dillon, W. P. *Diagnostic imaging of central nervous system radiation injury*. (Raven Press, 1991).

[52] Dequesada, I. M., Quisling, R. G., Yachnis, A. & Friedman, W. A. Can standard magnetic resonance

imaging reliably distinguish recurrent tumor from radiation necrosis after radiosurgery for brain metastases? A radiographic-pathological study. *Neurosurgery* **63**, 898-903 (2008).

[53] Taylor, J. S. *et al.* Clinical value of proton magnetic resonance spectroscopy for differentiating recurrent or residual brain tumor from delayed cerebral necrosis. Int. J. Radiat. Oncol. Biol. Phys. **36**, 1251-1261 (1996).

[54] Buchpiguel, C. A., Alavi, J. B., Alavi, A. & Kenyon, L. C. PET versus SPECT in distinguishing radiation necrosis from tumor recurrence in the brain. J. Nucl. Med. **36**, 159-164 (1995).

[55] Dowling, C. *et al.* Preoperative proton MR spectroscopic imaging of brain tumors: correlation with histopathologic analysis of resection specimens. AJNR. Am. J. Neuroradiol. **22**, 604-612 (2001).

[56] Tsuyuguchi, N. *et al.* Methionine positron emission tomography of recurrent metastatic brain tumor and radiation necrosis after stereotactic radiosurgery: is a differential diagnosis possible? J. Neurosurg. **98**, 1056-1064 (2003).

[57] Belohlávek, O., Simonová, G., Kantorová, I., Novotný, J. J. & Liscák, R. Brain metastases after stereotactic radiosurgery using the Leksell gamma knife: can FDG PET help to differentiate radionecrosis from tumour progression? Eur. J. Nucl. Med. Mol. Imaging **30**, 96-100 (2003).

[58] Hu, L. S. *et al.* Relative cerebral blood volume values to differentiate high-grade glioma recurrence from posttreatment radiation effect: direct correlation between image-guided tissue histopathology and localized dynamic susceptibility-weighted contrast-enhanced perfusio. Am. J. Neuroradiol. **30**, 552-558 (2009).

[59] Sugahara, T. *et al.* Posttherapeutic intraaxial brain tumor: the value of perfusion-sensitive contrast-enhanced MR imaging for differentiating tumor recurrence from nonneoplastic contrast-enhancing tissue. Am. J. Neuroradiol. **21**, 901-909 (2000).

[60] Barajas, R. F. *et al.* Distinguishing Recurrent Intra-Axial Metastatic Tumor from Radiation Necrosis Following Gamma Knife Radiosurgery Using Dynamic Susceptibility-Weighted Contrast-Enhanced Perfusion MR Imaging. *Am. J. Neuroradiol.* **30**, 367 LP – 372 (2009).

[61] Kim, D. Y., Kim, H. S., Goh, M. J., Choi, C. G. & Kim, S. J. Utility of intravoxel incoherent motion MR imaging for distinguishing recurrent metastatic tumor from treatment effect following gamma knife radiosurgery: initial experience. AJNR. Am. J. Neuroradiol. **35**, 2082-2090 (2014).

[62] Detsky, J. S. *et al.* Differentiating radiation necrosis from tumor progression in brain metastases treated with stereotactic radiotherapy: utility of intravoxel incoherent motion perfusion MRI and correlation with histopathology. J. Neurooncol. **134**, 433-441 (2017).

[63] Fayed, N., Morales, H., Modrego, P. J. & Pina, M. A. Contrast/Noise Ratio on Conventional MRI and Choline/Creatine Ratio on Proton MRI Spectroscopy Accurately Discriminate Low-Grade From High-Grade Cerebral Gliomas. Acad. Radiol. **13**, 728-737 (2006).

[64] Träber, F. *et al.* [1H-MR Spectroscopy of brain tumors in the course of radiation therapy: Use of fast spectroscopic imaging and single-voxel spectroscopy for diagnosing recurrence]. Rofo **174**, 33-42 (2002).

[65] Lichy, M. P. *et al.* [Metabolic imaging to follow stereotactic

radiation of gliomas -- the role of 1H MR spectroscopy in comparison to FDG-PET and IMT-SPECT]. Rofo **176**, 1114-1121 (2004).

[66] Plotkin, M. *et al.* 123 I-IMT SPECT and 1 HMR-Spectroscopy at 3.0T in the Differential Diagnosis of Recurrent or Residual Gliomas: A Comparative Study. J. Neurooncol. **70**, 49-58 (2004).

[67] Zeng, Q. S. *et al.* Multivoxel 3D proton MR spectroscopy in the distinction of recurrent glioma from radiation injury. J. Neurooncol. **84**, 63-69 (2007).

[68] Shah, R. *et al.* Radiation necrosis in the brain: Imaging features and differentiation from tumor recurrence. Radiographics **32**, 1343-1359 (2012).

[69] Chuang, M. T., Liu, Y. S., Tsai, Y. S., Chen, Y. C. & Wang, C. K. Differentiating radiation-induced necrosis from recurrent brain tumor using MR perfusion and spectroscopy: A meta-analysis. PLoS One **11**, (2016).

[70] Zhang, H. *et al.* Role of magnetic resonance spectroscopy for the differentiation of recurrent glioma from radiation necrosis: a systematic review and meta-analysis. Eur. J. Radiol. **83**, 2181-2189 (2014).

[71] Hollingworth, W. *et al.* A systematic literature review of magnetic resonance spectroscopy for the characterization of brain tumors. AJNR. Am. J. Neuroradiol. **27**, 1404-1411 (2006).

[72] Thompson, T. P., Lunsford, L. D. & Kondziolka, D. Distinguishing recurrent tumor and radiation necrosis with positron emission tomography versus stereotactic biopsy. in *Stereotactic and Functional Neurosurgery* vol. 73 9-14 (S. Karger AG, 1999).

[73] Deykin, D., Balko, C. & Isselbacher, K. J. Sugar and Amino Acid Transport by Cells in Culture — Differences between Normal and Malignant Cells. N. Engl. J. Med. **286**, 929-933 (1972).

[74] Lupi, A. *et al.* 18FDG-PET/CT in Traumatic Brain Injury Patients: The Relative Hypermetabolism of Vermis Cerebelli as a Medium and Long Term Predictor of Outcome. Curr. Radiopharm. **7**, 57-62 (2014).

[75] Segtnan, E. A., Hess, S., Grupe, P. & Høilund-Carlsen, P. F. 18F-fluorodeoxyglucose PET/computed tomography for primary brain tumors. PET Clinics vol. 10 59-73 (2015).

[76] Floeth, F. W. *et al.* Comparison of 18F-FET PET and 5-ALA fluorescence in cerebral gliomas. Eur. J. Nucl. Med. Mol. Imaging **38**, 731-741 (2011).

[77] Rachinger, W. *et al.* Positron Emission Tomography with O-(2-[18F] fluoroethyl)-l-tyrosine versus Magnetic Resonance Imaging in the Diagnosis of Recurrent Gliomas. Neurosurgery **57**, 505-511 (2005).

[78] Humbert, O. *et al.* 18F-DOPA PET/CT in brain tumors: impact on multidisciplinary brain tumor board decisions. Eur. J. Nucl. Med. Mol. Imaging **46**, 558-568 (2019).

[79] Yu, J. *et al.* Accuracy of 18F-FDOPA Positron Emission Tomography and 18F-FET Positron Emission Tomography for Differentiating Radiation Necrosis from Brain Tumor Recurrence. World Neurosurg. **114**, e1211–e1224 (2018).

[80] Palanichamy, K. & Chakravarti, A. Diagnostic and prognostic significance of methionine uptake and methionine positron emission tomography imaging in gliomas. *Frontiers in Oncology* vol. 7 (2017).

[81] Arora, G. *et al.* 99mTc-Methionine Hybrid SPECT/CT for Detection of Recurrent Glioma: Comparison with 18F-FDG PET/CT and

Contrast-Enhanced MRI. Clin. Nucl. Med. **43**, e132–e138 (2018).

[82] Qiao, Z. *et al.* Utility of dynamic susceptibility contrast perfusion-weighted MR imaging and 11 C-methionine PET/CT for differentiation of tumor recurrence from radiation injury in patients with high-grade gliomas. Am. J. Neuroradiol. **40**, 253-259 (2019).

[83] Takenaka, S. *et al.* Comparison of 11c-methionine, 11c-choline, and 18f-fluorodeoxyglucose-positron emission tomography for distinguishing glioma recurrence from radiation necrosis. Neurol. Med. Chir. (Tokyo). **54**, 280-289 (2014).

[84] Enslow, M. S. *et al.* Comparison of 18F-fluorodeoxyglucose and 18F-fluorothymidine PET in differentiating radiation necrosis from recurrent glioma. Clin. Nucl. Med. **37**, 854-861 (2012).

[85] Na, A., Haghigi, N. & Drummond, K. J. Cerebral radiation necrosis. Asia-Pacific Journal of Clinical Oncology vol. 10 11-21 (2014).

[86] Yoshii, Y. Pathological review of late cerebral radionecrosis. Brain Tumor Pathology vol. 25 51-58 (2008).

[87] Wang, Y. X. J. *et al.* Evolution of radiation-induced brain injury: MR imaging-based study. Radiology **254**, 210-218 (2010).

[88] Giglio, P. & Gilbert, M. R. Cerebral radiation necrosis. Neurologist vol. 9 180-188 (2003).

[89] Tye, K. *et al.* An analysis of radiation necrosis of the central nervous system treated with bevacizumab. J. Neurooncol. **117**, 321-327 (2014).

[90] Lubelski, D., Abdullah, K. G., Weil, R. J. & Marko, N. F. Bevacizumab for radiation necrosis following treatment of high grade glioma: A systematic review of the literature. Journal of Neuro-Oncology vol. 115 317-322 (2013).

[91] Chung, C., Bryant, A. & Brown, P. D. Interventions for the treatment of brain radionecrosis after radiotherapy or radiosurgery. *Cochrane Database of Systematic Reviews* vol. 2018 (2018).

[92] Levin, V. A. *et al.* Randomized double-blind placebo-controlled trial of bevacizumab therapy for radiation necrosis of the central nervous system. Int. J. Radiat. Oncol. Biol. Phys. **79**, 1487-1495 (2011).

[93] Tang, Y. *et al.* Effect of edaravone on radiation-induced brain necrosis in patients with nasopharyngeal carcinoma after radiotherapy: a randomized controlled trial. J. Neurooncol. **120**, 441-447 (2014).

[94] Chan, A. S., Cheung, M. C., Law, S. C. & Chan, J. H. Phase II Study of Alpha-Tocopherol in Improving the Cognitive Function of Patients with Temporal Lobe Radionecrosis. Cancer **100**, 398-404 (2004).

[95] Khan, M., Zhao, Z., Arooj, S. & Liao, G. Bevacizumab for radiation necrosis following radiotherapy of brain metastatic disease: a systematic review & meta-analysis. BMC Cancer **21**, 167 (2021).

[96] Dashti, S. R. *et al.* Targeted intraarterial anti-VEGF therapy for medically refractory radiation necrosis in the brain. J. Neurosurg. Pediatr. **15**, 20-25 (2015).

[97] Baroni, L. V. *et al.* Bevacizumab for pediatric radiation necrosis. Neuro-Oncology Pract. 7, 409-414 (2020).

[98] Wong, S. T. *et al.* Results of excision of cerebral radionecrosis: Experience in patients treated with radiation therapy

for nasopharyngeal carcinoma. J. Neurosurg. **113**, 293-300 (2010).

[99] Telera, S. *et al.* Radionecrosis induced by stereotactic radiosurgery of brain metastases: Results of surgery and outcome of disease. J. Neurooncol. **113**, 313-325 (2013).

[100] Williamson, R., Kondziolka, D., Kanaan, H., Lunsford, L. D. & Flickinger, J. C. Adverse radiation effects after radiosurgery may benefit from oral vitamin E and pentoxifylline therapy: A pilot study. Stereotact. Funct. Neurosurg. **86**, 359-366 (2008).

[101] Pasquier, D. *et al.* Hyperbaric oxygen therapy in the treatment of radio-induced lesions in normal tissues: A literature review. Radiotherapy and Oncology vol. 72 1-13 (2004).

[102] Rao, M. S., Hargreaves, E. L., Khan, A. J., Haffty, B. G. & Danish, S. F. Magnetic resonance-guided laser ablation improves local control for postradiosurgery recurrence and/or radiation necrosis. Neurosurgery **74**, 658-667 (2014).

[103] Chao ST, Ahluwalia MS, Barnett GH, et al. Challenges with the diagnosis and treatment of cerebral radiation necrosis. Int J Radiat Oncol Biol Phys. 2013 Nov 1;87(3):449-457.

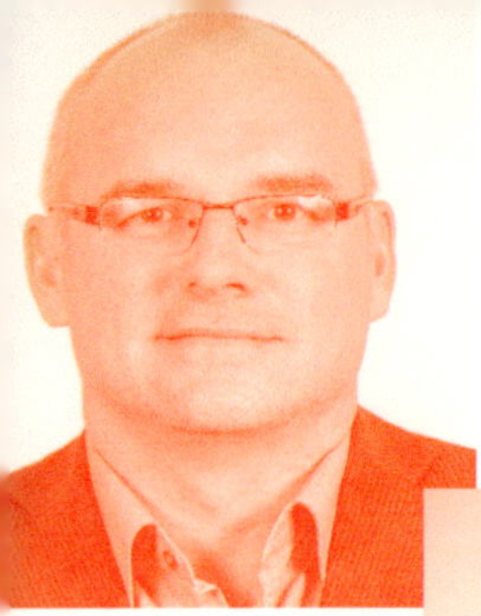
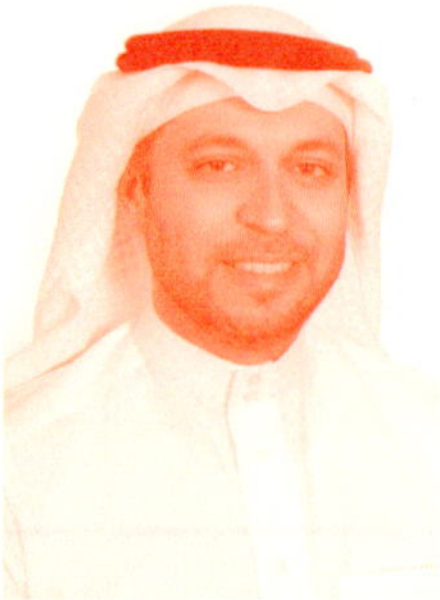
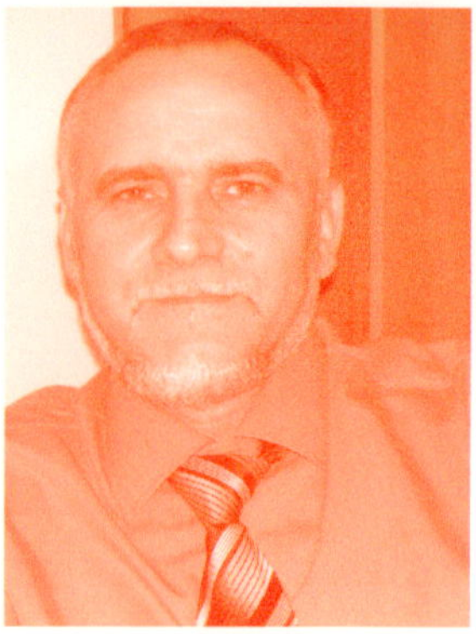
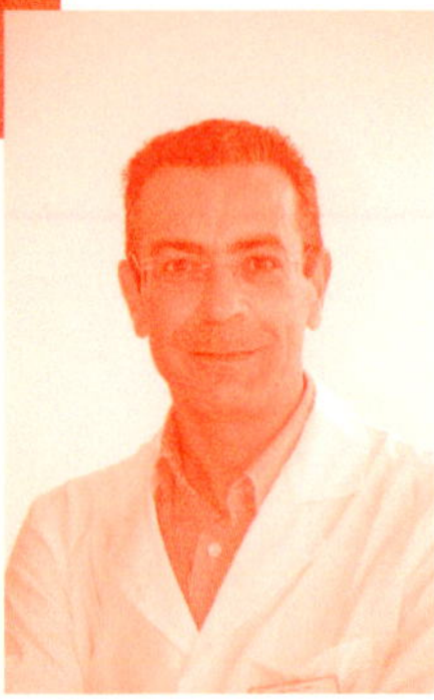
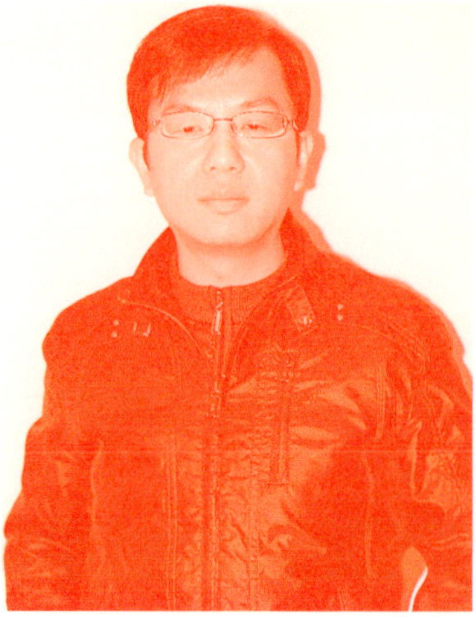
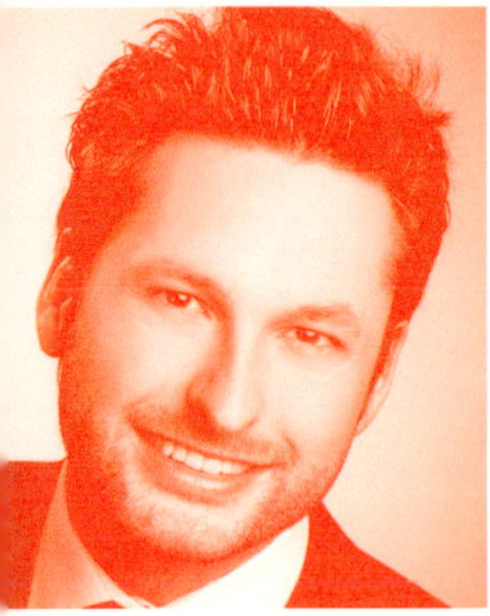
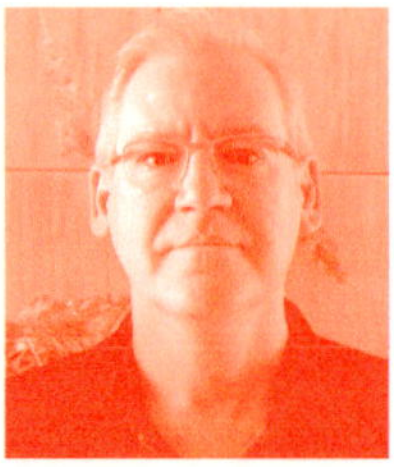

IntechOpen

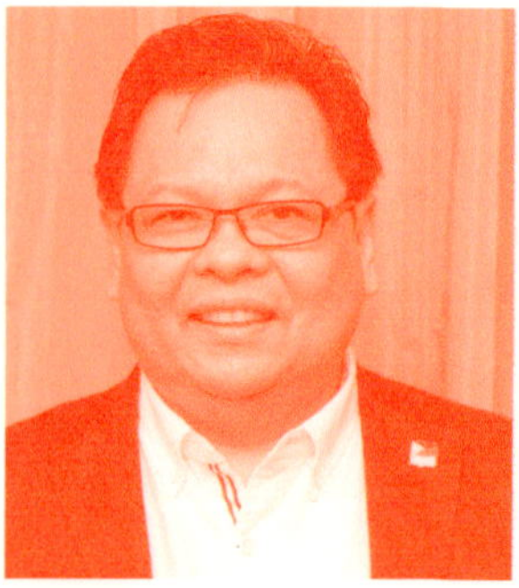
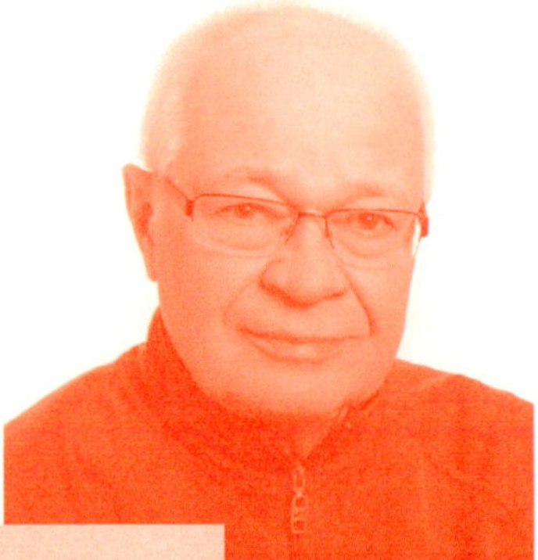
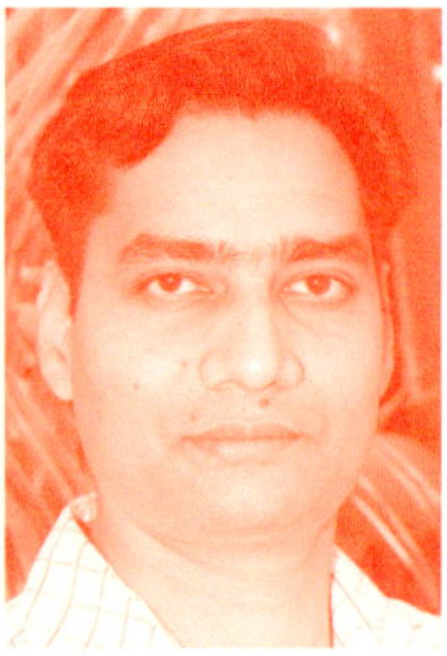
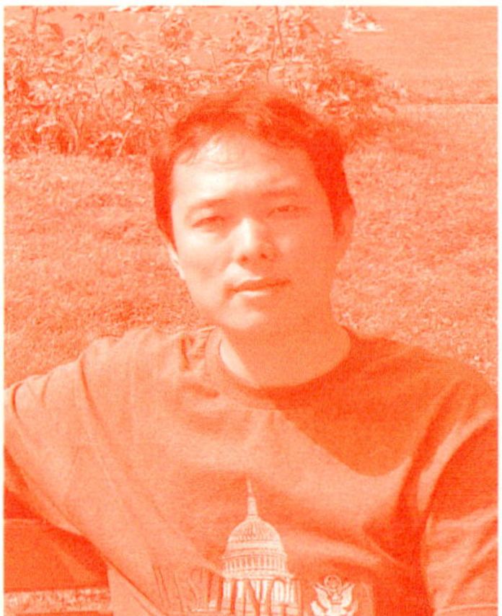
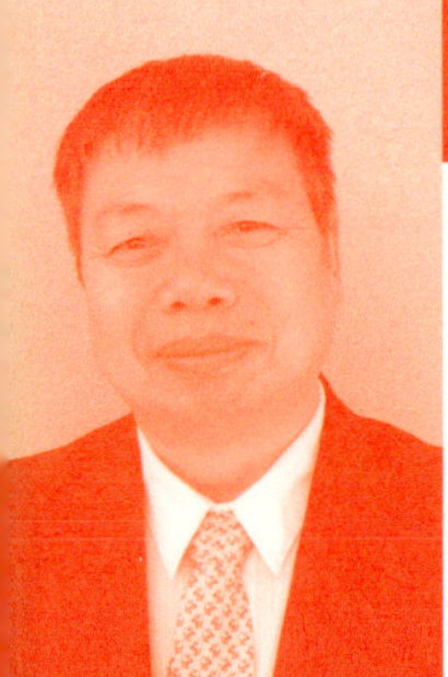
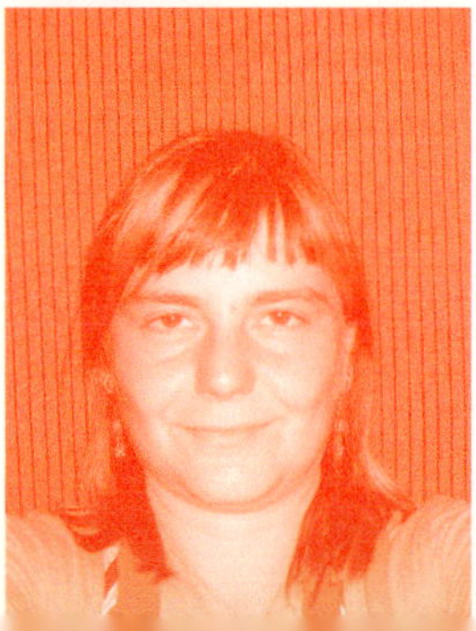